2010
YEAR BOOK OF
SURGERY®

The 2010 Year Book Series

Year Book of Anesthesiology and Pain Management™: Drs Chestnut, Abram, Black, Gravlee, Lien, Mathru and Roizen

Year Book of Cardiology®: Drs Gersh, Cheitlin, Elliott, Gold, Graham, and Suri

Year Book of Critical Care Medicine®: Drs Dellinger, Parrillo, Balk, Dorman, Dries, and Zanotti-Cavazzoni

Year Book of Dermatology and Dermatologic Surgery™: Dr Del Rosso

Year Book of Diagnostic Radiology®: Drs Osborn, Abbara, Birdwell, Elster, Manaster, Oestreich, Offiah, Rosado de Christenson, and Walker

Year Book of Emergency Medicine®: Drs Hamilton, Bruno, Handly, Mullin, Quintana, and Ramoska

Year Book of Endocrinology®: Drs Schott, Apovian, Clarke, Eugster, Ludlam, Meikle, Ovalle, Schinner, Schteingart, and Toth

Year Book of Gastroenterology™: Drs Talley, Dempsey, Harnois, Lange, Pearson, Picco, Rombeau, and Scolapio

Year Book of Hand and Upper Limb Surgery®: Drs Yao and Steinmann

Year Book of Medicine®: Drs Barker, Berney, Garrick, Gersh, Khardori, LeRoith, Talley, and Thigpen

Year Book of Neonatal and Perinatal Medicine®: Drs Fanaroff, Benitz, Donn, Neu, and Papile

Year Book of Neurology and Neurosurgery®: Drs Klimo and Rabinstein

Year Book of Obstetrics, Gynecology, and Women's Health®: Drs Dungan and Shulman

Year Book of Oncology®: Drs Thigpen, Arceci, Bauer, Byhardt, Gordon, and Lawton

Year Book of Ophthalmology®: Drs Rapuano, Cohen, Flanders, Hammersmith, Milman, Myers, Nelson, Penne, Pyfer, Sergott, Shields, and Vander

Year Book of Orthopedics®: Drs Morrey, Beauchamp, Huddleston, Swiontkowski, and Trigg

Year Book of Otolaryngology-Head and Neck Surgery®: Drs Sindwani, Balough, Franco, Gapany, and Mitchell

Year Book of Pathology and Laboratory Medicine®: Drs Raab, Parwani, Bejarano, and Bissell

Year Book of Pediatrics®: Dr Stockman

Year Book of Plastic and Aesthetic Surgery™: Drs Miller, Gosain, Gurtner, Gutowski, Ruberg, Salisbury, and Smith

Year Book of Psychiatry and Applied Mental Health®: Drs Talbott, Ballenger, Buckley, Frances, Krupnick, and Mack

Year Book of Pulmonary Disease®: Drs Barker, Jones, Maurer, Raza, Tanoue, and Willsie

Year Book of Sports Medicine®: Drs Shephard, Cantu, Feldman, Jankowski, Khan, Lebrun, Nieman, Pierrynowski, and Rowland

Year Book of Surgery®: Drs Copeland, Behrns, Daly, Eberlein, Fahey, Huber, Jones, Mozingo, and Pruett

Year Book of Urology®: Drs Andriole and Coplen

Year Book of Vascular Surgery®: Drs Moneta, Gillespie, Starnes, and Watkins

2010
The Year Book of SURGERY®

Editor-in-Chief
Edward M. Copeland III, MD
Distinguished Professor of Surgery, Department of Surgery, University of Florida, Gainesville, Florida

ELSEVIER
MOSBY

ELSEVIER
MOSBY

Vice President, Continuity: Kimberly Murphy
Editor: Ruth Malwitz
Production Supervisor: Donna M. Skelton
Electronic Article Manager: Emily Ogle
Illustrations and Permissions Coordinator: Dawn Vohsen

2010 EDITION

Composition by TNQ Books and Journals Pvt Ltd, India

Editorial Office:
Elsevier
1600 John F. Kennedy Blvd.
Suite 1800
Philadelphia, PA 19103-2899

International Standard Serial Number: 0090-3671
International Standard Book Number: 978-0-323-06847-5

Printed and bound in the United Kingdom
Transferred to Digital Print 2011

Editorial Board

Table of Contents

Journals Represented

Journals represented in this YEAR BOOK are listed below.

Acta Paediatrica
American Journal of Cardiology
American Journal of Clinical Nutrition
American Journal of Gastroenterology
American Journal of Infectious Diseases
American Journal of Pathology
American Journal of Surgery
American Journal of Transplantation
American Surgeon
Anesthesiology
Annals of Plastic Surgery
Annals of Surgery
Annals of Thoracic Surgery
Annals of Vascular Surgery
Archives of Otolaryngology Head & Neck Surgery
Archives of Surgery
British Journal of Surgery
Cancer
Cancer Research
Circulation
Clinical Cancer Research
Clinical Infectious Diseases
Critical Care Medicine
Diseases of the Colon and Rectum
European Journal of Endocrinology
European Journal of Vascular and Endovascular Surgery
Gastroenterology
Gastrointestinal Endoscopy
Injury
Intensive Care Medicine
Journal of Bone and Joint Surgery (British)
Journal of Burn Care & Research
Journal of Cardiothoracic and Vascular Anesthesia
Journal of Clinical Endocrinology & Metabolism
Journal of Clinical Neuroscience
Journal of Clinical Oncology
Journal of Investigative Dermatology
Journal of Parenteral and Enteral Nutrition
Journal of Pediatric Gastroenterology and Nutrition
Journal of Pediatric Surgery
Journal of Surgical Research
Journal of the American College of Surgeons
Journal of the American Medical Association
Journal of the National Cancer Institute
Journal of Thoracic and Cardiovascular Surgery
Journal of Thoracic Oncology
Journal of Trauma

Journal of Ultrasound in Medicine
Journal of Vascular Surgery
Lancet
Liver Transplantation
Molecular Medicine
Nature
Nephrology Dialysis Transplantation
Nephron Clinical Practice
New England Journal of Medicine
Pediatric Research
Plastic and Reconstructive Surgery
Stroke
Surgery
Surgical Endoscopy
Surgical Infections
Tissue Antigens
Transfusion
Transplantation
Transplantation Proceedings
World Journal of Surgery
Wound Repair and Regeneration

Standard Abbreviations

The following terms are abbreviated in this edition: acquired immunodeficiency syndrome (AIDS), cardiopulmonary resuscitation (CPR), central nervous system (CNS), cerebrospinal fluid (CSF), computed tomography (CT), deoxyribonucleic acid (DNA), electrocardiography (ECG), health maintenance organization (HMO), human immunodeficiency virus (HIV), intensive care unit (ICU), intramuscular (IM), intravenous (IV), magnetic resonance (MR) imaging (MRI), ribonucleic acid (RNA), and ultrasound (US).

Note

The Year Book of Surgery is a literature survey service providing abstracts of articles published in the professional literature. Every effort is made to assure the accuracy of the information presented in these pages. Neither the editors nor the publisher of the Year Book of Surgery can be responsible for errors in the original materials. The editors' comments are their own opinions. Mention of specific products within this publication does not constitute endorsement.

To facilitate the use of the Year Book of Surgery as a reference tool, all illustrations and tables included in this publication are now identified as they appear in the original article. This change is meant to help the reader recognize that any illustration or table appearing in the Year Book of Surgery may be only one of many in the original article. For this reason, figure and table numbers appear to be out of sequence within the Year Book of Surgery.

Dedication

James Matherson Seeger, MD

September 22, 1947 – October 21, 2009

The Editorial Board of the Year Book of Surgery dedicates this year's book to Dr Jim Seeger. Dr Seeger joined the Editorial Board in 1994 and served admirably as the Editor of the Vascular Surgery section until his untimely death in 2009. He was the consummate vascular surgeon and general surgeon whose chosen articles and commentaries were well suited to all general surgeons who are trained to do vascular surgery.

Dr Seeger joined the faculty of the University of Florida in 1982 and established the Division of Vascular Surgery. I had the pleasure of watching and supporting him as he developed one of the premier vascular surgery divisions in the country, complete with all the vascular techniques, sought-after fellowships, and a thriving research unit well funded with peer-reviewed resources. A lot can be said for spending an entire career at one institution, and Dr Seeger's successes here are a great example, for he received our most prestigious award, The Lifetime Achievement Award.

He was also Chief of Vascular Surgery at the Malcolm Randal Veterans Administration Hospital and had long-term Merit Review funding for his interest in endothelial cell seeding of arterial grafts. Later in life, he became interested in the reperfusion syndrome and made several important contributions in this field.

Jim was a member of the American Board of Surgery (Vascular Section), President of the Southern Association for Vascular Surgery and the Association of Program Directors in Vascular Surgery, and the Coeditor of the Journal of Vascular Surgery.

Dr Seeger was born on a farm in Welcome All, Georgia, graduated from Massachusetts Institute of Technology with a BS in Literature and Biology, returned home to matriculate through the Medical College of Georgia before completing both general surgery training under Dr Frank Moody at the University of Utah and vascular surgery training at Eastern Virginia Medical School.

We traveled together often. I would be reading a murder mystery and Dr Seeger would be reading some aspect of the cosmos theory. He was hardly a "book worm," for he was also an excellent sailor and golfer.

Dr Seeger is survived by his wife Carolyn, to whom he was married for 36 years. The untimely and unsuspected death of Dr Seeger left a tremendous hole in the Division of Vascular Surgery, in the hearts of everyone who knew him and in the Gainesville, Florida, community.

His favorite quote was from Thomas Campbell: "To live in the hearts we leave behind is not to die." Jim can rest easy that he fulfilled this mission in his life.

Edward M. Copeland, III, MD

Senior Editor, Year Book of Surgery

May 5, 2010

1 General Considerations

A Surgical Safety Checklist to Reduce Morbidity and Mortality in a Global Population

Haynes AB, for the Safe Surgery Saves Lives Study Group (Massachusetts General Hosp, Boston; et al)

N Engl J Med 360:491-499, 2009

Background.—Surgery has become an integral part of global health care, with an estimated 234 million operations performed yearly. Surgical complications are common and often preventable. We hypothesized that a program to implement a 19-item surgical safety checklist designed to improve team communication and consistency of care would reduce complications and deaths associated with surgery.

Methods.—Between October 2007 and September 2008, eight hospitals in eight cities (Toronto, Canada; New Delhi, India; Amman, Jordan; Auckland, New Zealand; Manila, Philippines; Ifakara, Tanzania; London, England; and Seattle, WA) representing a variety of economic circumstances and diverse populations of patients participated in the World Health Organization's Safe Surgery Saves Lives program. We prospectively collected data on clinical processes and outcomes from 3733 consecutively enrolled patients 16 years of age or older who were undergoing noncardiac surgery. We subsequently collected data on 3955 consecutively enrolled patients after the introduction of the Surgical Safety Checklist. The primary end point was the rate of complications, including death, during hospitalization within the first 30 days after the operation.

Results.—The rate of death was 1.5% before the checklist was introduced and declined to 0.8% afterward ($P = 0.003$). Inpatient complications occurred in 11.0% of patients at baseline and in 7.0% after introduction of the checklist ($P < 0.001$).

Conclusions.—Implementation of the checklist was associated with concomitant reductions in the rates of death and complications among patients at least 16 years of age who were undergoing noncardiac surgery in a diverse group of hospitals.

▶ I am impressed that the surgical checklist made the most difference in reducing complications in many of the same hospitals. Also, 3 of the hospitals did not routinely use preoperative antibiotics, and their use significantly reduced surgical site infections. Most of the hospitals did use the checklist items before the study, except none of the hospitals discussed the postoperative management among team members. To cite personal experience with a checklist, our institution uses each of the elements of the checklist except the discussion of the postoperative management. I can think of several instances where such a discussion would have prevented at least a minor, but annoying, complication for the patient. I doubt if many hospitals have thought of this postoperative strategy. So often, the same nursing and anesthesia teams that begin a case are not the same individuals who finish it. The constant during the operation is the surgical team, at least in this country. However, an entirely different team may assume the care in the recovery room, and then again in the intensive care unit. At each change of venue for the patient, a verbal discussion among the fore and aft teams might further reduce complication rates, especially now with the ever-increasing fragmentation of the care of a single patient.

The drop in complications, especially the serious ones, is impressive. I hope this information is disseminated via all practical channels, both globally and nationally.

E. M. Copeland, MD

A survey of academic surgeons: Work, stress, and research

Chokshi NK, Simeone DM, Chari RS, et al (Children Hosp Los Angeles, CA; Univ of Michigan, Ann Arbor; Vanderbilt Univ Med Ctr, Nashville, TN)

Surgery 146:462-468, 2009

Background.—An academic surgeon's workweek is divided among patient care, administrative duties, education, and research. The time available for research activities may change as a surgeon's career evolves. We sought to determine involvement of academic surgeons in research and to assess how this research endeavor was affected by demographic and workplace characteristics.

Methods.—We constructed a survey to explore the following 4 domains: demographics, time allotment, research activities, and effects of stressors. We distributed the survey to members of the Society of University Surgeons. In addition to performing descriptive statistics, we defined an active researcher as someone with a funding source who devoted 15% or more work hours to research. Using this definition, we performed statistical analyses to assess the significance of independent variables on research. Stress factors were evaluated on a Likert scale with responses ranging from 1 (not at all) to 5 (extremely).

Results.—We received 314 completed surveys (response rate 23%). Of the respondents, 274 (87%) stated that they were involved in some kind of research activity; however, only 143 (46%) were active researchers. Using univariate logistic regression analysis, younger respondents and surgeons who practiced for more than 10 years were more likely to be active researchers (odds ratio [OR]: 1.93, confidence interval [CI]: 1.51–2.46 and OR: 2.06, CI: 1.64–2.59, respectively). Males were less likely than females to be active researchers (OR: 0.32, CI: 016–0.67); however, by multivariate analysis, we found that the "years in practice" of an active researcher was the most significant predictor of research activity, whereas age and sex were not. In regard to stress, most respondents reported scores of 1–3 for all 7 stressors, which is consistent with minimal to moderate stress.

Conclusion.—Academic surgeons are involved actively in research; however, this involvement decreases as other professional responsibilities increase. To optimize the surgical research environment, departments should invest time and resources in young investigators to prevent them from decreasing their research activities.

▶ There have been surveys of academic surgeons for my entire career. They basically all have come to the same conclusion. Successful research begets more successful research, and department chairs should create more time for young investigators. Why have the results of these surveys always reached the same conclusions? Because individuals who are going to do basic research are going to do it regardless of the amount of protected time allocated to faculty members. Interest in basic research is engendered during medical school, and those interested in it seek out residencies that provide the appropriate mentoring. Such mentors often come from funded basic scientists within a surgical department or through collaboration with basic scientists in other departments. These residents now trained in a basic science discipline are sought after by chairs seeking such a faculty member, and by definition, they should be given the time and resources to pursue their research interests.

Unfortunately, these research-trained surgeons too often are hired into a surgical department that can only give lip service to basic research because of lack of space, of funding, or of no understanding of basic research from the leadership. When such occurs, the young faculty member becomes more clinically orientated within the department or leaves for other practice opportunities. They usually do not change schools in search of more fertile ground and, thus, are lost to the research community.

Yes, we do need to train more surgical scientists as all of the surveys have shown, but seldom mentioned is the effort that should be made to keep those whom we have trained interested and committed to basic research. A surgical department that cannot support a clinical scientist should not attempt to do so. Many broken promises to promising young faculty members have occurred over the failure to admit to the above.

E. M. Copeland, MD

Access to emergency operative care: A comparative study between the Canadian and American health care systems

Krajewski SA, Hameed SM, Smink DS, et al (Univ of British Columbia, Vancouver, Canada; Brigham and Women's Hosp, Ctr for Surgery and Public Health, Boston, MA; et al)

Surgery 146:300-307, 2009

Background.—Canada provides universal health insurance to all citizens, whereas 47 million Americans are uninsured. There has not been a study comparing access to emergency operative care between the 2 countries. As both countries contemplate changes in health care delivery, such comparisons are needed to guide health policy decisions. The purpose of this study is to determine whether or not there is a difference in access to emergency operative care between Canada and the United States.

Methods.—All patients diagnosed with acute appendicitis from 2001 to 2005 were identified in the Canadian Institute for Health Information database and the US Nationwide Inpatient Sample. Severity of appendicitis was determined by ICD-9 codes. Patients were further characterized by age, gender, insurance status, race, and socioeconomic status (SES; income). Univariate and multivariate analyses were performed to determine the odds of appendiceal perforation at different levels of SES in each country.

Results.—There were 102,692 Canadian patients and 276,890 American patients with acute appendicitis. In Canada, there was no difference in the odds of perforation between income levels. In the United States, there was a significant, inverse relationship between income level and the odds of perforation. The odds of perforation in the lowest income quartile were significantly higher than the odds of perforation in the highest income bracket (odds ratio, 1.20; 95% confidence interval, 1.16–1.24).

Conclusion.—The results suggest that access to emergency operative care is related to SES in the United States, but not in Canada. This difference could result from the concern over the ability to pay medical bills or the lack of a stable relationship with a primary care provider that can occur outside of a universal health care system.

▶ Interestingly, we are moving toward a universal health care system, whereas Canada is evaluating an increase in privatization of a current universal health care system. Such seems odd in countries that abut each other, have somewhat the same social and ethical standards, and should have leaders of somewhat equal intellect. Multiple studies have shown easier access to medical care for more routine medical needs favors the United States' system. The topic at hand, however, is emergency care of patients with an acute surgical disease not related to trauma.

Perforation rates are in the 30% to 35% range in both countries regardless of insurance status. The lowest perforation rates are among the insured United States patients (28.6%) and the self-pay patients (29.7%). This latter group is of particular interest and may represent the citizens among the 47 million uninsured in this country who elect to be uninsured, ie, those who get sick infrequently and can afford it when they do.

My question has nothing to do with insurance status. Is a perforation rate of almost one-third of patients diagnosed with appendicitis an acceptable rate? I think not. Then there is a problem with patient education, health care access, and/or diagnostic abilities in both countries. I expect the problem is the lack of a patient-selected, private physician whom the patient is comfortable calling for what could be a non-emergent problem, such as gastroenteritis. A culture has been created in both countries that physicians do not want to be bothered unless there is a true emergency. If I am right, we have a sad situation that might be impossible to reverse regardless of insurance status.

E. M. Copeland, MD

An observational study of surgery-related activities between nurses and surgeons during laparoscopic surgery

Zheng B, Taylor MD, Swanström LL (Legacy Health System, Portland, OR)

Am J Surg 197:497-502, 2009

Background.—In the operating room (OR), nurse-surgeon coordination is essential to the success of a surgery.

Methods.—This observational field study was conducted in the OR for selected laparoscopic surgeries to record surgery-related activities (SRAs) performed by the scrub nurses with different levels of OR experience. Those SRAs performed without instruction were defined as anticipatory movements.

Results.—The scrub nurse spent 74% of OR time watching surgery and 35% of OR time performing SRAs. The intermediate skill nurses watch surgeon on 76% of the OR time and they performed 16 counts of anticipatory movements per procedure. Experienced nurses spent shorter amount of OR time (72%) watching surgery but they performed more anticipatory movements (20 counts) than the intermediate skill nurses. With basic cases, experienced and intermediate-skill nurses performed equal amounts of anticipatory movements; however, when assisting in complex cases, the experienced nurses performed significantly more anticipatory movements (24 counts) than the intermediate-skill nurses (16 counts).

Conclusions.—Experienced nurses develop sophisticated cognition during their careers in the OR, which allows them to maintain their involvement with the surgical team consistently. The anticipatory movement and the eye gaze are 2 valuable behavioral markers for assessing team performance.

▶ The results of this study seem grossly obvious; however, in the 2 hospitals in which I have spent my entire career, the obvious was not the standard. The prevailing thought of the nursing leadership was that the operating room (OR) nurses should be well qualified to do all the procedures done in the OR. This philosophy leads to OR nurses being, at most, average in all cases, and expert in none. Both hospitals eventually went to OR teams that would be constant from day to day, but it took a long time for the wake-up call to occur.

In a hospital with a residency program, this continuity is even more important. Surgeons have different approaches to the same procedure. For example, I am left-handed, and it is nice to have my left-handed needle holders on the table. Positioning of the patient is another "quirk" that surgeons have, especially for procedures such as a low anterior resection. "Your" nurse knows the eccentricities and can speed the setup of the case along rather than frequently having to show or explain this part of the operation to a new resident. Surgeons need to feel comfortable in the OR, and having "my" nurse there is the foremost thing in making me comfortable.

While on the subject, I have never understood why the person with the nursing degree is the circulator and the person scrubbed is a technical trainee. Is counting sponges and retrieving equipment from another room more important than having a nurse who can anticipate your next move during an operation? I guess the answer is yes, at least in our hospital.

E. M. Copeland, MD

Attitudes, Training Experiences, and Professional Expectations of US General Surgery Residents: A National Survey

Yeo H, Viola K, Berg D, et al (Yale Univ School of Medicine, New Haven, CT; et al)

JAMA 302:1301-1308, 2009

Context.—General surgery residency programs are facing multiple pressures, including attracting and retaining residents. Despite the importance of resident perspectives in designing effective responses to these pressures, understanding of residents' views is limited.

Objective.—To profile US general surgery residents; characterize resident attitudes, experiences, and expectations regarding training; and examine differences by sex and training year.

Design, Setting, and Participants.—Cross-sectional study of all general surgery residents completing a survey in January 2008 following administration of the American Board of Surgery In-Training Examination.

Main Outcome Measures.—Resident satisfaction; perceived supports, strains and concern; career motivations; and professional expectations.

Results.—Of 5345 categorical general surgery residents, 4402 (82.4%) responded, representing 248 of 249 surgical residency programs. Most respondents expressed satisfaction with training (3686 [85.2%]; 95% confidence interval [CI], 84.1%-86.3%) and supportive peer relationships (3433 [84.2%]; 95% CI, 83.1%-85.3%). However, residents also reported unmet needs and apprehensions about training and careers. Worry that they will not feel confident performing procedures independently was reported by 1185 (27.5%; 95% CI, 26.2%-28.8%), while 2681 (63.8%; 95% CI, 62.4%-65.3%) reported that they must complete specialty training to be competitive. Perceptions of program support differ, with men more likely than women to report that their program provides support (2188 [74.5%] vs 895 [65.6%]; $P < .001$), and that they can turn to faculty when having difficulties (2193 [74.5%] vs 901 [66.4%]; $P < .001$). Reports of having considered leaving training in the prior year differed significantly across years ($P < .001$), highest in postgraduate year 2 (19.2%) and lowest in postgraduate year 5 (7.2%).

Conclusions.—General surgery residents' attitudes, experiences, and expectations regarding training reflect both high levels of satisfaction and sources of strain. These factors vary by sex and training year.

▶ A lot of surveys have been done on this subject during the past 6 years and I have reported the findings on several of them. I have made predictions as to the outcome of the new training paradigm, and now the surveys are available to see if I was right.

This is the best of all the surveys to date. The participants were a trapped audience having just completed the American Board of Surgery In-Training Examination (ABSITE). Consequently, the participation was 82%, whereas in most surveys attaining 30% to 40% participation is considered a success. There could be some skewing of the responses because the participants had just completed an examination that might have had some positive or negative effects on the responses. For the most part, however, the responses were quite favorable and probably are reflective of the responses from residents if the same survey had been conducted before the introduction of the 80-hour work week.

The feeling of lack of confidence to do the required procedures of a general surgical practice and the need to become a general surgery subspecialist to be a competitive, competent and secure surgeon are the new findings generated by this survey and were 2 of the consequences of the 80-hour work week that I predicted. In my 21 years as a chairman on a department of surgery (1982-2003), 33% of the graduating residents became cardiothoracic, colorectal, or plastic surgeons. The remainder practiced general surgery and were evenly divided between private and academic practice. These numbers are changing dramatically as indicated by this survey. A shortage of general surgeons will soon be upon us. The fear is for rural areas, but urban areas need general surgeons also.

E. M. Copeland, MD

Does Surgical Quality Improve in the American College of Surgeons National Surgical Quality Improvement Program: An Evaluation of All Participating Hospitals

Hall BL, Hamilton BH, Richards K, et al (John Cochran Veterans Affairs Med Ctr, St Louis, MO; Olin Business School at Washington Univ in St Louis, MO; American College of Surgeons, Chicago, IL; et al)
Ann Surg 250:363-376, 2009

Background/Objective.—The National Surgical Quality Improvement Program (NSQIP) has demonstrated quality improvement in the VA and pilot study of 14 academic institutions. The objective was to show that American College of Surgeons (ACS)-NSQIP helps all enrolled hospitals.

Methods.—ACS-NSQIP data was used to evaluate improvement in hospitals longitudinally over 3 years (2005–2007). Improvement was defined as reduction in risk-adjusted "Observed/Expected" (O/E) ratios between periods with risk adjustment held constant. Multivariable logistic regression-based adjustment was performed and included indicators for procedure groups. Additionally, morbidity counts were modeled using a negative binomial model, to estimate the number of avoided complications.

Results.—Multiple perspectives reflected improvement over time. In the analysis of 118 hospitals (2006–2007), 66% of hospitals improved risk-adjusted mortality (mean O/E improvement: 0.174; $P < 0.05$) and 82% improved risk adjusted complication rates (mean improvement: 0.114; $P < 0.05$). Correlations between starting O/E and improvement (0.834 for mortality, 0.652 for morbidity), as well as relative risk, revealed that initially worse-performing hospitals had more likelihood of improvement. Nonetheless, well-performing hospitals also improved. Modeling morbidity counts, 183 hospitals (2007), avoided ~9598 potential complications: ~52/hospital. Due to sampling this may represent only 1 of 5 to 1 of 10 of the true total. Improvement reflected aggregate performance across all types of hospitals (academic/community, urban/rural). Changes in patient risk over time had important contributions to the effect.

Conclusions.—ACS-NSQIP indicates that surgical outcomes improve across all participating hospitals in the private sector. Improvement is reflected for both poor- and well-performing facilities. NSQIP hospitals appear to be avoiding substantial numbers of complications, improving care and reducing costs. Changes in risk over time merit further study.

▶ I have been fortunate to be a member of the leadership of the American College of Surgeons (ACS) from the inception of National Surgical Quality Improvement Program (NSQIP) until the present. This is a landmark article showing that participating in the program does improve quality of care in the private community. The improvement is demonstrated over time and for hospitals of all sizes. The data are derived from patient records of each hospital. This process makes the program somewhat labor intensive and requires a financial investment by the individual participating hospitals. The patient records are sampled and the data cannot yet be applied to an individual surgeon. This capability, however, will soon be available.

The next question is, So what? There will be measures of outcomes (ie, quality of care), and these outcomes measures will be tied to reimbursement. NSQIP has not been embraced by the hospitals across the country, including the hospital where I work, ostensibly because of the annual investment that is required to run the program. This investment is essentially the salary of the data collector. I find this reticence by some hospitals to be a "head in the sand" approach, especially now when the identification of poor quality has no downside, and improvement can be made without penalty.

I am in favor of reimbursement based on quality of outcomes. I am not in favor of the outcomes measures being devised by bureaucrats hired by governmental agencies. I will give an example. There was a suggestion that reimbursement for colectomy be based on the recovery of an appropriate number of lymph nodes in the pathologic specimen. Treatment for locally advanced rectal cancer includes preoperative chemoradiation therapy because of the improvement in survival with such regimens. Frequently there are very few lymph nodes recovered in the specimens because of this initial treatment. Basing reimbursement on recovery of lymph nodes would possibly eliminate neoadjuvant therapy from the treatment of rectal cancer.

Best the private sector look to the ACS-NSQIP for quality measures, at least for surgeons, because the program has surgical input.

E. M. Copeland, MD

Health Plan Use of Board Certification and Recertification of Surgeons and Nonsurgical Subspecialists in Contracting Policies

Freed GL, Dunham KM, Singer D (Univ of Michigan, Ann Arbor)

Arch Surg 144:753-758, 2009

Objectives.—To characterize the role of board certification in general surgeon, surgical specialist, and nonsurgical subspecialist credentialing and contracting policies and to examine possible variation among different types of health plans.

Design.—Telephone survey conducted from October 27, 2006, through March 30, 2007.

Setting.—Health plans across the United States.

Participants.—Health plan credentialing personnel from a random sample of 223 health plans stratified by enrollment size, plan type, Medicaid enrollment, and tax status.

Main Outcome Measures.—Proportion of health plans that require specialty board certification at initial contract or at some point during association with the plan and health plan requirements for recertification.

Results.—Of 223 health plans, 9 were ineligible, and credentialing personnel completed the telephone survey in 176, which resulted in an overall response rate of 82%. More than 60% of the health plans in this study did not require surgical specialists, general surgeons, or nonsurgical subspecialists ever to be board certified to contract with the plan. Approximately two-thirds of respondents reported that they did not require surgeons (65%) or nonsurgical subspecialists (63%) with time-limited board certification to recertify in their specialty. More than half of the health plans reported that they made exceptions to their board certification policies based on geographic or network need.

Conclusions.—Most health plans did not use specialty board certification to assess surgeon and nonsurgical subspecialist competence.

▶ As a United States citizen, I find the results of this survey demoralizing, especially having spent so much time in voluntary organizations (American Board of Surgery and the American College of Surgeons) that have patient safety as the primary mission. As Chairman of the American Board of Surgery from 1990-1991, I was surprised to find that the Joint Commission on Hospital Accreditation did not require at least board eligibility to gain access to the operating room. The only requirement was that hospitals have a credentialing committee or a medical board that determined surgical privileges of an individual. This requirement remains the same today, almost 20 years later, although most hospitals now require board eligibility, but do so voluntarily.

For smaller communities the hospital may be the major driving force of the local economy. For the hospital, surgically related income is the financial driving force. Because the medical boards of these hospitals are made up of successful local people, the success of the hospital could be tied to the success of the businesses of the board members. This situation creates a possible conflict of interest between the board and the quality of care the hospital provides. In other words a subpar surgeon may be better than no surgeon at all from their financial standpoint, even though another health care facility may be in close proximity. No help will come from the hospital administrators because their salary is also somewhat dependent on a financially successful surgical service.

Now we find from this article that more than half of the health plans do not require board certification for plan participation. We are setting up for the perfect storm: 1) fewer general surgeons are available; 2) reimbursement for those who are available will soon come from hospitals; 3) the financial viability of the hospital, the administrators, and possibly the community businesses rely on surgical services; 4) there are dwindling requirements for general surgeons to be credentialed or paid by health plans; and 5) graduates of offshore medical schools will fill the physician void predicted to occur in the next few years.

The health care crisis of today is one of expense and access. In the future we can add quality to that list.

E. M. Copeland, MD

Impact of sleep deprivation on medium-term psychomotor and cognitive performance of surgeons: Prospective cross-over study with a virtual surgery simulator and psychometric tests

Lehmann KS, Martus P, Little-Elk S, et al (Charité–Campus Benjamin Franklin, Berlin; et al)

Surgery 147:246-254, 2010

Background.—Despite recent work hour restrictions, 24-hour calls remain an important part of patient care. The aim of this study was to assess the impact of 24-hour night calls on the psychomotor and cognitive skills of surgeons with a virtual surgery simulator (VSS) and psychometric tests. We hypothesized that sleep loss impairs surgical skills and concentration performance.

Methods.—Seventeen surgery residents (test group) and 13 medical students (reference group) performed a 5-day training program on the VSS. The test group was then assessed during a night call on 4 test points (8 AM and 4 PM on the on-call day, 8 AM on the postcall day, and 8 AM on the recovery day) to assess the effects of sleep loss on these surgery residents. The reference group performed the same tests but without a night call.

Results.—The training resulted in a homogenous performance level for both groups. The average time for the test group was 26 minutes. The analysis between rested and sleep-deprived participants (6.5 ± 0.9 vs 2.9 ± 1.4 hours of night sleep) in the on-call part showed no performance differences. No impairment was found for the VSS and the cognitive tests within the test group between the start of the working day and the start of the postcall day after the night of relative sleep loss. The subgroup analysis showed no significant differences regarding the amount of night sleep and laparoscopic experience.

Conclusion.—No performance impairment was found for surgeons with a VSS and standardized cognitive tests after a night of relative sleep loss. Although there is no doubt that sleep deprivation ultimately impairs human functioning, typical surgical skills do not necessarily deteriorate with a limited amount of sleep loss under clinical conditions.

▶ The debate about the effects of sleep loss on technical and cognitive functions continues. Frankly, I think these skills relate to the individual being tested rather than sleep loss. It is well known that some people do quite well with 4 hours of sleep and others require 8 hours to function up to their potential. I am in the latter group, but have never noticed sleep deprivation to affect either cognitive or technical skills after sleep deprivation for 24 to 36 hours. I crash when I am off call, but not during it. Likewise a 15-minute power nap is quite refreshing.

I like the results of this study because the results agree with my bias. There are several problems. Sleep was available if time allowed, and the time to measure is better at 36 hours rather than at 24 hours. The ideal call schedule is every third or fourth night, and the resident will work the next day

(32-36 hours). Surgical residents are highly motivated to actively participate in an operative procedure. The operative word here is "actively." I could fall asleep holding a retractor after a good night's sleep!!

On 24 hours, off 24 hours or longer is fine for an acute care service like the emergency room or, possibly, the trauma service. Otherwise the lessons learned from continuity of care should dictate that residents be around to see the fruits of their labor.

E. M. Copeland, MD

Implementation of Resident Work Hour Restrictions is Associated With a Reduction in Mortality and Provider-Related Complications on the Surgical Service: A Concurrent Analysis of 14,610 Patients

Privette AR, Shackford SR, Osler T, et al (Univ of Vermont, Burlington; et al)
Ann Surg 250:316-321, 2009

Objective.—To determine the effect of implementation of work hour restrictions on the rates of morbidity, mortality, and provider-related complications in surgical patients and to determine the incremental personnel costs associated with implementation.

Summary Background Data.—In 2003, the Accreditation Council for Graduate Medical Education enacted resident work hour restrictions (RWHR) to improve patient safety by decreasing errors attributed to resident fatigue. There are no quantitative data on surgical patients to validate whether this objective has been achieved and, if so, at what cost.

Methods.—Retrospective observational cohort analysis of data gathered concurrently with patient care for 30 days after admission or surgical intervention before implementation (prerestriction: July 2001–June 2003) and after (postrestriction: July 2005–June 2007). Main outcome measures: mortality, surgical complications, percentage of complications judged to be provider-related, and incremental personnel costs (salary and fringe of providers).

Results.—A total of 14,610 patients were admitted during the 2 periods. Compared with the prerestriction period, there was a significant reduction in the percentage of complications attributed to providers (pre: 48.3%; post: 38.6%, $P < 0.001$) and a significant reduction in mortality rate (pre: 1.9%; post: 1.1%, $P = 0.002$) in the postrestriction period. Postrestriction the clinical care hours provided by attending surgeons increased significantly and was associated with a 1250% increase in the RVU-82 billing modifier ("no qualified resident available") from 523 RVUs pre-RWHR to 6542 post-RWHR. There was an increase in annual personnel costs postrestriction of $1.466 million.

Conclusions.—Implementation of RWHR was associated with reduced provider-related complications and mortality suggesting improved patient safety. This was likely due to several factors including reduced resident fatigue and greater attending involvement in clinical care.

▶ This study should serve as a benchmark for the cost benefit and the patient-outcome benefit of the resident work hour restrictions (WHR). The bottom line in this report is a reduced mortality rate in the postWHR period. First of all, many studies have a halo effect, meaning that the expected outcome can bias the investigator. There is no indication that there was a halo effect here. The most likely explanation is the increase in faculty member involvement, especially in continuity of care. The reverse is also probably true, that is, a reduction in reliance on resident care. What is not known is the level of faculty member care in the preWHR period, although it seems to be more than appropriate as defined by the authors. The number of operations done by the senior residents decreased, but remained adequate as determined by the American Board of Surgery. Was the participation by the resident in the operative case diminished? In other words, was the case done primarily by the faculty member in the postWHR period to better insure a favorable outcome because the resident would not be primarily responsible for the postoperative care? The answer to this question in my practice is yes.

Nevertheless, we have the results from one institution that demonstrates rather clearly that mortality has been reduced concomitant with the reduction in work hours, and probably as a result of the new patient care paradigms put in place because of the WHR.

The authors are to be congratulated on the thoroughness with which they report the data and the excellence of the discussion. This report could, however, become an example for those zealots in favor of WHR on surgical services, and without the zealots having read anything but the abstract. This is one of those articles that finds itself referenced by a lot of authors without these authors ever having read the article.

E. M. Copeland, MD

Influence of Double-Gloving on Manual Dexterity and Tactile Sensation of Surgeons

Fry DE, Harris WE, Kohnke EN, et al (Northwestern Univ Feinberg School of Medicine, Chicago, IL; Manchester Univ, England; Virginia Hand Ctr, Richmond, VA; et al)

J Am Coll Surg 210:325-330, 2010

Background.—Double-gloving in the performance of surgical procedures has been demonstrated to reduce the frequency of blood contact with the hands of members of the surgical team. Concerns persist that double-gloving can compromise the dexterity and tactile sensitivity of the surgeon.

Study Design.—Fifty-three surgeons and surgeons-in-training volunteered at the Clinical Congress of the American College of Surgeons and were studied using the Purdue Pegboard test and a standard 2-point discrimination test to compare no gloves, a single pair of gloves, and double-gloving on manual dexterity and tactile sensitivity. Categorical and continuous variables were identified, general linear prediction models were computed, and the influence of glove status was analyzed as an independent variable. Monte Carlo simulation was employed to validate conclusions.

Results.—Gender, specialty, and handedness did not affect prediction models. Glove status did not affect dexterity performance scores ($p = 0.57$) after accounting for the influence of age on score variation ($p < 0.001$). Comparing ulnar and radial surfaces of the index finger for 2-point discrimination, no difference was detected between trials ($p < 0.66$), nor was an interaction effect detected with glove status ($p = 0.40$). Monte Carlo simulations validated the apparent absence of differences.

Conclusions.—Double-gloving does not have a substantial impact on manual dexterity or tactile sensitivity when compared with no gloves or single-gloving in this study.

▶ The thickness of the gloves and the tightness of fit obviously will affect the data collected in this study. In today's world, most gloves are well suited for comfort and appropriate thickness to allow for double-gloving. The results of this study eliminate tactile sensation and dexterity as reasons to not double glove. No doubt, double-gloving is a matter of preference and perception. Good studies have demonstrated the added safety of wearing double gloves. Knife cuts and needle penetrations are reduced, as is the inoculum of an undesirable agent into the skin of the surgeon.

In my experience, a double glove allows for a better margin of error for penetration of the skin. Most possible penetrations are quite superficial and require the surgeon to investigate the integrity of the glove to determine whether it has been violated. In such cases, double glove will better insure intact integrity. Obviously, blood under the glove is proof of integrity violation, but tactile sensation of a possible violation is not. It is these tactile sensations that are most common for a surgeon to test the integrity of the gloves.

E. M. Copeland, MD

Is Routine Postoperative Chest X-Ray Necessary after Fluoroscopic-Guided Subclavian Central Venous Port Placement?

Brown JR, Slomski C, Saxe AW (Michigan State Univ College of Human Medicine, Lansing)

J Am Coll Surg 208:517-519, 2009

Background.—Two uncommon but serious complications after subclavian central venous port (SCVP) placement are pneumothorax (PNX) and malposition of the catheter. Chest x-rays (CXR) are commonly obtained after SCVP placement to identify these complications, but their use is controversial.

Study Design.—We performed a retrospective review of SCVP placements to establish the incidence of PNX or catheter malposition identified exclusively by postprocedure CXR.

Results.—Between July 1, 2001, and June 30, 2006, 205 patients underwent elective SCVP placement. Although 4 patients (2%) sustained a PNX, none was identified by routine postprocedure CXR. Postprocedure clinical symptoms (3 to 72 hours later) prompted repeat CXR, which identified the PNX. Five patients (2.4%) had catheter malposition recognized by intraoperative fluoroscopy and corrected intraoperatively. No malpositioned catheters were identified on postprocedure CXR.

Conclusions.—In our study, incidence of PNX after SCVP placement was low, and PNX was not detected by intraoperative fluoroscopy or by routine postprocedure CXR. We conclude that the practice of routine postprocedure CXR after SCVP placement is not necessary and should be replaced with diagnostic chest radiography only if symptoms develop.

▶ I respectfully disagree with the conclusion of the authors. I was at the University of Pennsylvania when Stanley Dudrick and Douglas Wilmore described the proper management of subclavian catheters, and over the years have placed a large number of these catheters. In my experience, the postinsertion chest film will identify a pneumothorax, even if the film is done by portable technique. The authors have been lucky that a significant pneumothorax has not developed, especially in a patient who is treated as an outpatient without confirmation of catheter placement and of the absence of a pneumothorax.

In fact, the 2 most important indications for a postinsertion chest film are as follows: (1) an outpatient who could suffer a delayed pneumothorax and not have access to a health care facility (for example, while driving home to a distant site) and (2) when failure to insert the catheter occurs on 1 side and the surgeon is going to attempt to place the catheter in the opposite subclavian vein. I have seen a bilateral pneumothorax from bilateral attempts to place a subclavian catheter. It was almost fatal. A chest film should be done to rule out a pneumothorax on the ipsilateral side before proceeding to the contralateral side. When a catheter cannot be inserted, the surgeon will almost always make several attempts to access the subclavian vein before moving to the opposite side. It is in just this circumstance that a pneumothorax is most likely to develop.

Accurate catheter placement in the middle of the subclavian vein, especially for stiff catheters, is quite important. In a septic patient, a catheter tip that touches the tricuspid valve can create a nidus for infection on the valve surface. A catheter that gains access to either internal mammary vein will result in substernal pain, mimicking a heart attack. If the catheter is not removed the vein will burst because the solutions today are infused under pressure from a pump. Large amounts of infused fluid can accumulate in the pleural space, in an amount that can result in a shift of the mediastinal structures. I could go on, but I think I have made my point.

E. M. Copeland, MD

Mortality in Medicare Patients Undergoing Surgery in July in Teaching Hospitals

Englesbe MJ, Fan Z, Baser O, et al (Univ of Michigan, Ann Arbor)
Ann Surg 249:871-876, 2009

Objective.—To determine whether operative mortality rates at teaching hospitals in the United States are higher in July, the start of the academic year.

Summary Background Data.—Surgical patients at teaching hospitals often worry about the involvement of inexperienced physician trainees in their care.

Methods.—This retrospective cohort study included all Medicare recipients undergoing 1 of 7 diverse inpatient procedures at teaching hospitals between 2003 through 2006 (N = 320,216). Teaching status was defined both by membership in the United States Council of Teaching Hospitals and by hospital ratio of trainees to beds. We compared operative mortality rates in July relative to all other months, adjusting for potentially confounding patient characteristics. The main outcome measure was operative mortality (before discharge or within 30 days of procedures).

Results.—Adjusted operative mortality rates were no higher in July than in other months combined for all procedures, including coronary artery bypass grafting, carotid endarterectomy, repair of nonruptured abdominal aortic aneurysms, colectomy, pancreatectomy, esophagectomy, and repair of hip fracture. Trend analysis revealed no significant monthly or seasonal variation in operative mortality rates.

Conclusions.—Operative mortality rates do not decline as surgical trainees acquire more experience during the academic year. With respect to mortality, July is a safe month to have major surgery in teaching hospitals in the United States.

▶ The common misconception has been that July is a month with higher surgical mortality rates because of new residents who are often unfamiliar with the hospital systems. I am glad to see a large cohort study from the Medicare database that disproves this notion. Likewise, the operations with the highest mortality and morbidity rates were studied. In fact, July could be a month to have an operation by me in an academic center. On my service, I usually put the most accomplished chief resident in the initial 3-month rotation and the least accomplished one on the last 3-month rotation. The least accomplished chief resident would have 9 more months of training before finishing the residency on my service. The improvement during the residency for the chiefs is dramatic in some cases. One of the joys of an academic career is watching the maturation of a surgeon in training. Another reason that July might be the preferable month is because the faculty member must be more involved in all aspects of surgical care, simply because the residents are a year older and have new and sometimes unfamiliar responsibilities. I took the most accomplished chief resident first because I had the least amount of time to give one-on-one training.

The University of Florida has been blessed with excellent young people who have been motivated to be the best they can. There are some residents, however, who do not mature either technically or judgmentally as fast as others, and there was the occasional complaint about a certain resident's lack of progress. My job was to remind the faculty members that we are paid to train residents, so go and do it.

Rarely, there is a resident who does not have the technical capability to become a competitive surgeon. These residents need to be identified as quickly as possible so they can transfer into a specialty in which they can excel (and make a living!). No one should be finished who will be noncompetitive. This is a major disservice to the individual and to the patients with whom the individual may come in contact.

E. M. Copeland, MD

Residential Segregation and Access to Surgical Care by Minority Populations in US Counties

Hayanga AJ, Kaiser HE, Sinha R, et al (Univ of Michigan Health System, Ann Arbor; Johns Hopkins Bloomberg School of Public Health, Baltimore, MD)

J Am Coll Surg 208:1017-1022, 2009

Background.—Minority groups in the US have comparatively poorer access to a range of health care services. Access can be considered a function of opportunity and use and can vary with the level of segregation within a county. We hypothesized that with varying levels of segregation, increasing the proportion of the minority population within a county was accompanied by decreasing levels of access to surgical care.

Study Design.—A cross-sectional analysis was performed on data from the 2004 Area Resource File. Each county in the US was categorized into one of three levels: most, moderately, or least segregated, using the Isolation Index. Multivariable linear regression analysis was performed to examine the association between access to surgical services and proportion of minority population with varying levels of segregation adjusting for socioeconomic and health characteristics.

Results.—In the most segregated counties, each percentage point increase in Hispanic or African-American population was associated with a statistically significant decrease in outpatient surgery volume ($p < 0.0001$), ambulatory surgical facilities ($p < 0.0001$), and number of general surgeons ($p < 0.0001$). In the least segregated counties, these associations showed no statistical significance. A significant increase ($p < 0.0001$) in the volume of emergency medical visits was associated with increasing proportions of African-American and Hispanic populations within the most segregated counties.

Conclusions.—In the most segregated counties, an increase in the African-American or Hispanic population was associated with a decrease

in the availability and use of surgical services and an increase in emergency visits after adjustment for socioeconomic and health characteristics.

▶ Over the years I have selected many articles from the group at Michigan who are interested in health policy. I select them because they are excellent, and this article is one of the best. I hope that President Obama has someone from the group at Michigan on his health policy staff. The President clearly gets misinformation from someone. An example was his statement at a town hall meeting at which he said that reimbursement for a surgeon who performs an amputation of the leg is $50 000.00. The point was to diagnose and treat diabetes to limit the need for amputations and, thus, save money. I don't doubt that the total costs for an amputation approaches $50 000; however, the reimbursement for the surgeon is about $750 max, and this is a global fee. The bulk of the remainder goes to the facility. Facility costs are driving the cost of health up, not physician reimbursement. The hospital is reimbursed by the diagnostic-related group system (DRG), which allows unbundling of patients' bills. A patient who was recently dead on arrival (DOA) at an emergency room generated a facility bill of $15 000 simply to pronounce the unfortunate victim DOA.

No one seems to care about facility costs. Two years ago the average salary for a hospital CEO was $973 000.[1] Salaries for the COO and CFO were less, but not by much. All of this money comes from the health care reimbursement system, which collects from the facility side of reimbursement.

Limited access to health care is not limited to African Americans, Hispanics, and Asians. There are Caucasians with limited access to health care also. There are counties in central Northwest Florida in which the residents are almost exclusively white, have little access to health care, and have a low income. I have long been a supporter of universal health care, at least to eliminate the economic issues and possibly to attract physicians to practice in these areas. The money to enact universal health care probably already exists in the system if insurance and hospital executives were willing to have smaller salaries, and insurance companies would accept a lower profit margin. Insurance premiums go up and reimbursement to subscribers goes down. Somehow I don't think this is the American way.

E. M. Copeland, MD

Reference

1. Special Feature Article. *Modern Health Care*. July 2008: 53.

Should All Duty Hours Be the Same? Results of a National Survey of Surgical Trainees

Moalem J, Salzman P, Ruan DT, et al (Univ of Rochester Med Ctr, NY; Brigham and Women's Hosp, Boston, MA; et al)

J Am Coll Surg 209:47-54, 2009

Background.—Although duty hours regulations (DHR) were introduced as a measure to improve patient safety and graduate medical education, new evidence suggests that the opposite might be happening. This study was designed to assess surgery resident perceptions of the impact that DHR have had on their education, the number of hours they believed would be ideal for their training, and to evaluate the effect of seniority on these opinions.

Study Design.—An Internet-based survey was electronically distributed to all Resident and Associate members of the American College of Surgeons.

Results.—Of 599 respondents, 247 (41%) believed that DHR were an important barrier to their education, and 266 (44%) believed that the ideal work week should have 80 to 100 hours. These two opinions were highly correlated, and were increasingly voiced with increased resident experience. Senior residents were more likely to view DHR as an important barrier to their education whether or not they were general surgery residents or were trained in small, medium, or large programs.

Conclusions.—A large subset of surgery residents, particularly senior residents, considered DHR an important barrier to their education and expressed a desire to work longer hours than restrictions allow. These findings suggest that strict and uniform DHR do not allow for optimal training of residents at different levels who have disparate educational goals and needs. Introducing some flexibility into senior residents' limitations should be considered.

▶ I have reviewed other articles looking at the effect of work hours restriction on resident training since the inception of the mandate in 2003. The initial reports were that the restrictions were welcomed by the junior residents, but were considered onerous by the senior residents. The senior residents then had begun their residency under the "old" system, and were annoyed by any work hours restrictions. They saw continuity of care and surgical case numbers eroding. The question was what would the junior residents who embraced work hours restrictions think when they became senior residents? This article addresses this question directly.

Most of the respondents in this survey began their residency at the time of the initiation of work hours restrictions. As they progressed through their training, and the time for them to become competitive as a competent surgeon approached, the greater the criticisms of the work hours restrictions have become. I had not predicted this outcome. I thought that those residents indoctrinated into the 80-hour workweek at the outset would continue to embrace it throughout their residencies and carry that work ethic into practice. I am happy that I appear to be wrong. Had I been right, shift hour mentality with multiple "hand-offs" would have become the standard of practice, and patient ownership and continuity of care would be a thing of the past. Patient care would deteriorate to the point that a problem with surgical training would have been identified and the culprit would have been work hours restrictions with all the coincident negative effects on resident training so well enumerated in this article. This process of realization of the problem would have taken years.

Now it appears, at least from this study, that surgical residents regardless of specialty realize that their training has not given them the confidence to proceed outside the training environment. Resident work hours restrictions took hold because the concept was embraced by residents. If residents realize the fallacy of the concept, it will be revised much quicker, and the quality of patient care will not be diminished by lack of appropriate knowledge and experience.

E. M. Copeland, MD

Stress and Burnout Among Surgeons: Understanding and Managing the Syndrome and Avoiding the Adverse Consequences

Balch CM, Freischlag JA, Shanafelt TD (Johns Hopkins Med Inst, Baltimore, MD; Mayo Clinic, Rochester, MN)

Arch Surg 144:371-376, 2009

Training for and practicing surgery are stressful endeavors. Studies involving national samples of surgeons from surgical subspecialty societies and graduates of surgical training programs suggest that burnout rates among surgeons range from 30% to 38%. These statistics indicate that a substantial number of our colleagues are struggling with personal and professional distress at a level that should be of concern to all surgeons.

▶ All physicians delay short-term goals to attain a long-term goal. Short-term goals may be income, marriage, children, and participation in leisure activities such as golf, fishing, hunting, cooking, etc. I am somewhat describing myself, but to my knowledge, have never experienced burnout. Why? I have been more successful than I ever imagined. Medicine, as a profession, is even better than I expected. Studies show that 80% of people work 8 hours a day to support their activities in the other 16 hours. I am one of the other 20% who work more than 8 hours a day and go home to rest to be able to fully enjoy the next day's work. Your work should be your hobby, especially if you are a surgeon. Osler once said that medicine is a jealous mistress, meaning your work is constantly drawing you back to it.

An overriding reason for burnout is that medicine did not meet expectations and/or goals were set too high to be obtained. Chairs of departments should be trained to recognize the prevailing traits of students and residents who may experience burnout later in life. Some of these traits are lack of interest, technical inability, anger, poor patient relationships, demanding family needs, poor organizational skills, and a greater interest in outside activities than surgical training. A person with these traits should be in another profession, or if in medicine, avoid a potentially stressful surgical discipline. Never train a resident who cannot be competitive as a surgeon in his local environment.

The 80-hour workweek was instituted to meet the needs of individuals with some of the possible burnout traits. A problem with the study of burnout is no comparative data with a previous generation of surgeons. Dr Balch and his colleagues are to be congratulated for providing a baseline for the immediate past generation of surgeons who were trained before institution of the 80-hour workweek. Ten years from now it will be interesting to see the rates of burnout.

E. M. Copeland, MD

The Independent Physician — Going, Going...

Isaacs SL, Jellinek PS, Ray WL (San Francisco)

N Engl J Med 360:655-657, 2009

Despite the current focus on expanding health insurance coverage, relatively little attention has been paid to the future of the physicians who provide care for the insured and uninsured alike — specifically, to their ongoing migration from independent solo or small-group practices to larger-group practices, where they are often employees. This trend and its consequences for the care of patients and the practice of medicine have scarcely been explored.

The percentage of U.S. physicians who own their own practice has been declining at an annual rate of approximately 2% for at least the past 25 years. Although the decline is unquestionable, the percentage of physicians currently remaining in independent practice is unknown. For 2001, the most recent year for which data are available from the three usual sources, the American Medical Association (AMA) has estimated the proportion at 61.5% and the Center for Studying Health System Change (CSHSC) puts it at 55.9%, whereas the Census Bureau's Current Population Survey calculates it at only 29.3%.

▶ The reasons for migration to employee status are the desire of the recent graduates from medical school to have a better lifestyle than their predecessors. This makes sense because approximately 50% of medical students today are women. Childbirth and motherhood still remain in their domain. Men, also, are seeking a better lifestyle. The 80-hour workweek for training plays directly into this lifestyle desire.

Salaried positions are becoming more attractive because work hours are predictable, and the salaries offered by hospitals are now very attractive, especially for physicians that rely heavily on hospital services to make a living, ie, general surgeons. The reimbursement system in place today, primarily driven by the federal government via Medicare and Medicaid, has the majority of the money accumulating on the hospital side through facility and technical fees. Therefore, the money to pay high salaries exists to pay physicians just as it does to pay hospital administrators (the average salary of whom is approaching a million dollars a year).

The reimbursement system will be responsible for the elimination of the solo and small group surgical practices. On the medical side, hospitalists have freed up the internists to concentrate on increasing volume in their private offices by relieving them of the need to admit and, in some instances, round on their patients.

For those specialties that can be practiced in an outpatient facility, such as plastic, orthopedic, and ophthalmologic surgery and endoscopy, the physicians can, for now, collect the facility and technical fee along with the physician fee.

The problem that I see with this new paradigm is a potential failure for anyone to take pride of ownership of the patients' longitudinal care. If I am right, patients are in for a rude awakening, at least until they get accustomed to the new system of patient care. Who knows, patients may not care. Certainly in obstetrical practices, women have not complained about multiple obstetricians participating in the care of one patient.

E. M. Copeland, MD

The Present and Future Use of Physician Extenders in General Surgery Training Programs: One Response to the 80-Hour Work Week

Pezzi C, Leibrandt T, Suryadevara S, et al (Abington Memorial Hosp, Abington, PA)

J Am Coll Surg 208:587-591, 2009

Background.—The aim of this study was to assess the use of physician extenders (PEs) in general surgery residency programs.

Study Design.—We surveyed the program directors in surgery for the number of chief residents, PEs on general surgery services, PE duties, whether PEs were hired in response to Accreditation Council for Graduate Medical Education work-hour restrictions, plans to hire additional PEs, and program type. Data were analyzed using the Student's *t*-test; p values are two-tailed and considered significant if <0.05.

Results.—There were 163 programs (65%) that responded, (87 university, 70 nonuniversity, and 6 military programs), with a total of 689 graduating chief residents per year. One hundred sixty programs use 840 PEs (median, 3.5 PEs per program; mean, 5.3 PEs per program, 2 PEs per chief resident). One hundred twenty-seven programs (79%) use at least 1 PE (range 1 to 50 PEs); 93 programs (57%) hired 513 (61%) PEs in response to work-hour restrictions. Before 2003, the mean number of PEs per program was 2.0; after 2003, there were 5.3 per program ($p = 0.0001$). Most common uses of PEs included taking histories and physicals (84%), seeing consults (58%), first-assisting (52%), and seeing patients in the emergency department (47%). Forty-seven of 162 (29%) programs plan to hire more PEs in the next 3 years, 76 programs (47%) would like to, but are unsure of funding; 23 programs (14%) are not planning to increase the total, and 16 programs (10%) are unsure. With available funding, 431 additional PEs may be hired in the next 3 years, for a total of 1,271 PEs in 163 programs, or an average of 7.8 PEs per program and 1.8 PEs per chief resident.

Conclusions.—PEs have been hired in large numbers to assist on general surgery teaching services, with most hired in response to Accreditation Council for Graduate Medical Education work-hour restrictions, and most of their duties are intended to aid resident education. Almost 80% of programs currently use PEs; 76% would like to hire more. Currently 1.2 PEs are used per graduating chief resident; this could increase to 1.8 PEs per chief resident in the next 3 years.

▶ The conclusion from this study is that physician extenders (PEs) are a benefit to the educational experience of surgical residents by reducing "scut work" from the daily schedule of the resident. Because most of the PEs were hired in response to the work hours restrictions imposed by the Accreditation Council for Graduate Medical Education, the interpretation of the work hours restrictions would appear to be of great benefit to resident education. Yet the most common use of PEs was seeing consults, first assisting and evaluating patients in the emergency room. As I recall, these duties were the responsibility of junior residents, and considered in the past to be an important and integral part of their surgical education. The questionnaire was limited in its scope, with only a few choices for PE utilization, and this limitation may be the reason the utilizations clustered around the above-listed activities.

Another use of PEs is to replace the residents in the clinic and to perform the task of evaluating the patients on the floor while the team is in the OR. This duty would include the gathering of data needed for daily afternoon rounds. These 2 uses result in the residents not participating in the diagnosis and decision-making that takes place neither in the clinic nor in the decisions necessary for postoperative management. Part of the postoperative management is making treatment decisions based on the data collected from the daily studies done for the patient. The residents may find themselves as observers on afternoon rounds because the PEs have the data and know what occurred during the day. The attending physician needs only to communicate with the PEs, and then assign duties to the resident who is not required to go home.

There is the possibility in a university program for the PE to work up the patient in the clinic—first assisting during the procedure, then discharging the patient from the hospital, and finally, providing postoperative follow-up in the clinic. I know this, because for the last 4 years of my practice this scenario is exactly what happened. It didn't seem to bother anyone, residents or faculty members, so I relaxed and enjoyed the experience. It was just like being in private practice.

E. M. Copeland, MD

Trauma and Surgical Critical Care Workforce in the United States: A Severe Surgeon Shortage Appears Imminent

Cohn SM, Price MA, Villarreal CL (Univ of Texas Health Science Ctr, San Antonio)

J Am Coll Surg 209:446-452, 2009

Background.—We conducted a survey to determine the state of the trauma and critical care workforce and compensation for such surgeons.

Study Design.—We sent questionnaires to 460 directors of Level I and Level II trauma centers in the US to gather information about their current and expected resource needs and compensation packages.

Results.—We received responses from 117 directors (25%). Midlevel faculty mean salary was \$282,000 ± \$85,000; with a mean bonus of \$33,000 ± \$34,000; and a mean trauma call stipend of \$1,690 ± \$900. Mean of the yearly representative value units of work was 7,845 ± 3,154. An average of 1.7 ± 1.4 trauma surgeon positions per center are currently unfilled (mean vacancy duration of 19 ± 20 months), with another 1.2 ± 0.5 full-time equivalents expected to retire within 3 years. A mean of 0.9 ± 0.9 additional positions are expected to be added within the next 3 years because of the growing workload. By 2012, the US might have 1,500 unfilled trauma surgeon positions (with 2,250 occupied).

Conclusions.—Trauma and critical care surgeons in the US are clinically busy and well compensated for their efforts, but a severe shortage of surgeons in this specialty appears imminent.

► The purpose of this article was 2-fold: 1) to examine the potential shortfall in the number of trauma and critical care (TCC) surgeons in the immediate future, and 2) to see if compensation was a reason for the shortfall. The latter is not the case because TCC surgeons are well compensated.

I have chosen to include this article because I have written that the new general surgeon in the immediate future will be the TCC surgeon. With the shortage predicted by this study, patients with general surgical urgent diseases have a major problem with access to health care. I was not aware of this shortfall because I don't attend many of the meetings of trauma surgeons. We have had a level I trauma service for 6 years (because I retired as chairman) and have 12 trauma surgeons. Six years ago we had no trauma surgeons, the general surgeons on our faculty, to include the specialties of surgical oncology and laparoscopic and breast surgery took call every ninth night—not a heavy burden. Individuals in these categories were trained general surgeons, and patients with trauma and urgent surgical diseases received excellent care when compared with the care they receive currently when only the TCC surgeons take night call. Now the specialty general surgeons take no night call!!

I had felt relatively comfortable with the flight to lifestyle-friendly general surgery specialties until I read this article.

E. M. Copeland, MD

Use of Board Certification and Recertification in Hospital Privileging: Policies for General Surgeons, Surgical Specialists, and Nonsurgical Subspecialists

Freed GL, Dunham KM, Singer D (Univ of Michigan, Ann Arbor)

Arch Surg 144:746-752, 2009

Objectives.—To better understand the relationship between board certification and credentialing policies for surgeons and nonsurgical subspecialists and to examine possible variation in use of board certification among different types of hospitals.

Design, Setting, and Participants.—Telephone survey conducted from November 14, 2006, through March 16, 2007, of the privileging personnel among a random sample of 235 nonchildren's hospitals stratified by teaching status, bed size, metropolitan statistical area, system affiliation, and tax status.

Main Outcome Measures.—Proportion of hospitals that require specialty board certification to gain privileges and hospital requirements for recertification.

Results.—Of 235 hospitals, 11 were ineligible and 183 completed the telephone interview, resulting in an overall response rate of 82%. Approximately one-third of hospitals did not require surgeons and nonsurgical subspecialists ever to be board certified to receive hospital privileges. Among the 109 hospitals that required certification at some point, only 5 (5%) required surgeons and 3 (3%) required nonsurgical subspecialists to be board certified at the point of initial privileging. More than three-fourths of hospitals had exceptions to their certification policies for surgeons and 84 (77%) had them for nonsurgical subspecialists. Eighty-two percent of all hospitals and two-thirds of hospitals whose policies required recertification allowed surgeons and nonsurgical subspecialists to retain privileges when their board certification expired.

Conclusion.—Most hospitals do not consistently use board certification to ensure physician competence at their institutions.

▶ This well-designed study gives a very specific overview of the importance of board certification by a member of the American Board of Medical Specialist (ABMS). All of the surgical boards, such as the American Board of Surgery, are members. To sit for certification by an ABMS board member an individual must have completed a residency approved by the appropriate Residency Review Committee (RRC) of the Accreditation Council for Graduate Medical Education (ACGME). Common sense would dictate that a patient would prefer to be the patient of someone who had met these requirements and that these requirements had been substantiated by the hospital to which the patient is admitted. The former is true, but, as pointed out by this survey, the latter is not. In fact, the correlates with not requiring board certification by a hospital were small size, rural location, and for-profit status. These correlates were not necessarily interrelated. What was not studied was the need for hospital financial viability, which may correlate with each of these variables.

The ABMS member organizations have always stressed patient safety, and in that effort now require both recertification and maintenance of certification (MOC), an intermediate step between the times of certification and recertification. This survey found that the correlations for not insisting on recertification correlated with large size, urban location, and not-for-profit status. In other words, small, rural, and for-profit hospitals needed to attract the doctors initially, whereas large, urban, and not-for-profit hospitals needed to keep the doctors that had already been attracted, possibly because of the competitive nature of their demographic environment.

None of the above addresses MOC, which predictably may be ignored entirely. Why then do the members of the ABMS go to the trouble of establishing these quality parameters of physicians' capabilities if hospitals are allowed to ignore them? I am allowed to ask this question because I spent many uncompensated hours as a member of the American Board of Surgery and was the Chairman in 1990-1991. If you lose privileges in one hospital just go practice in another one!!

E. M. Copeland, MD

Use of Locum Tenens Surgeons to Provide Surgical Care in Small Rural Hospitals

Doty B, Andres M, Zuckerman R, et al (Bassett Healthcare, Cooperstown, NY)

World J Surg 33:228-232, 2009

Background.—Too few general surgeons practice in rural American communities, and many hospitals in the smallest rural areas do not have a surgeon. Therefore, it is likely that some small rural hospitals are using alternative arrangements to provide surgical care, including hiring locum tenens surgeons. We describe the degree to which small rural hospitals are using locum tenens surgeons to provide surgical services.

Methods.—Administrators at 129 small rural hospitals were surveyed by telephone. The survey instrument was comprised of questions asking whether the hospital provides surgical services, if the hospital has recruited a surgeon, whether the hospital uses locum tenens surgeons and if so for what purposes.

Results.—A total of 76% of surveyed rural hospitals have offered surgical services during the past 5 years. In all, 56% of hospitals providing surgical care have recruited a surgeon during the past 5 years. Of those who have been unsuccessful in their search, 30% have considered using a locum tenens surgeon, and 20% have done so.

Conclusions.—Given the difficulty of recruiting surgeons to practice in rural America, it is critical to develop strategies to address this problem. Although using locum tenens surgeons may allow rural hospitals to offer surgical services, the quality of surgical care could be compromised. Other means for delivering surgical services at rural hospitals that cannot recruit or retain a surgeon should be explored to ensure that rural residents have access to high quality surgical care.

▶ The disclaimers made by the authors of this unique article may be accurate because only 76% of potential respondents answered the questionnaire, and the administrators in these hospitals may have been the ones most interested in surgical care or the lack thereof. Nevertheless with the upcoming shortage of surgeons trained in the United States, the problem may not be just for rural hospitals, as defined by the authors, but also for small urban hospitals, especially if the hospital is the only one in the community.

A hospital in a small community is one of the most important drivers of the local economy. It provides jobs, needs laundry facilities, and other resources that are of value to the local economy. These hospitals have boards made up of local business people who are interested in the health of the hospital. Because surgical services may make up a significant portion of the profit margins of these hospitals, board members are not interested in a failure of the surgical service. Such motivation could result in an even greater dependence on locum tenens physicians.

The other option is to not require board certification to use the OR. This solution allows for foreign trained physicians who have not qualified to take the American Board of Surgery examination to practice the discipline, or a potentially less desirable situation whereby a physician has qualified for the exam but has failed multiple times to pass it. In this setting, a United States-trained board-certified surgeon, as a locum tenens may be the more desirable solution.

I create a scenario where the hospital remains profitable because of surgical services, the board members feel successful and possibly fuel their OWN local businesses, but the inhabitants of the local community may have inferior surgical care.

E. M. Copeland, MD

2 Trauma

A Genomic Score Prognostic of Outcome in Trauma Patients

Warren HS, and The Inflammation and the Host Response to Injury Large Scale Collaborative Research Program (Massachusetts General Hosp, Charlestown; et al)

Mol Med 15:220-227, 2009

Traumatic injuries frequently lead to infection, organ failure, and death. Health care providers rely on several injury scoring systems to quantify the extent of injury and to help predict clinical outcome. Physiological, anatomical, and clinical laboratory analytic scoring systems (Acute Physiology and Chronic Health Evaluation [APACHE], Injury Severity Score [ISS]) are utilized, with limited success, to predict outcome following injury. The recent development of techniques for measuring the expression level of all of a person's genes simultaneously may make it possible to develop an injury scoring system based on the degree of gene activation. We hypothesized that a peripheral blood leukocyte gene expression score could predict outcome, including multiple organ failure, following severe blunt trauma. To test such a scoring system, we measured gene expression of peripheral blood leukocytes from patients within 12 h of traumatic injury. cRNA derived from whole blood leukocytes obtained within 12 h of injury provided gene expression data for the entire genome that were used to create a composite gene expression score for each patient. Total blood leukocytes were chosen because they are active during inflammation, which is reflective of poor outcome. The gene expression score combines the activation levels of all the genes into a single number which compares the patient's gene expression to the average gene expression in uninjured volunteers. Expression profiles from healthy volunteers were averaged to create a reference gene expression profile which was used to compute a difference from reference (DFR) score for each patient. This score described the overall genomic response of patients within the first 12 h following severe blunt trauma. Regression models were used to compare the association of the DFR, APACHE, and ISS scores with outcome. We hypothesized that patients with a total gene response more different from uninjured volunteers would tend to have poorer outcome than those more similar. Our data show that for measures of poor outcome, such as infections, organ failures, and length of hospital stay, this is correct. DFR scores were associated significantly with adverse outcome, including multiple organ failure, duration of ventilation, length of hospital stay, and infection rate. The association remained significant after adjustment for injury severity as measured by APACHE or ISS. A single score representing changes in gene expression in peripheral blood leukocytes within hours of severe blunt injury is associated with adverse clinical outcomes that develop later in the hospital course. Assessment of genome-wide gene expression provides useful clinical information that is different from that provided by currently utilized anatomic or physiologic scores.

▶ A major finding of the analysis was that even after controlling for the degree of physiologic dysfunction (using the APACHE II or ISS scores), higher DFR scores were associated with poor outcome. This finding strongly suggests that there is information relating to clinical outcome that is contained in the measurement of gene expression that is not captured by current scoring systems. It also raises the possibility that some combination of initial genomic and physiologic scores could provide useful prognostic information about patient outcomes that is superior to each score alone. There are several limitations to the present study: First, the number of patients in each of the analysis groups was relatively small. The small numbers precluded sufficient power to detect association with infrequent outcomes such as death. Second, the statistical associations with some outcomes of the DFR score were weaker in the second group of 79 patients. Third, as with many studies of gene expression in peripheral blood leukocytes, the results reflect changes in gene expression in the entire population of leukocytes in peripheral blood. Different results might be obtained when exploring subpopulations of leukocytes.

D. W. Mozingo, MD

Complication Rates among Trauma Centers

Ang DN, Rivara FP, Nathens A, et al (Univ of Washington, Seattle; St Michael's Hosp, Toronto, Ontario, Canada; et al)
J Am Coll Surg 209:595-602, 2009

Background.—The goal of this study was to examine the association between patient complications and admission to Level I trauma centers (TC) compared with nontrauma centers (NTC).

Study Design.—This was a retrospective cohort study of data derived from the National Study on the Costs and Outcomes of Trauma (NSCOT). Patients were recruited from 18 Level I TCs and 51 NTCs in 15 regions encompassing 14 states. Trained study nurses, using standardized forms, abstracted the medical records of the patients. The overall number of complications per patient was identified, as was the presence or absence of 13 specific complications.

Results.—Patients treated in TCs were more likely to have any complication compared with patients in NTCs, with an adjusted relative risk (RR) of 1.34 (95% CI, 1.03, 1.74). For individual complications, only the urinary tract infection RR of 1.94 (95% CI, 1.07, 3.17) was significantly higher in TCs. TC patients were more likely to have 3 or more complications (RR, 1.83; 95% CI, 1.16, 2.90). Treatment variables that are surrogates for markers of injury severity, such as use of pulmonary artery catheters, multiple operations, massive transfusions (> 2,500 mL packed red blood cells), and invasive brain catheters, occurred significantly more often in TCs.

Conclusions.—Trauma centers have a slightly higher incidence rate of complications, even after adjusting for patient case mix. Aggressive treatment may account for a significant portion of TC-associated complications. Pulmonary artery catheter use and intubation had the most influence on overall TC complication rates. Additional study is needed to provide accurate benchmark measures of complication rates and to determine their causes.

▶ The American College of Surgeons developed criteria for defining trauma centers and for regionalizing trauma care in the mid-1970s. They then began the evaluation process for designating and verifying trauma centers in 1987. Today, 190 centers in the United States have been designated as level 1 trauma centers. A slower than expected rate of adoption of organized trauma systems in the United States was partly from the lack of evidence to support their effectiveness. Recent publications have shown that designated level 1 trauma centers substantially improve overall survival and outcomes for subgroups of patients when compared with nontrauma centers. This study evaluates the complication rates at level 1 trauma centers compared with nontrauma centers and finds the interesting result that the rate is slightly higher at level 1-designated centers, possibly as a result of more aggressive care and more liberal use of invasive procedures. The major difficulty in comparing these centers is controlling for patient comorbidities and severity of injury.

D. W. Mozingo, MD

Early Predictors of the Need for Emergent Surgery to Control Hemorrhage in Hypotensive Trauma Patients

Kaiser M, Ahearn P, Nguyen X-M, et al (Univ of California, Orange; Univ of California, Irvine)

Am Surg 75:986-990, 2009

Twenty-five to 30 per cent of hypotensive trauma patients require an emergent surgery, however, we have no reliable means to quickly determine that need. Our goal was to determine, via retrospective review, parameters available within minutes of arrival that predict the need for emergent surgery to control hemorrhage in hypotensive trauma patients. Inclusion criterion was initial systolic blood pressure (SBP) < 90 mm Hg in the emergency department (ED). Patients who were dead on arrival or underwent ED thoracotomy were excluded. Emergent surgery was defined as sternotomy, thoracotomy, laparotomy, or major neck vascular repair on day of admission. Potential clinical predictors were analyzed in a binary logistic regression model. Six hundred and thirty-nine hypotensive patients were identified and 193 excluded, leaving 446 with a mean age of 33 ± 19 years and Injury Severity Score of 22 ± 17. Thirty-two per cent suffered penetrating trauma, 30 per cent needed emergent surgery, and 19 per cent died. Independent predictors were: prolonged extrication (odds ratio (OR) 2.3), no loss of consciousness (OR 2.8), intubation (OR 1.7), central line placement (OR 1.7), and blood transfusion (OR 2.1, all $P < 0.05$). We concluded that hypotensive trauma patients without head injuries who require prolonged extrication, intubation, central venous access, and blood transfusion in the ED are more likely to need emergent surgery.

▶ Trauma surgery has become an increasingly nonoperative specialty; however, strong indications for emergency surgical intervention remain. This has resulted in many studies exploring the appropriate criteria for triage to a trauma center, trauma team activation, and the presence of a trauma surgery attending at the time of arrival. The challenge facing many trauma surgeons is to determine in a timely fashion which patients will benefit from emergency surgical intervention.

Advanced Trauma Life Support guidelines assume that hypotension in trauma patients correlates to class III hemorrhage or greater or at least a 30% total blood volume loss. Previous studies have shown that hypotensive trauma patients having a systolic blood pressure less than 90 mm Hg are more likely to require surgery for control of ongoing hemorrhage, but less than half of hypotensive trauma patients will actually require emergent operative intervention.

The objective of this study was to determine a set of parameters available within minutes of arrival to the trauma center that predict the need for emergency surgery to control hemorrhage in hypotensive patients. The investigators identified that hypotensive trauma patients without head injuries who required prolonged extrication, intubation, insertion of a central venous catheter, and blood transfusion in the emergency department more likely need early surgical intervention to control hemorrhage.

D. W. Mozingo, MD

Expedited Treatment of Lower Extremity Gunshot Wounds

Sadjadi J, Cureton EL, Dozier KC, et al (Univ of California San Francisco-East Bay, Oakland)

J Am Coll Surg 209:740-745, 2009

Background.—Patients with isolated lower extremity gunshot wounds are currently admitted for observation and often undergo angiography. We hypothesized that if such patients have a normal ankle-brachial index (ABI), they can be discharged safely from the emergency department without invasive imaging or admission.

Study Design.—We retrospectively reviewed the records of hemodynamically stable patients with isolated lower extremity gunshot wounds seen at our urban, university-based trauma center and who were discharged from the emergency department. Evaluation consisted of determining which patients were hemodynamically normal, had no fractures, and had an ABI ≥0.9. Patients with an ABI <0.9 underwent CT angiography. We then applied this practice algorithm prospectively, adding evaluation of high probability proximity wounds by ultrasonography or CT angiography to rule out missed injuries.

Results.—The retrospective review identified 182 patients who met our criteria. None had bleeding, limb ischemia, or limb loss. The specificity of the evaluation in the retrospective study to predict safe discharge was 100%, with a negative predictive value of 98%. There were 90 patients in the prospective study. Bleeding, limb ischemia, or limb loss did not develop in any patient. The prospective algorithm for predicting safe discharge home had a 100% positive predictive value and 98% negative predictive value. Using this algorithm, costs were $992 per patient. If every patient received ultrasonography or CT angiography, it would have been $1,135 or $4,632, respectively, per patient.

Conclusions.—Hemodynamically normal patients with lower extremity gunshot wounds without fracture and an initial ABI ≥0.9 can be

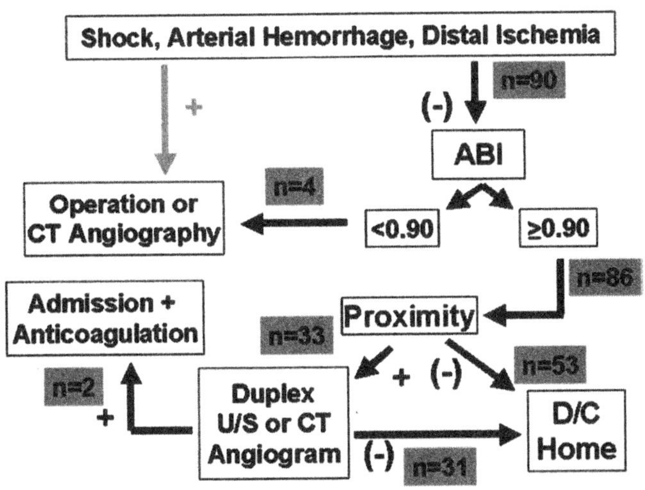

FIGURE 2.—Flow chart depicting the results of applying the evaluation algorithm in the prospective study of 90 patients with isolated gunshot wounds to the leg who were hemodynamically stable. The algorithm also includes evaluation of the proximity to the bullet trajectory to vascular structures based on location of the entrance and exit wounds. ABI, ankle-brachial index; D/C, discharge; U/S, ultrasonography. (Reprinted from Sadjadi J, Cureton EL, Dozier KC, et al. Expedited treatment of lower extremity gunshot wounds. *J Am Coll Surg*. 2009;209:740-745, with permission from the American College of Surgeons.)

discharged safely from the emergency department without additional diagnostic imaging, potentially saving health care costs (Fig 2).

▶ Traditional practice assumes that nonoperative management of lower extremity gunshot wounds requires patients to be admitted to the hospital for observation with or without angiography for trajectories close to major vessels to diagnose clinically occult vascular injuries. Angiography is also expensive and not without complications. Because of the reported efficacy of the physical examination alone, the authors of this article hypothesized that patients with isolated gunshot injury to the lower extremity who are hemodynamically normal with a normal ankle-brachial index, and no fracture, can be discharged safely from the emergency department without being admitted for observation and without obtaining additional diagnostic imaging. Their prospective treatment algorithm is included as Fig 2. The cost savings of this approach is substantial, and the accuracy of the patient triage is impressive. One major concern, however, is the lack of long-term follow-up.

D. W. Mozingo, MD

Extreme Thrombocytosis in Trauma Patients: Are Antiplatelet Agents the Answer?

Saadi Z, Inaba K, Barmparas G, et al (Univ of Southern California, Los Angeles; et al)

Am Surg 75:1020-1024, 2009

The purpose of this study was to review the incidence of extreme thrombocytosis (ExT) (platelet count 1,000,000/μL or greater) in trauma patients and to examine the role of antiplatelet agents in its treatment. The Los Angeles County Medical Center trauma registry was used to obtain injury demographics, medications, and daily platelet counts for injured patients 16 years of age or older admitted between July 2005 and February 2008. Of 6,985 total trauma patients admitted during the study period, 95 developed ExT (1.4%). Average age was 29 years (range, 16–63 years), 89 per cent were male, 44 per cent had penetrating trauma, and mean Injury Severity Score was 24 (range, 1–57). Of the 95 patients with ExT, 41 were treated with aspirin (43%) and 54 were not (57%). The two groups did not differ with regard to basic demographics, injury patterns, vitals on admission, or splenectomy rate (34 *vs* 20%, $P = 0.13$). After adjusting for maximum platelet counts and duration of ExT, there was no difference between the treated and untreated groups in terms of mortality, complications, and intensive care unit or hospital lengths of stay. The incidence of ExT is approximately 1.4 per cent in trauma patients. Antiplatelet therapy does not affect ExT patient outcome. Further prospective studies are warranted.

▶ The purpose of this study was to determine the incidence of extreme thrombocytosis in the trauma population along with the complication rate and to examine whether a course of antiplatelet therapy administered to patients with this condition had any effect on outcomes. Detecting abnormally high values in patients who do not have a clonal hematologic disease is a phenomenon known as secondary or reactive thrombocytosis. It is known that reactive thrombocytosis can be associated with the presence of tissue damage, infection, malignancy, or splenectomy.

However, a theoretically expected increase in vaso-occlusive complications has not been documented. Findings from several studies support a lower incidence of these events compared with patients with myelodysplastic syndromes who have a similar increase in platelet counts.

The authors of this selection term these patients the platelet millionaires—those who have platelet counts that exceed 1 000 000/mL. These patients, also known as patients with extreme thrombocytosis, are often treated with antiplatelet therapy in the setting of a surgical intensive care unit. However, there is no evidence showing any benefit to this practice in this patient population.

D. W. Mozingo, MD

Hospital Performance in Caring for Injured Patients: Does the Type of Injury Make a Difference?

Glance LG, Mukamel DB, Meredith W, et al (Univ of Rochester School of Medicine, NY; Univ of California, Irvine, UK; Wake Forest School of Medicine, Winston-Salem, NC; et al)

Arch Surg 144:1121-1126, 2009

Objective.—To determine whether quality measures based on injury-specific models provide a different perspective about relative hospital rankings compared with a single outcome measure based on all trauma patients.

Design.—We customized the Trauma Mortality Probability Model to create separate injury-specific models for patients who sustained blunt trauma, gunshot wounds, pedestrian trauma, or motor vehicle accident trauma.

Setting.—This analysis was conducted using the National Trauma Data Bank. We limited the study to hospitals with 250 or more trauma admissions per year, which coded more than 90% of patients.

Patients.—The final data set included 54 859 patients admitted to 44 hospitals.

Main Outcome Measures.—We performed hospital-level analyses to examine the correlation between hospital risk-adjusted mortality measures based on all trauma patients vs quality measures based on injury-specific measures.

Results.—The analysis of the intraclass correlation coefficients suggests fair-to-substantial agreement (0.39-0.68) between the hospital-adjusted odds ratios based on all patients vs odds ratios based on specific injuries. κ Analysis demonstrated poor-to-fair agreement between hospital categorical quality measures (high, intermediate, and low quality) when hospital quality was based on outcomes for all trauma patients vs specific subgroups of patients (0.0-0.38). However, none of the hospitals classified as high quality, based on data from all trauma patients, was found to be low quality for any specific injury populations.

Conclusion.—A single composite measure based on all injured patients may not capture all the differences in hospital quality across different populations of injured patients.

▶ Previous studies have shown that outcomes across high-risk surgery, such as coronary artery bypass grafting and valve surgery, are correlated because hospital structural variables and process measures that impact 1 procedure may also impact outcomes for related procedures. The authors of this selection sought to determine if this was also true for trauma care. They report the extent to which hospital performance for patients with specific injuries correlates with overall trauma outcomes.

Injury-specific outcome reports provide information that is not available in a single outcome measure based on all trauma patients. The added expense of production of injury-specific reports is small when compared with the cost of data collection and is justified by the added opportunities for quality improvements that may result from providing hospitals more specific information on trauma outcomes.

The authors should be commended for developing a trauma mortality probability design that would create a more injury-specific model. This modification could translate into a better tracking mechanism for quality measures that could, in turn, create initiatives for better outcomes.

D. W. Mozingo, MD

Impact of joint theater trauma system initiatives on battlefield injury outcomes

Eastridge BJ, Costanzo G, Jenkins D, et al (United States Army Inst of Surgical Res, Ft Sam Houston, TX; United States Air Force Willford Hall Med Ctr, San Antonio, TX; et al)

Am J Surg 198:852-857, 2009

Introduction.—The US military forces developed and implemented the Joint Theater Trauma System (JTTS) and Joint Theater Trauma Registry (JTTR) using US civilian trauma system models with the intent of improving outcomes after battlefield injury.

TABLE 2.—Impact of Evidence-Based Clinical Practice Guidelines

	Pre-CPG	Post-CPG	*P*	CPG Compliance
Burn resuscitation-associated abdominal compartment syndrome mortality (burn CPG)	36%	18%	<.05	94%
Hypothermia on presentation (hypothermia CPG)	7%	1%	<.05	84%
Massive transfusion mortality (≥10 U RBCs/24 h) (damage control resuscitation CPG)	32%	20%	<.05	85%

RBCs = red blood cells.

Methods.—The purpose of this analysis was to elaborate the impact of the JTTS. To quantify these achievements, the JTTR captured mechanism, acute physiology, diagnostic, therapeutic, and outcome data on 23,250 injured patients admitted to deployed US military treatment facilities from July 2003 through July 2008 for analysis. Comparative analysis to civilian trauma systems was done using the National Trauma Data Bank (NTDB).

Results.—In contrast to civilian trauma systems with an 11.1% rate of penetrating injury, 68.3% of battlefield wounds were by penetrating mechanism. In the analyzed cohort, 23.3% of all patients had an Injury Severe Score (ISS) ≥16, which is similar to the civilian rate of 22.4%. In the military injury population, 66% of injuries were combat-related. In addition, in the military injury group, 21.8% had metabolic evidence of shock with a base deficit ≥5, 29.8% of patients required blood transfusion, and 6.4% of the total population of combat casualties required massive transfusion (>10 U red blood cells/24 hours). With this complex and severely injured population of battlefield injuries, the JTTS elements were used to recognize and remedy more than 60 trauma system issues requiring leadership and advocacy, education, research, and alterations in clinical care. Of particular importance to the trauma system was the implementation and tracking of performance improvement indicators and the dissemination of 27 evidence-based clinical practice guidelines (CPGs). In particular, the damage control resuscitation guideline was associated with a decrease in mortality in the massively transfused from 32% pre-CPG to 21% post-CPG. As evidence of the effectiveness of the JTTS, a mortality rate of 5.2% after battlefield hospital admission is comparable to a case fatality rate of 4.3% reported in an age-matched cohort from the NTDB.

Conclusions.—JTTS initiatives contributed to improved survival after battlefield injury. The JTTS has set the standard of trauma care for the modern battlefield using contemporary systems-based methodologies.

▶ The concept of developing trauma management clinical practice guidelines was popularized by the Eastern Association for the Surgery of Trauma in the late 1990s.

Extrapolation of this concept to include combat trauma clinical practice guidelines is a novel development for the Joint Theater Trauma System because little data were available previously from large-scale military conflicts. The authors were able to show the impact of evidence-based trauma care guidelines by demonstrating improvements in outcome for burn resuscitation, damage control resuscitation mortality, and hypothermia prevention following injury (Table 2). These Joint Theater Trauma System initiatives have contributed significantly to improved survival after battlefield injury in a real-time manner. There have always been many important contributions to the field of surgery that have developed through wartime experience; however, the theater-wide implementation of these trauma practice clinical management guidelines is precedent setting. The authors and all of those physicians and care providers that implemented and followed these guidelines should be commended for their efforts to improve combat casualty care for our soldiers.

D. W. Mozingo, MD

Increased number of coagulation products in relationship to red blood cell products transfused improves mortality in trauma patients

Shaz BH, Dente CJ, Nicholas J, et al (Emory Univ School of Medicine, Atlanta, GA)

Transfusion 50:493-500, 2010

Background.—Recent data from military and civilian centers suggest that mortality is decreased in massive transfusion patients by increasing the transfusion ratio of plasma and platelet (PLT) products, and fibrinogen in relationship to red blood cell (RBC) products during damage control resuscitation and surgery. This study investigates the relationship of plasma:RBC, PLT:RBC, and cryoprecipitate:RBC transfusion ratios to mortality in massively transfused patients at a civilian Level 1 trauma center.

Study Design and Methods.—Demographic, laboratory, transfusion, and outcome data were collected prospectively from February 1, 2007, to January 31, 2009, and retrospectively from February 1, 2005, to January 31, 2007, on all injured patients who underwent massive transfusion (defined as ≥10 RBC products within 24 hr). Mortality was analyzed in relation to the plasma:RBC, PLT:RBC, and cryoprecipitate:RBC transfusion ratios using both univariate and multivariate analyses.

Results.—A total of 214 patients received massive transfusion secondary to traumatic injury. High versus low transfusion ratios were associated with improved 30-day survival: plasma:RBC 59% versus 44%, $p = 0.03$; PLT:RBC 63% versus 33%, $p < 0.01$; and cryoprecipitate:RBC 66% versus 41%, $p < 0.01$. By multivariable stepwise logistic regression analysis, increased plasma:RBC ($p = 0.02$) and PLT:RBC ($p = 0.02$), and decreased age ($p = 0.02$), ISS ($p < 0.01$) and total RBCs ($p = 0.03$) were statistically associated with improved 30-day survival.

Conclusions.—In the civilian setting, plasma, PLT, and cryoprecipitate products significantly increased 30-day survival in trauma patients. Future prospective randomized clinical trials are required to determine the optimal transfusion ratios.

▶ Early trauma-related mortality is usually secondary to head injury or hemorrhage, while late mortality is secondary to multiorgan failure or infection. In addition, massive transfusion predicts a higher mortality rate in trauma patients. In those patients receiving 10 or more red blood cell (RBC) units in their hospital stay, mortality approaches 40%, and in patients who receive 50 or more units of blood products, a mortality rate of 57% has been reported. It

A

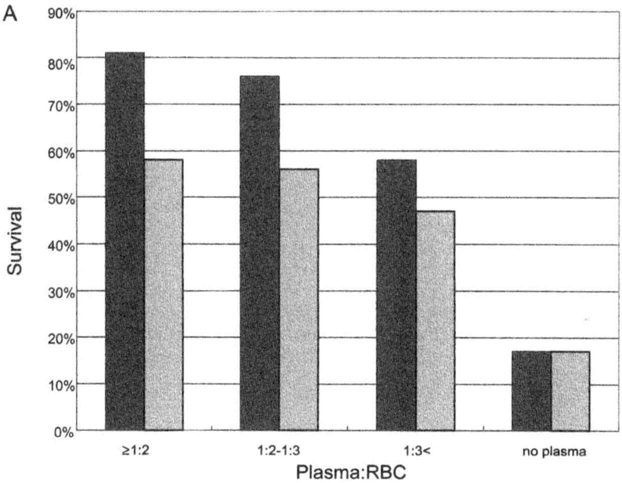

B

Plasma:RBC	≥1:2	1:2-1:3	1:3<	no plasma
n	86	66	38	24
24-hour survival	81%	76%	58%	17%
30-day survival	58%	56%	47%	17%
ISS(ave)	30	26	27	27
Penetrating	47%	44%	47%	50%
MTP	81%	56%	47%	29%

C

Plasma:RBC	n	MTP	24-hour survival	30-day survival	ISS (ave±SD)	Penetrating
high	100	79%	80%	59%	29 ±12	49%
low	114	46%	58%	44%	27 ±14	44%
		p<0.01	p<0.01	p=0.03	p=0.46	p=0.45

FIGURE 1.—Plasma:RBC product transfusion ratios effect on patient survival. (A) Survival versus ratio. (■) 24-hour survival; (□) 30-day survival. (B) Patient characteristics in each ratio group. (C) Patient outcome and characteristics in high (one or more plasma per two RBC products) versus low (less than one plasma per two RBC products) transfusion group. Ave = average. (Courtesy of Shaz BH, Dente CJ, Nicholas J, et al. Increased number of coagulation products in relationship to red blood cell products transfused improves mortality in trauma patients. *Transfusion.* 2010;50:493-500.)

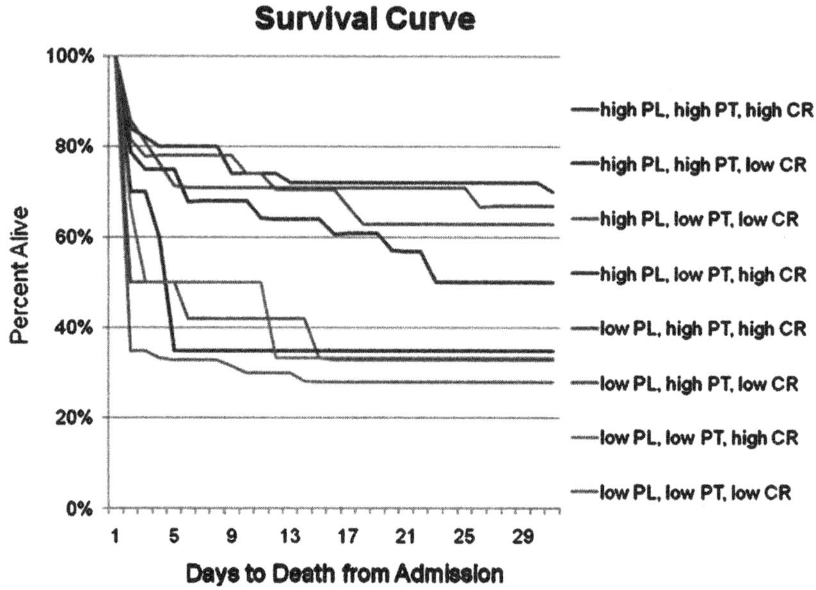

FIGURE 4.—Survival curves for the eight groups: 1) high plasma, high PLT, high cryoprecipitate (n = 50); 2) high plasma, high PLT, low cryoprecipitate (n = 28); 3) high plasma, low PLT, low cryoprecipitate (n = 12); 4) high plasma, low PLT, high cryoprecipitate (n = 10); 5) low plasma, high PLT, high cryoprecipitate (n = 21); 6) low plasma, high PLT, low cryoprecipitate (n = 27); 7) low plasma, low PLT, high cryoprecipitate (n = 6); and 8) low plasma, low PLT, low cryoprecipitate (n = 60). High versus low ratio groups determined as a ratio of 0.5 or more versus less than 0.5. CR = cryoprecipitate; PL = plasma; PT = PLT. (Courtesy of Shaz BH, Dente CJ, Nicholas J, et al. Increased number of coagulation products in relationship to red blood cell products transfused improves mortality in trauma patients. *Transfusion.* 2010;50:493-500.)

has been described in recent years that the ratio of blood products transfused affects mortality both in the military and in the civilian setting.

In 2005, surgeons, anesthesiologists, hematologists, transfusion medicine specialists, and others developed guidelines for transfusion practices following massive blood loss during a symposium held at the US Army Institute of Surgical Research. These guidelines suggested that plasma:RBC:platelets (PLTs) be administered in a 1:1:1 ratio for massive transfusion in the severely injured patient.[1] This ratio corrects the coagulation factor loss resulting from early transfusion of crystalloids and packed RBCs. In this selection, the authors have shown an improvement in survival with even higher plasma:RBC, PLT:RBC, and cryoprecipitate: RBC transfusion ratios. Figs 1 and 4 demonstrate the increasing effect of these ratios on mortality following major trauma and hemorrhage. Additional prospective studies will be required to define the optimal ratio, but I suspect that a combination mimicking fresh whole blood would be the intuitive choice.

D. W. Mozingo, MD

Initial Implementation of an Acute Care Surgery Model: Implications for Timeliness of Care

Britt RC, Weireter LJ, Britt LD (Eastern Virginia Med School, Norfolk)

J Am Coll Surg 209:421-424, 2009

Background.—In July 2007, we introduced an acute care surgery service to an academic department of surgery staffed in a prearranged, dedicated rotation by critical care-trained surgeons to address all emergency department, inpatient, and transfer consultations. This study is designed to evaluate the impact on patient care and describe the case-mix experienced.

Study Design.—A retrospective review was done of a prospectively collected database encompassing all patients evaluated. Diagnosis, operations performed, and times of operations were recorded.

Results.—Eight hundred sixty-one patients were evaluated. Four hundred ten patients (47.6%) had 500 operations; 368 (72.8%) were performed in the operating room and 132 (26.2%) at the bedside. Respiratory failure and malnutrition (n = 130), soft-tissue infection (n = 115), abdominal pain (n = 97), biliary (n = 94), bowel obstruction (n = 78), diseases of the colon (n = 49), and appendicitis (n = 46) were the most common diseases seen. The most common operations performed included incision and drainage (n = 61); tracheostomy or percutaneous gastrostomy, or both (n = 125); cholecystectomy (n = 53); appendectomy (n = 41); colectomy (n = 34); and complex abdominal wound care (n = 43). In the year before implementation, 55.4% of emergent procedures were performed between 7:30 am and 5:30 pm, compared with 70% after implementation (p = 0.0002). Procedures performed after 5:30 pm decreased from 44.6% to 30%.

Conclusions.—Implementation of an acute care surgery service has been positive in terms of facilitating the ability to provide more timely care by increasingly using the daytime operating room and providing a breadth of consultative and operative experience to the participating academic surgeons and trainees.

▶ Limited access to high-quality emergency surgical care is a growing problem in the United States, with multiple factors contributing to this problem. A shortage of surgeons, diminishing reimbursement, increasing numbers of uninsured patients, disruption of elective surgical practice, and lifestyle issues are just some of the factors relating to the lack of enthusiasm for covering emergency surgical cases.

Increased subspecialization by general surgeons with subsequent reluctance in providing expert care for emergency cases has also limited the availability of the emergency general surgeon.

With continued population growth and a disproportionate increase in the number of elderly patients combined with the staggering predictions of physician workforce shortages, the outlook for the provision of emergency surgical care is bleak, at best. Trauma surgery has also changed recently, with an increasing trend for nonoperative management of injuries and a considerable shortage of physicians interested in providing trauma care. Factors contributing to a lack of interest in the specialty of trauma include lack of operative cases, lifestyle concerns, and impact on elective practice, among others.

The acute care surgery model, integrating trauma, critical care, and emergency surgery has been proposed as a means to both entice surgeons to continue to provide emergency care and improve the quality of care provided to their patients. The authors of this selection introduced an acute care surgery service to an academic department of surgery as many others have done throughout the country. At these authors' institution, they were able to separate the acute care surgery service from the trauma service during the business workday, but emergency surgery and trauma remained an integrated service for nights and weekends to maintain a reasonable call schedule. Hospital and departmental support for these types of services is crucial to maintain these programs.

D. W. Mozingo, MD

Isolated Rollover Mechanism Does Not Warrant Trauma Center Evaluation

Haan JM, Glassman E, Hartsock R, et al (R. Adams Cowley Shock Trauma Ctr Univ of Maryland, Baltimore)

Am Surg 75:1109-1111, 2009

Significant resources are expended on the assessment of trauma patients who arrive at the trauma center based solely on mechanism of injury. We hypothesized that rollover motor vehicle crashes (ROMVC) are not an independent predictor for trauma center care. All patients seen between January 1, 2001, and December 31, 2005, involved in a ROMVC, were reviewed. Patients with any confounding factors were removed, leaving those transported to the trauma center based on mechanism only. Five hundred sixty-nine patients were transported to our center for the mechanism of ROMVC. Of the 569 patients, 369 (65%) were evaluated and discharged with minimal Injury Severity Score and regional Abbreviated Injury Scale scores. Of the remaining 200 (35%) patients admitted, 130 required surgery, predominantly for closed extremity and facial fractures. Six patients required immediate surgery for life-threatening injuries: 3 splenectomies, 1 subdural evacuation, and 2 vascular repairs (1.1%). Of the remaining 123 (4.2%) patients requiring surgery, 24 required urgent surgery (2 craniotomies, 9 laparotomies, and 13 spinal fixations). None of the patients with spinal injury had neurologic deficit. Eight patients were admitted to the intensive care unit for neurologic monitoring (1.4%). Only 6.7 per cent benefited from initial Trauma Triage Criteria. Therefore, ROMVC is not an independent predictor of the need for trauma center evaluation or admission. The majority of these patients could be safely evaluated and treated at nontrauma centers or transferred later.

▶ Significant resource commitments are required to maintain trauma systems in general and individual trauma centers in particular. The use of emergency medical service (EMS) systems and trauma centers is expensive and costly from a public health standpoint. Better justification is needed for patients requiring evaluation at a trauma center versus a regional hospital. Most EMS systems use a decision tree accounting for trauma mechanism, patient physiological status, and physical findings as well as medical history to determine those patients requiring evaluation at a trauma center. Because significant resources are used in trauma center evaluation and care, appropriate triage is critical to optimize the use of these limited resources. In patients who are triaged due to mechanism of injury only, defined by accident events rather than the patient's physiological status, the need for trauma center evaluation is less clear. In this selection, the authors noticed a high number of patients being transported to their trauma center for the accident mechanism. Many of these patients were found to have minimal or no injuries and, in fact, could have been safely evaluated in the nontrauma center setting. This occurred most commonly in asymptomatic patients transported for rollover mechanism only. Using a statewide trauma registry to evaluate the hospital course and evaluation of available EMS records for prehospital injury mechanism and physiologic detail, the authors examined the impact of mechanism only on patient transfers on trauma center resource utilization.

They clearly demonstrated that rollover mechanism, in isolation, is not an indication for evaluation at a trauma center. In the current setting of decreasing resources and increasing demands on trauma systems, continuing evaluation and revision of trauma center referral protocols is essential.

D. W. Mozingo, MD

Morphine Use after Combat Injury in Iraq and Post-Traumatic Stress Disorder

Holbrook TL, Galarneau MR, Dye JL, et al (Naval Health Res Ctr, San Diego, CA)

N Engl J Med 362:110-117, 2010

Background.—Post-traumatic stress disorder (PTSD) is a common adverse mental health outcome among seriously injured civilians and military personnel who are survivors of trauma. Pharmacotherapy in the aftermath of serious physical injury or exposure to traumatic events may be effective for the secondary prevention of PTSD.

Methods.—We identified 696 injured U.S. military personnel without serious traumatic brain injury from the Navy–Marine Corps Combat Trauma Registry Expeditionary Medical Encounter Database. Complete data on medications administered were available for all personnel selected.

The diagnosis of PTSD was obtained from the Career History Archival Medical and Personnel System and verified in a review of medical records.

Results.—Among the 696 patients studied, 243 received a diagnosis of PTSD and 453 did not. The use of morphine during early resuscitation and trauma care was significantly associated with a lower risk of PTSD after injury. Among the patients in whom PTSD developed, 61% received morphine; among those in whom PTSD did not develop, 76% received morphine (odds ratio, 0.47; $P<0.001$). This association remained significant after adjustment for injury severity, age, mechanism of injury, status with respect to amputation, and selected injury-related clinical factors.

Conclusions.—Our findings suggest that the use of morphine during trauma care may reduce the risk of subsequent development of PTSD after serious injury.

▶ Post-traumatic stress disorder (PTSD) is an important mental health outcome among critically injured civilian and military survivors of trauma and burns. Increasing recognition of the profound and protracted detrimental effects on general health and quality of life when PTSD develops in the aftermath of serious physical injury or exposure to traumatic events has made its prevention a focus of research-related outcomes.

Prevention of PTSD with pharmacotherapy in the post-trauma period is an evolving area of research.

Current knowledge of the pathogenesis and neurobiology of PTSD provides a strong theoretical basis for the role of pharmacotherapy in the secondary prevention of PTSD after major trauma.

The primary goal of this therapy is to inhibit memory consolidation and the associated conditioned response to fear after a person sustains a traumatic event. Similar findings have been described in children with burn injuries. The findings in this study heighten our awareness of the need to provide analgesia (and probably anxiolysis) following major trauma. These results also point to the need to define the best preventive agents from our pharmacologic arsenal.

D. W. Mozingo, MD

Motorcycle Helmets Save Lives, But Not Limbs: A National Trauma Data Bank Analysis of Functional Outcomes After Motorcycle Crash

Crompton JG, Oyetunji T, Stevens KA, et al (The Johns Hopkins Univ School of Medicine, Baltimore, MD; Howard Univ College of Medicine, Washington, DC)

J Surg Res 158:1-5, 2010

Background.—The incidence of motorcycle fatalities over the last 10 y has nearly doubled. There is considerable evidence that motorcycle helmets save lives, but there are little data regarding the impact that helmets have on functional outcomes after a motorcycle crash. The

TABLE 3.—Proportion of Patients with Unadjusted Functional Deficits in Helmeted and Non-Helmeted Riders Involved in a Motorcycle Collision in the National Trauma Data Bank

	Helmeted ($n = 17,207$) %	Non-Helmeted ($n = 5532$) %
Speech*	4.9	7.5
Locomotion*	49.2	43.8
Feeding*	9.8	12.1

*$P < 0.05$.

objective of this study was to determine the difference between helmeted and non-helmeted motorcyclists in the odds of developing a functional deficit at discharge in three domains: speech, locomotion, and feeding.

Methods.—Reviewed cases in the National Trauma Databank v7.0 involved in motorcycle collisions. Multiple logistic regression was used to analyze the effect of helmets on mortality and functional outcomes, adjusting for age, race, gender, insurance status, anatomic and physiologic injury severity, and head injury.

Results.—The adjusted odds of mortality (0.75; 95% CI 0.65–0.86) and functional deficits in speech (0.82; 95% CI 0.69–0.97), locomotion (1.19; 95% CI 1.11–1.29), and feeding (0.96; 95% CI 0.84–1.08) among helmeted riders was compared with non-helmeted motorcyclists with equivalent injuries.

Conclusion.—Helmeted motorcyclists are less likely to die and develop a deficit in speech after a motorcycle collision. These data support that motorcycle helmets are important in preventing functional deficits related to head injury (Table 3).

► It is well known that motorcycle helmets save lives. Recent Cochrane review concluded that helmets reduce the risk of death and head injury in riders who crash. The National Highway Traffic Safety Administration estimates that a non-helmeted rider is 40% more likely to incur a fatal head injury and 15% more likely to sustain a nonfatal injury than a helmeted motorcyclist. Little evidence evaluates the impact that helmets have on functional outcomes after a motorcycle crash. The authors questioned whether functional deficits in speech, locomotion, and feeding represent significant morbidity associated with motorcycle collisions. Table 3 is included describing these outcomes. These conditions potentially result in long-term medical expenditures and loss of years of potential productivity. There were no previous studies using large databases to evaluate this potential outcome of motorcycle crashes.

The legally mandated use of helmets is currently a commonly debated topic in the context of the repeal of helmet laws in several states. There is compelling evidence to suggest that outcomes such as mortality after motorcycle crashes have increased in states that have repealed the law because fewer riders are wearing helmets than previously. This study adds to that evidence by evaluating long-term deficits in a large database of trauma patients.

D. W. Mozingo, MD

Pulmonary Embolism and Deep Venous Thrombosis in Trauma: Are They Related?

Velmahos GC, Spaniolas K, Tabbara M, et al (Massachusetts General Hosp and Harvard Med School, Boston)

Arch Surg 144:928-932, 2009

Hypothesis.—Pulmonary embolism (PE) and deep venous thrombosis (DVT) in trauma are related.

Design.—Retrospective review of medical records.

Setting.—Academic level I trauma center.

Patients.—Trauma patients who underwent computed tomographic pulmonary angiography (CTPA) with computed tomographic venography (CTV) of the pelvic and proximal lower extremity veins over a 3-year period (January 1, 2004, to December 31, 2006) were reviewed. Data on demographics, injury type and severity, imaging findings, hospital length of stay, and mortality were collected.

Main Outcome Measures.—Pulmonary embolism and DVT.

Results.—Among 247 trauma patients undergoing CTPA/CTV, PE was diagnosed in 46 (19%) and DVT in 18 (7%). Eighteen PEs were central (main or lobar pulmonary arteries), and 28 PEs were peripheral (segmental or sub-segmental branches). Pulmonary embolism occurred within the first week of injury in two-thirds of patients. Seven patients with PE (4 femoral, 2 popliteal, and 1 iliac) had DVT. Pulmonary embolism was central in 5 patients and peripheral in 2 patients. No significant differences were noted in any of the examined variables between patients with PE having DVT and those not having DVT.

Conclusions.—Few patients with PE have DVT of the pelvic or proximal lower extremity veins. Pulmonary embolism may not originate from these veins, as commonly believed, but instead may occur de novo in the lungs. These findings have implications for thromboprophylaxis and, particularly, the value of vena cava filters.

▶ The authors of this selection question whether there is a true relationship between the development of a deep venous thrombosis (DVT) and a pulmonary embolism (PE), theorizing that a primary thrombus could form in the pulmonary circulation initially. The results of the study support that DVT and PE may be temporally related; however, because there is a chance that the entire thrombus may dislodge from the deep veins and travel to the lungs, attempts to make both diagnoses concurrently may lead to erroneous conclusions. There was also no mechanism proposed for their hypothesis that clots may form initially in the lungs.

This study raises more questions than it answers, but the question of timing and anatomic location of the thrombus is a good one and deserves further study.

D. W. Mozingo, MD

The "July Phenomenon": Is Trauma the Exception?

Schroeppel TJ, Fischer PE, Magnotti LJ, et al (Univ of Tennessee Health Science Ctr, Memphis)

J Am Coll Surg 209:378-384, 2009

Background.—The concept of increased medical errors in July, secondary to new residents (the "July phenomenon"), often receives considerable attention without supporting evidence. A recent study reported a 41% increase in mortality during July and August in general surgery patients. The objective of this study was to determine if a July phenomenon existed in a Level I trauma center with an attending present at all times.

Study Design.—A retrospective cohort study was conducted at an academic, tertiary Level I trauma center. Blunt trauma patients admitted during a 5-year period were compared for differences in outcomes by month and quarter. Chi-square and analysis of variance were used for categorical and continuous variables where appropriate. Linear regression was used to examine the effect of month on ventilator support days, ICU days, and minutes in the resuscitation room. Multivariable linear regression was used to examine the effect of month and quarter on mortality.

Results.—A total of 12,525 patients were analyzed by month and 14,798 patients were analyzed by quarter. Overall, 68% were men and 32% women, with a mean age of 39.5 years. Mean Injury Severity Score was 12.4. Mean 24-hour transfusion requirement was 0.5 U. Mean emergency department Glasgow Coma Scale score was 14. Multivariable logistic regression failed to show month or quarter of the year to be an independent predictor of mortality after adjusting for age, Injury Severity Score, emergency department Glasgow Coma Scale score, and 24-hour transfusion requirement ($c = 0.97$). Linear regression failed to show any monthly variation on ventilator-support days, ICU days, or minutes in the resuscitation room.

Conclusions.—The July phenomenon does not exist at this Level I trauma center with in-hospital attending supervision.

▶ The suspicion of increased medical errors occurring in July has long existed in medical lore, popular press, and the minds of the general public. The influx of new graduates from medical and nursing schools occurs in relatively large numbers. Previous studies have failed to show the existence of changes in the outcomes relative to the new graduates starting in July of each new academic year. Previous studies have suggested that the cost of health care is higher earlier in the year at teaching hospitals, but the quality of care is no different throughout the year. A recent study, however, reported a 41% increase in mortality in general surgery patients in July and August. This study was done using a large surgical outcomes database, but information on supervision of residents was not available. Level I trauma centers represent a different cohort of patients within the surgical subspecialties. Many trauma centers have injury-specific treatment algorithms, clinical pathways, and constant attending coverage and participation, which should eliminate the variables in care provided by new residents. The authors of this selection hypothesized that in a large urban level I trauma center with constant attending supervision, the July phenomenon would not be found.

Multivariable linear regression of 12 286 patients analyzed by month and 14 559 patients analyzed by quarter of the year during a 5-year period failed to show any variation in the quality of care indicators examined in this study. Although some may still question the presence of quality being compromised early in each academic year, these data analyzed in this selection show no evidence that such a phenomenon exists.

D. W. Mozingo, MD

Trauma and Surgical Critical Care Workforce in the United States: A Severe Surgeon Shortage Appears Imminent

Cohn SM, Price MA, Villarreal CL (Univ of Texas Health Science Ctr, San Antonio)

J Am Coll Surg 209:446-452, 2009

Background.—We conducted a survey to determine the state of the trauma and critical care workforce and compensation for such surgeons.

Study Design.—We sent questionnaires to 460 directors of Level I and Level II trauma centers in the US to gather information about their current and expected resource needs and compensation packages.

Results.—We received responses from 117 directors (25%). Midlevel faculty mean salary was $282,000 ± $85,000; with a mean bonus of $33,000 ± $34,000; and a mean trauma call stipend of $1,690 ± $900. Mean of the yearly representative value units of work was 7,845 ± 3,154. An average of 1.7 ± 1.4 trauma surgeon positions per center are currently unfilled (mean vacancy duration of 19 ± 20 months), with another 1.2 ± 0.5 full-time equivalents expected to retire within 3 years. A mean of 0.9 ± 0.9 additional positions are expected to be added within the next 3 years because of the growing workload. By 2012, the US might have 1,500 unfilled trauma surgeon positions (with 2,250 occupied).

Conclusions.—Trauma and critical care surgeons in the US are clinically busy and well compensated for their efforts, but a severe shortage of surgeons in this specialty appears imminent (Table 3).

▶ The number of applicants for available fellowships in trauma and surgical critical care has not grown considerably during the past 15 years, even though the number of available fellowship positions have increased considerably. The number of surgeons currently pursuing training in surgical critical care fellowships is only approximately two-thirds as large as it was during the peak period in the early 1990s, shortly after board certification became available. Only about half of the surgical critical care fellowship positions are filled each year.

TABLE 3.—Compensation Paid to Surgeons at US Trauma Centers in 2007

Variable	All Trauma Centers		
	Salary		Bonus*
Assistant professor	238 ± 70		34 ± 23
Associate professor	282 ± 85		43 ± 34
Full professor	294 ± 73		41 ± 27
Service chief	328 ± 95		47 ± 34
ARNP	80 ± 13		—
PA	82 ± 13		—
Call pay† per 24 hours		1.7 ± 0.9	

All values are given in thousands of dollars ($) as mean ± SD. Note that data from Level I and Level II trauma centers were essentially the same for all providers.

ARNP, advanced registered nurse practitioner; PA, physician assistant.

*Bonuses were paid at only 40% of responding institutions.

†Call stipends were paid at only 66% of responding institutions.

The results of this survey demonstrate that there is a shortage of trauma and surgical critical care surgeons in the United States, even though such practitioners receive generous financial compensation.

Directors of level I and level II trauma centers reported that these centers are currently supported by an average of 5 trauma and critical care surgeons, but that 4 additional surgeons per site will be needed within the next 3 years. The total compensation for a trauma and critical care surgeon taking an average of 6 calls per month (assuming that surgeons received a salary plus both a bonus and an on-call pay) ranged from a mean of $400 000 for entry-level faculty members to nearly $500 000 (Table 3) for service directors. The American Association of Medical Colleges (AAMC) tracks the salaries of university physicians, but the salaries reported specifically exclude bonus pay and on-call pay, which can easily make up 40% or more of a trauma surgeon's total compensation.

D. W. Mozingo, MD

Use of a modified chitosan dressing in a hypothermic coagulopathic grade V liver injury model

Bochicchio G, Kilbourne M, Kuehn R, et al (Univ of Maryland, Baltimore; Walter Reed Army Med Ctr, Washington, DC)

Am J Surg 198:617-622, 2009

Background.—Exsanguination from hepatic trauma is exacerbated by the lethal triad of acidosis, coagulopathy, and hypothermia. We evaluated the application of a modified chitosan dressing in a hypothermic coagulopathic model of grade V liver injury.

Methods.—Subject swine underwent induced hypothermic coagulopathy followed by standardized grade V liver injuries. A modified chitosan dressing was applied and compared with standard packing.

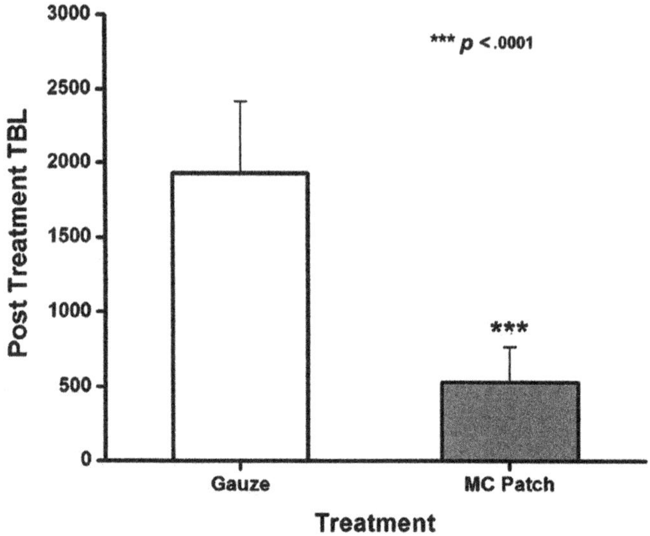

FIGURE 3.—Total post-treatment blood loss (TBL) between modified chitosan (MC) patch group and standard gauze packing group. (Reprinted from Bochicchio G, Kilbourne M, Kuehn R, et al. Use of a modified chitosan dressing in a hypothermic coagulopathic grade V liver injury model. *Am J Surg.* 2009;198:617-622, with permission from Elsevier.)

Results.—Pretreatment temperature, activated clotting time, and blood loss were similar between groups. Post treatment blood loss was significantly less and resuscitation mean arterial pressure were significantly greater in the modified chitosan group ($P < .0001$ and $P < .018$, respectively). Mean fluid resuscitative volume was significantly less in the modified chitosan group ($P < .0056$). Hemostasis was achieved on average 5.2 minutes following modified chitosan and never achieved with standard packing. At 1 hour post injury, all treatment animals survived compared with half of controls.

Conclusions.—Modified chitosan dressings provide simple rapid treatment of life-threatening liver injuries (Fig 3).

▶ Exsanguination is the leading cause of death on the battlefield and a major cause of death in civilian trauma. Hemorrhage may be compounded by hypothermia, acidosis, and coagulopathy; this lethal triad has been shown to increase mortality in both civilian and military injuries. There has been a recent major research effort toward the development of advanced hemostatic agents that are capable of stopping major hemorrhage. Such agents under development include liquid fibrin sealants, which require longer preparatory time and are somewhat difficult in their mixing ability and delivery procedures.

They tend also to require a temperature-controlled environment before application, which may limit their ability to be used in an emergency trauma setting. There are also hemostatic powders and a variety of dry dressings. These agents are developed mostly for external application and control of hemorrhage. The authors of this selection describe an experiment wherein one of these dry dressings was used to augment packing control of a grade V hepatic injury in a porcine model of injury. Significantly less blood loss was observed (Fig 3). This may be a particularly good application of this technology, in light of the difficulty in controlling bleeding in major hepatic injury. The questions remaining to be answered relate to potential toxicity when used intraperitoneally and to the ease and timing of the removal of this type of packing.

D. W. Mozingo, MD

Use of Leukoreduced Blood Does Not Reduce Infection, Organ Failure, or Mortality Following Trauma

Englehart MS, Cho SD, Morris MS, et al (Oregon Health & Science Univ, Portland)
World J Surg 33:1626-1632, 2009

Background.—Leukoreduced (LR) blood has been demonstrated to reduce morbidity and mortality in high-risk surgical patients, but not in trauma patients. The objective of the present study was to determine the effect of LR blood on morbidity and mortality. We hypothesized that the use of LR blood does not improve outcome in trauma patients.

Methods.—This study was a retrospective cohort analysis of trauma patients transfused at a level 1 Trauma Center from 2001 to 2004. Between 2002 and 2003, LR blood was transfused. Prior to that time and subsequent to it, non-leukoreduced (NLR) blood was transfused. This created two historical comparison groups. Data collected included patient demographics, units of blood transfused, intensive care unit (ICU) and hospital days, ventilator days, injury severity score (ISS), mortality, presence of acute respiratory distress syndrome (ARDS), and infectious complications. A multiple organ dysfunction syndrome (MODS) score was calculated.

Results.—The distribution of patients was as follows: 284 patients received only NLR blood, 153 received only LR blood, and 58 received at least one unit of each. The mean ISS was similar (NLR: 26, LR: 24; $P > 0.1$). No differences were seen between groups in units transfused (6.2 vs. 5.5), number of ICU days (8.2 vs. 9.0), number of hospital days (16.9 vs. 18.6), number of ventilator days (6.1 vs. 5.7), incidence of ARDS (8.3% vs. 8.5%), MODS score (5.5 vs. 5.9), mortality rate (15.1% vs. 15.7%), or infection rate (36% vs. 30%) ($P > 0.1$).

Conclusions.—This study represents the largest series comparing trauma patients who received either LR or standard blood transfusions. The use of LR blood does not improve outcome in trauma patients.

► Critically ill trauma patients are frequently transfused with packed red blood cells (PRBCs). Blood transfusion in trauma patients has been demonstrated to be an independent predictor of mortality, length of hospital stay, and infection independent of the severity of injury.

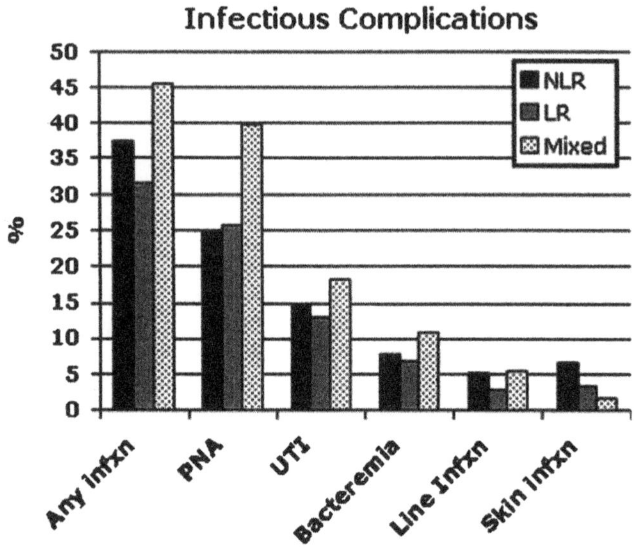

FIGURE 2.—Infectious complications. * $P < 0.05$. *PNA* pneumonia, *UTI* urinary tract infection. (With kind permission from Springer+Business Media: Englehart MS, Cho SD, Morris MS, et al. Use of leukoreduced blood does not reduce infection, organ failure, or mortality following trauma. *World J Surg*. 2009;33:1626-1632.)

Allogeneic blood transfusion is associated with numerous additional complications—febrile nonhemolytic transfusion reactions, transfusion-related acute lung injury, viral transmission, and transfusion-related immunologic alterations. Donor leukocytes present in the allogeneic blood have been implicated as a potential cause of these complications.

Proposed mechanisms include induction of T-cell anergy in the recipient, decreased natural killer cell function, altered ratio of T helper to T suppressor cells, and soluble proinflammatory cytokines produced by leukocytes during storage. Leukoreduced (LR) blood has been demonstrated to reduce morbidity and mortality in high-risk surgical patients but not in trauma patients. This study represents the largest series in the literature to date concerning outcomes following transfusion of LR blood over standard PRBCs. Preferential transfusion of LR blood did not significantly affect the incidence of infection (Fig 2), organ failure, transfusion reaction, intensive care unit (ICU) or hospital length of stay, ventilator days, or mortality. The universal use of LR blood may not be beneficial in the trauma population and may add unnecessary costs to the patient and the blood bank. One limitation of the study was that there was no control for the age of the blood transfused, as this may also contribute to the subsequent complications following trauma and blood transfusion.

D. W. Mozingo, MD

Western Trauma Association Critical Decisions in Trauma: Nonoperative Management of Adult Blunt Hepatic Trauma

Kozar RA, Moore FA, Moore EE, et al (Univ of Texas Health Science Ctr at Houston; The Methodist Hosp, Houston, TX; Denver Health Med Ctr, CO; et al)

J Trauma 67:1144-1149, 2009

This is a recommended algorithm of the Western Trauma Association for the management of blunt hepatic injuries. Because there are no published prospective randomized trials, the recommendations are based on available published prospective, observational, and retrospective data and expert opinion of Western Trauma Association members. The algorithm and accompanying text represent safe and reasonable treatment strategies that could be followed at most trauma centers. We recognize that there will be variability in decision making and institutional and patient-specific factors that may warrant deviation from the recommended algorithm. We encourage institutions to use this algorithm as a basis to develop institution-specific protocols. The algorithm contains letters, which correspond to the text. Their purpose is to explain the critical factors affecting decisions and to guide the reader through the algorithm. References to support each step are inserted as appropriate. Specific areas where published data are lacking are mentioned as potential topics for future studies.

▶ Extensive experience in the nonoperative management of blunt hepatic injuries has accrued over the past 20 years resulting in the publication of a number of practice guidelines based mostly on individual centers' experience.

Published, prospective randomized trials, as the authors of this selection have identified, do not exist. The authors provide an algorithm based on published data and expert opinions on the management of adult patients sustaining blunt hepatic injuries. A detailed analysis and rationale for each step of the rather complex algorithm is provided that greatly enhances its use. It also transforms into a great teaching tool for surgical residents.

In an editorial comment following the publication by Leon Pachter, the following 4 excellent points are made:

1. Hemodynamic instability in the patients with isolated hepatic injuries should prompt operative intervention.
2. The scanner is not the appropriate venue to triage hemodynamically unstable patients.
3. The use of diagnostic peritoneal aspiration is an invaluable tool in patients unstable with a negative FAST.
4. Isolated high-grade injuries (IV–V), which meet inclusion criteria, can successfully be managed nonoperatively.

The guidelines presented in this algorithm are evidence based and presented clearly. They are also presented in a format that could be edited easily if new information, particularly of that relating to the presence of angiographic blushing, becomes available to refine our treatment strategies.

D. W. Mozingo, MD

Operative vs nonoperative management of blunt pancreatic trauma in children

Wood JH, Partrick DA, Bruny JL, et al (Univ of Colorado Health Science Ctr, Aurora)

J Pediatr Surg 45:401-406, 2010

Purpose.—The aim of this study was to evaluate the outcome of nonoperative vs operative management of blunt pancreatic trauma in children.

Methods.—Retrospective review of pancreatic injuries from 1995 to 2006 at an urban level I regional pediatric trauma center.

Results.—Forty-three children with pancreatic injury were included in the analysis. Injuries included grade I (n = 18), grade II (n = 6), grade III (n = 17), and grade IV (n = 2). For grade II to IV injuries, patients managed operatively (n = 14) and nonoperatively (n = 11) had similar lengths of stay and rates of readmission, despite increased pancreatic complications (PCs) in the nonoperative cohort (21% vs 73%; $P = .02$). There was a trend toward increased non-PCs in patients managed with resection ($P = .07$). Twelve patients underwent successful diagnostic endoscopic retrograde cholangiopancreatography in which duct injury was identified. In this group, nonoperative management was pursued in 6 patients but was associated with increased rates of PC (86% nonoperative vs 29% operative; $P = .02$).

Conclusions.—Operative management of children with grades II to IV pancreatic injury results in significantly decreased rates of PCs but fails to decrease length of stay in the hospital, possibly as a result of non-PCs. Endoscopic retrograde cholangiopancreatography may serve as a useful diagnostic modality for guiding operative vs nonoperative management decisions.

▶ Although the incidence of pancreatic injury in children sustaining blunt abdominal trauma is low, management of these injuries remains a challenge. Ongoing debate about the optimal approach for treating pancreatic injuries continues, with some advocating early operative intervention and others suggesting that a nonoperative approach is best. This study from a single institution was selected because it provides a detailed discussion of this problem and logically sorts patients into operative and nonoperative categories.

A number of limitations of the study have been noted; however, several conclusions about the management of pancreatic trauma in children can be made. The data suggest that operative management results in significantly decreased rates of pancreatic complications but fails to decrease the length of hospital stay. Conversely, pancreatic complications are associated with increased length of stay and increased need for additional drainage procedures. This discrepancy implies that the morbidity associated with pancreatic resection may offset the gains made by avoidance of pancreatic complications.

D. W. Mozingo, MD

3 Burns

A multicenter clinical trial of recombinant human GM-CSF hydrogel for the treatment of deep second-degree burns

Zhang L, Chen J, Han C (Zhejiang Univ College of Medicine, Hangzhou, China; The Third Affiliated Hosp, Wenzhou, China)

Wound Repair Regen 17:685-689, 2009

Wound healing is a complex and dynamic biological process. The efficacy and safety of a recombinant human granulocyte-macrophage colony-stimulating factor (rhGM-CSF) hydrogel to promote deep-second-degree burn wound healing is evaluated in this study. In this multicenter, randomized, double-blind, and placebo-controlled clinical trial, 90 patients with deep second-degree burns were randomly assigned into two groups. Complete healing time and percentage of wound healing at different time points were observed and side effects were recorded. A statistically significant difference was noted at each time point ($p < 0.01$). No side effects were observed. These results suggest that

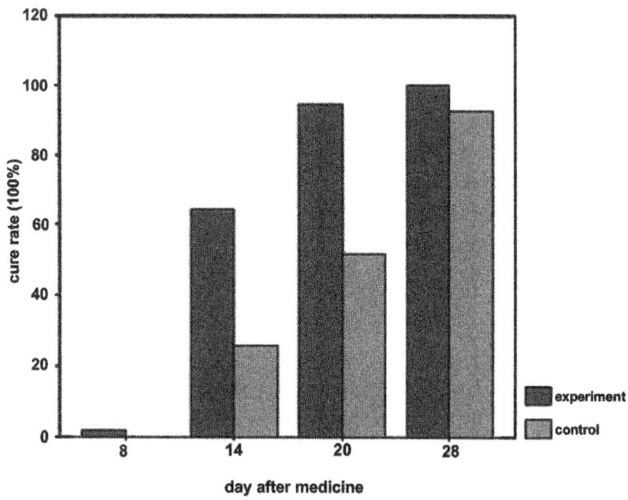

FIGURE 1.—The cure rate in different days. (Reprinted from Zhang L, Chen J, Han C. A multicenter clinical trial of recombinant human GM-CSF hydrogel for the treatment of deep second-degree burns. *Wound Repair Regen.* 2009;17:685-689, with permission from the Wound Healing Society.)

rhGM-CSF hydrogel can significantly accelerate deep second-degree burn wound healing and is considered to be safe.

▶ This study showed that a topical application of an rhGM-CSF hydrogel to superficial and deeper deep second-degree burns achieved a significantly higher total effectiveness rate on day 8 (60.70%) compared with the control (18.50%). Subsequently, the cure rate on day 20 was 94.60% in the treatment group and only 51.85% in the control group. Finally, on day 28, the cure rate was 100% in the treatment group and 92.59% in the control group (Fig 1). Thus, rhGM-CSF hydrogel plays an important therapeutic role in deep second-degree burns.

No adverse reactions were observed, and the possibility of adverse events was very low. In conclusion, rhGM-CSF hydrogel therapy could play a role in the future treatment of deep second-degree burns. Estimates of cost of treatment versus delay in return to normal function would be important to consider. Also, little is known about the application to larger surface areas of burn, and adverse reactions might become more likely.

D. W. Mozingo, MD

A Novel TGF-Beta Antagonist Speeds Reepithelialization and Reduces Scarring of Partial Thickness Porcine Burns

Singer AJ, Huang SS, Huang JS, et al (Stony Brook Univ, NY; Saint Louis Univ, MO)

J Burn Care Res 30:329-334, 2009

Scar formation after thermal injury is common and results in significant aesthetic and functional impairment. Transforming growth factor beta (TGF-β) plays a significant role in scar formation. We tested the hypothesis that a novel TGF-β peptantagonist would reduce scar formation and wound contraction in partial thickness burns by using a randomized controlled experiment. The subjects include two domestic pigs (20–25 kg). Forty burns were created on the animal's dorsum using an aluminum bar preheated to 80°C and applied for 20 seconds resulting in a partial thickness thermal burn extending half way down the dermis. Burns were treated every other day for 1 week, then twice weekly for 3 weeks with a topical TGF-β antagonist or its vehicle. Full thickness biopsies were obtained from all burns at 7, 10, and 14 days after injury. The wounds were completely excised after 28 days for histological assessment. Wound sections were stained with H&E and evaluated by a dermatopathologist masked to treatment assignment for reepithelialization and depth of scar formation. We also determined the number of wounds at 28 days that healed with contracted, hour-glass shaped scars. Data were compared with χ^2 and *t*-tests. Twenty burns were treated with TGF-β antagonist and 20 with control vehicle. TGF-β antagonist increased the percentage of completely reepithelialized wounds at 14 days

(90 vs 45%, $P=.002$) and reduced the percentage of contracted wounds (35 vs 65%, $P=.02$) and full thickness scars (10 vs 60%, $P=.002$) at 28 days. Treatment of partial thickness porcine burns with the TGF-β antagonist speeds reepithelialization and reduces scar formation and wound contraction in partial thickness porcine burns.

▶ Scar formation after burn injury is common and may result in significant aesthetic disfigurement and functional impairment. Effective methods to prevent or reduce scarring are still needed, as only limited progress has been made in this area. Transforming growth factor (TGF) beta 1 is a pluripotent peptide involved in wound healing and scar contraction. TGF beta 1 is released by degranulating platelets at the site of injury and affects a wide range of wound healing processes, including the inflammatory response, angiogenesis, re-epithelialization, extracellular matrix deposition, and wound remodeling. Keloid-derived keratinocytes express more TGF-beta 1, thus further stimulating extracellular matrix synthesis by both normal and keloid fibroblasts. Wounds that are treated with neutralizing antibodies to TGF-beta 1 have a lower inflammatory response, reduced extracellular matrix deposition, and reduced cutaneous scarring in animal studies.

In this selection, the authors used a partial thickness burn injury in swine to study a novel TGF-beta 1 antagonist and its effect on burn wound healing. This treatment accelerated wound re-epithelialization and reduced wound contraction and scar depth (Fig 2 in the original article). Treatments such as this could have great implications in the care of burn patients since there have been no recent significant advances in the battle against scarring.

D. W. Mozingo, MD

American Burn Association Practice Guidelines for Prevention, Diagnosis, and Treatment of Ventilator-Associated Pneumonia (VAP) in Burn Patients

Mosier MJ, Pham TN (Univ of Washington Burn Ctr, Seattle; Harborview Med Ctr, Seattle, WA)

J Burn Care Res 30:910-928, 2009

The purpose of this guideline is to review the available published literature on ventilator-associated pneumonia (VAP) as it pertains to the burn patient. It provides an evidence-based recommendation for the prevention, diagnosis, and treatment of VAP in adult burn patients. This guideline is designed to assist all healthcare providers caring for adult burn patients with suspected VAP. Summary recommendations were made using the following grading scale: grade A—supported by at least one well-designed prospective trial with clear-cut results; grade B—supported by several small prospective trials with a similar conclusion; and grade C—supported by a single small prospective trial, retrospective analyses, cases studies, and expert opinions based on investigators' practices.

▶ This selection is included because it summarizes in detail the current knowledge base for smoke inhalation injury and ventilator-associated pneumonia in patients with burns. Despite its common occurrence, no clinical gold standard exists for the diagnosis of ventilator-associated pneumonia in any patient population. Others have created guidelines for the prevention and management of ventilator-associated pneumonia; however, establishing the diagnosis of ventilator-associated pneumonia can be particularly difficult in the patient with burns where other causes of pulmonary dysfunction, namely smoke inhalation injury, systemic inflammation, and pulmonary edema, not only predisposes the patient to postinjury pneumonia but also may obscure its diagnosis. Traditionally, ventilator-associated pneumonia is suspected if the patient has clinical findings suggesting infection, including fever, purulent sputum, leukocytosis or leukopenia, and decreased oxygenation along with a new or worsening infiltrate on chest radiograph. Unfortunately, no consensus exists on which combination of findings yields an accurate diagnosis of ventilator-associated pneumonia, and many patients with the clinical diagnosis of pneumonia may have noninfectious etiologies for their clinical findings.

Fever, leukocytosis, or leukopenia infiltrates from smoke inhalation injury in the absence of pulmonary infection and decreased blood oxygenation are often present in the patient with burns, making the utilization of the Centers for Disease Control (CDC) guidelines for the diagnosis difficult.

D. W. Mozingo, MD

An assessment of acute kidney injury with modified RIFLE criteria in pediatric patients with severe burns

Palmieri T, Lavrentieva A, Greenhalgh D (Shriners Hosp for Children Northern California, Sacramento; Papanikolau General Hosp, Thessaloniki, Greece)
Intensive Care Med 35:2125-2129, 2009

Objective.—To apply the modified pediatric RIFLE criteria for severity of acute kidney injury (AKI) to pediatric burn ICU patients and to evaluate the overall incidence of AKI, risk factors for AKI and influence of AKI on outcome.

Design.—Retrospective, descriptive cohort study.

Setting.—10-bed burn PICU facility.

Patients.—All consecutive patients with a burn injury of 10% or more of total body surface area percentage (TBSA, %) admitted during a 2 year period.

Measurements and Results.—Data of 123 patients were studied. The incidence of AKI was 45.5%. Patients with AKI tended to have higher mortality than those without AKI ($p = 0.057$). All nonsurvivors attained pRIFLE AKI by combination of serum creatinine and urine output criteria.

Patients with a more severe form of AKI (Failure and Injury) as well as patients with late AKI had more episodes of sepsis as compared to patients with early AKI and the Risk category of AKI. Logistic regression analysis indicated that PRISM score and TBSA were the independent risk factors for acute kidney injury in pediatric burn patients; the presence of sepsis and septic shock were the independent risk factors for the Failure class of AKI.

Conclusion.—We observed a high incidence of AKI in the burn PICU population. Sepsis seems to contribute to the development of the Failure class of AKI. Maximum Failure class of AKI is associated with high mortality.

▶ Acute kidney injury (AKI) has been associated with increased mortality, lengthened hospital stay, and increased health care resource utilization and costs in critically ill patients. A consensus definition of AKI using the RIFLE criteria was proposed by the Acute Dialysis Quality Initiative working group. Recently, a modified version of the RIFLE criteria for pediatric patients (pRIFLE) was developed and a mortality of 60% in children with AKI was reported.

Although some studies have applied the RIFLE classification system in adult patients with burn, its usefulness in pediatric burn patients has not been evaluated.

The aim of this study was to determine the incidence and characteristics of burned children with AKI using the pRIFLE criteria to identify risk factors for AKI and to evaluate the association between AKI and outcomes in children with burns. In this study, the investigators observed a higher incidence of AKI in the burn ICU population. Sepsis seemed to contribute to the development of the failure class of AKI, and maximum failure class of AKI is associated with high mortality. This study did not demonstrate a drug-related effect on AKI as did other studies, and is somewhat limited by the small number of subjects compared with other studies.

D. W. Mozingo, MD

Are topical antimicrobials effective against bacteria that are highly resistant to systemic antibiotics?

Neely AN, Gardner J, Durkee P, et al (Shriners Hosps for Children, Cincinnati, OH)

J Burn Care Res 30:19-29, 2009

An increasing number of bacteria are resistant to multiple systemic antibiotics. The purpose of this study was to determine if topical antimicrobials are still effective against multi-drug resistant organisms (MDROs). MDROs, including *Acinetobacter*, *Pseudomonas*, *Klebsiella*, *Staphylococcus*, and *Enterococcus*, were collected from four burn hospitals. The sensitivity of 47 MDROs to 11 commonly used topical agents (mafenide acetate, nystatin, mafenide + nystatin, silver nitrate, Dakin's, polymyxin B, neomycin, polymyxin + neomycin, silver sulfadiazine, bacitracin, silver sulfadiazine + bacitracin) was tested using the agar well diffusion assay and compared with the sensitivity of 27 non-MDROs of similar genera. Overall 88% of the tests of the non-MDROs showed susceptibility to the topicals compared with 80% for the MDROs ($P < .05$). Specific findings included: all of the gram-positive non-MDROs were sensitive to bacitracin compared with only 67% of the MDROs ($P < .05$); 74% of the non-MDROs were sensitive to neomycin vs 26% of the MDROs ($P < .01$). Even for the susceptible isolates, the zones of inhibition were smaller for the MDROs than for the non-MDROs ($P < .002$), indicating decreased susceptibility of the MDROs. Specifically, while the MDRO Acinetobacter were sensitive to most of the topicals, the zones of inhibition for silvadene, silvadene + bacitracin, neomycin, and neomycin + polymyxin were significantly smaller ($P < .001$) for the Acinetobacter MDROs than the non-MDROs. Although many topicals are still effective against some MDROs, MDROs are more resistant to topicals than are non-MDROs. Some treatment assumptions based historically on the efficacy of topical antimicrobial agents against non-MDROs need to be re-evaluated for MDROs.

► Topical antimicrobial agents that are commonly used in the care of patients with burns remain very effective against nonmultiple drug-resistant organism (MDRO) bacterial strains. The non-MDRO data presented in this selection are consistent with topical testing susceptibility data that were generated in the past when multiple drug-resistant strains were not as prevalent. The new data in this article demonstrate that the topical antimicrobial agents that were so effective against non-MDRO bacteria were significantly less effective against the newer MDRO strains and are included in this review.

Resistance to topical agents should be reassessed periodically as the resistance to systemic antimicrobials increases.

D. W. Mozingo, MD

Burn Hazards of the Deployed Environment in Wartime: Epidemiology of Noncombat Burns from Ongoing United States Military Operations

Kauvar DS, Wade CE, Baer DG (United States Army Inst of Surgical Res, Fort Sam Houston, TX)

J Am Coll Surg 209:453-460, 2009

Background.—Service in the deployed military environment carries risks for accidental (noncombat-related) burns. Examining these risks can assist in the development of military burn prevention measures. This study endeavored to examine noncombat burn epidemiology in the context of similar civilian data.

Study Design.—We performed a retrospective cohort study of consecutive casualties evacuated from operational military theaters in Iraq and Afghanistan to the sole tertiary military burn center in the US. Military

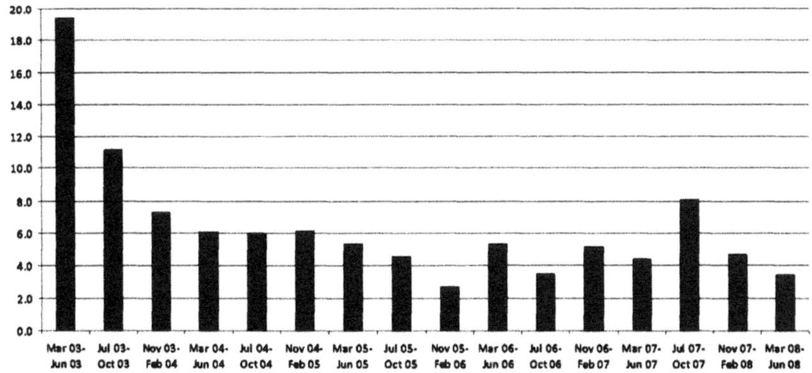

FIGURE 2.—Noncombat burns/100,000 troops at risk for 16 periods of 4-months each, from March 2003 to June 2008. (Reprinted from Kauvar DS, Wade CE, Baer DG. Burn hazards of the deployed environment in wartime: epidemiology of noncombat burns from ongoing United States military operations. *J Am Coll Surg*. 2009;209:453-460, with permission of the American College of Surgeons.)

data were compared with database samples of the US population from the American Burn Association and the Centers for Disease Control and Prevention.

Results.—The main causes of the 180 noncombat burns seen from March 2003 to June 2008 were waste burning, fuel mishaps, and unintentional ordinance detonations. Overall prevalence of noncombat burns was 19.5 burns/100,000 person-years lived. If causes specific to military operations are removed, military prevalence was 13.0/100,000. More than one-third of noncombat burns occurred in the first year of the study; a period of stability followed. A similar US population had an accidental burn prevalence of 7.1/100,000 from 2003 to 2007. Burn size, presence of inhalation injury, and burn center mortality were not different from those in a similar civilian cohort.

Conclusions.—Deployed service members have a greater risk of unintentional burns than a similar civilian cohort does. This is in part because of the specific dangers of military activities. More attention to deployed military burn prevention is needed, especially early in combat support operations (Fig 2).

▶ The authors of this study have demonstrated that service members deployed to a military environment in support of combat operations have a baseline risk of burn injury that exceeds by a factor of 2 to 3 the risk faced by a similar population in the United States. This increased risk appears to be closely determined by the specific requirements of their environment. Resources developed in a maturing combat theater seem to result in reduced noncombat burn risks, include the development of centralized power plants to replace portable fueled generators and the use of chemical toilets and the installation of sanitary sewer systems to eliminate waste burning (Fig 2).

Emphasis on safe procedures and the wearing of protective clothing during high-risk activities remains indicated in attempts to reduce the incidence and impact of noncombat military burn injuries. This well-designed review of injury patterns will likely serve to reduce noncombat-related burn injury by raising awareness of the most preventable causes of burn in this setting.

D. W. Mozingo, MD

Escharotomy and Decompressive Therapies in Burns

Orgill DP, Piccolo N (Brigham and Women's Hosp, Boston, MA; Pronto Socorro para Queimaduras, Goiânia, Brazil)

J Burn Care Res 30:759-768, 2009

Experienced clinicians treating burns recognize the need for escharotomy and decompressive therapies. The burning process causes the integument to become stiff, and the underlying tissues can swell during the fluid resuscitation process. We reviewed the literature that supports the current clinical practice of decompressive therapies following burn injury.

▶ Full-thickness circumferential burns of the extremity result in an inelastic eschar that leads to ready compression of nerves and blood vessels during the fluid resuscitation phase of burn care when fluid accumulates in the extracellular space. Pressure within the compartment increases and may eventually lead to ischemia and necrosis of the tissues within. Untreated, the consequence can be amputation, tissue loss, infection, or a painful muscle contracture. In the chest and abdomen, large areas of burn can prevent the normal expansion of skin during respiration. Hemodynamic or respiratory compromise often results.

This practice guideline is included in this year's selections because it represents the most up-to-date evidence-based information available on this important aspect of burn care. The report also identifies knowledge deficiencies that would indicate the need for future research including the following:

1. Development of more sensitive clinical tools or bedside technology to diagnose tissue ischemia before rhabdomyolysis has evolved.
2. Determination of threshold values for muscle and nerve ischemia.
3. Determination of the biomechanical properties of eschar and modeling tissue pressure and release criteria.
4. Comparing prophylactic escharotomy versus escharotomy performed based on objective measurements.

D. W. Mozingo, MD

Influence of Nebulized Unfractionated Heparin and *N*-Acetylcysteine in Acute Lung Injury After Smoke Inhalation Injury

Miller AC, Rivero A, Ziad S, et al (State Univ of New York Downstate Med Ctr and Kings County Hosp Ctr, Brooklyn; Univ of South Florida, Tampa; Univ of Maryland Baltimore County; et al)

J Burn Care Res 30:249-256, 2009

To determine whether the combination of aerosolized unfractionated heparin and *N*-acetylcystine reduces 28-days mortality and lung injury scores (LISs) in adult patients with smoke inhalation injury requiring mechanical ventilation. The study was a single-center retrospective study with historical control. The authors included 30 mechanically ventilated adult subjects who were admitted within 48 hours of their bronchoscopy confirmed smoke inhalation injury over a 5-year period. The experimental group was treated with nebulized heparin sulfate, *N*-acetylcystine, and albuterol sulfate. Controls received ventilation support and albuterol sulfate. The authors calculated acute physiology and chronic health evaluation (APACHE)-III scores on admission in addition to daily LIS for 7 days. The experimental group was divided into five APACHE-III subgroups and matched with inhalation lung injury patients in the historical control

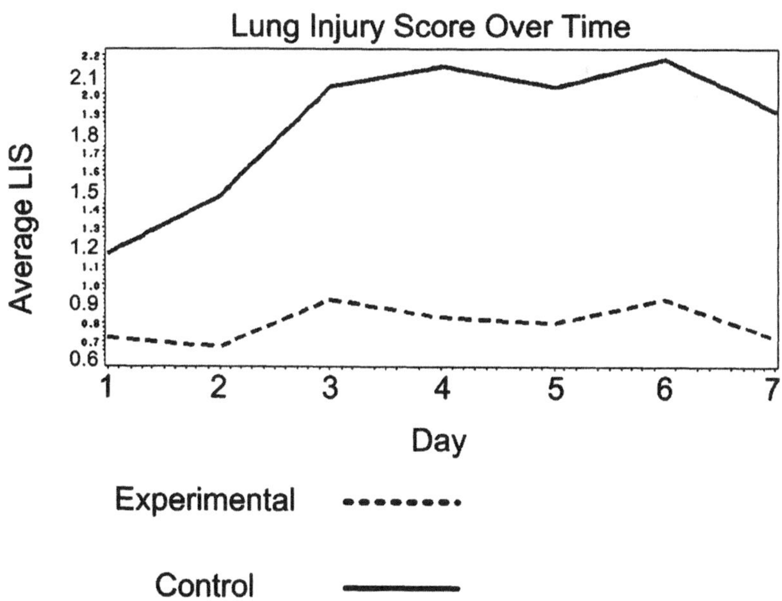

FIGURE 3.—Longitudinal graphical representation of average lung injury score plotted as a function of hospital day. The experimental group (*dashed line*) displays a persistently lower lung injury score than the control group (*solid line*). Additionally, the average lung injury score does not rise significantly for the experimental group (as opposed to the controls) for the duration of the first week postinjury. (Reprinted from Miller AC, Rivero A, Ziad S, et al. Influence of nebulized unfractionated heparin and *N*-acetylcysteine in acute lung injury after smoke inhalation injury. *J Burn Care Res*. 2009;30:249-256, with permission from the American Burn Association.)

group. There was no significant difference in initial APACHE-III scores or LISs between groups ($\alpha = 0.05$) upon entry to the study. The experimental group showed significant improvement in LISs, respiratory resistance and compliance measurements, and hypoxia scores as compared with controls throughout the duration of the study. There was a statistically significant survival benefit in the experimental group that was most pronounced in patients with APACHE-III scores >35. Survival for the control vs experimental group was 0.5714 ± 0.1497 vs 0.9375 ± 0.0605, respectively, (risk ratio −0.0055; 95% confidence interval −0.0314–0.0204; hazard ratio 1.003; number needed to treat 2.7). The use of aerosolized unfractionated heparin and *N*–acetylcystine attenuates lung injury and the progression of acute respiratory distress syndrome in ventilated adult patients with acute lung injury following smoke inhalation (Fig 3).

▶ This selection was chosen because it presents evidence that the combined effects of nebulized heparin sulfate, *N*-acetylcysteine, and albuterol sulfate significantly improve pulmonary function, decrease lung injury score (Fig 3), decrease respiratory resistance, and improve survival in adult patients with smoke inhalation injury requiring mechanical ventilation. This is likely due to the inhibition of airway fibrin clot formation by the heparin, mucolysis by *N*-acetylcysteine, and bronchodilation by albuterol sulfate. The combined effects of these treatments are believed to be the prevention of airway obstruction, improvement of ventilation, minimization of ventilation/perfusion mismatch, decreased neutrophil chemotaxis, and superoxide release, thereby diminishing peroxynitrate formation and subsequent endothelial injury and vascular permeability. The authors' results show a significant decrease in morbidity and mortality. This has significant potential implications with regard to the treatment of smoke inhalation injury.

Validation through a larger prospective study is needed.

D. W. Mozingo, MD

Intensive insulin therapy confers a similar survival benefit in the burn intensive care unit to the surgical intensive care unit

Gibson BR, Galiatsatos P, Rabiee A, et al (Johns Hopkins Bayview Med Ctr, Baltimore, MD)

Surgery 146:922-930, 2009

Background.—In contrast to the benefits of intensive insulin therapy (IIT) in the surgical intensive care unit (SICU), its benefits in the burn ICU (BICU) remain unclear. Furthermore, IIT and tight glycemic control has received little attention in elderly ICU patients.

Methods.—We evaluated the normalization of blood glucose level with IIT in BICU and SICU patients. From October 2006 to July 2007, 970 patients were admitted to our BICU and our SICU. A total of 79 of these patients met criteria for initiation of IIT, 37 of who required IIT

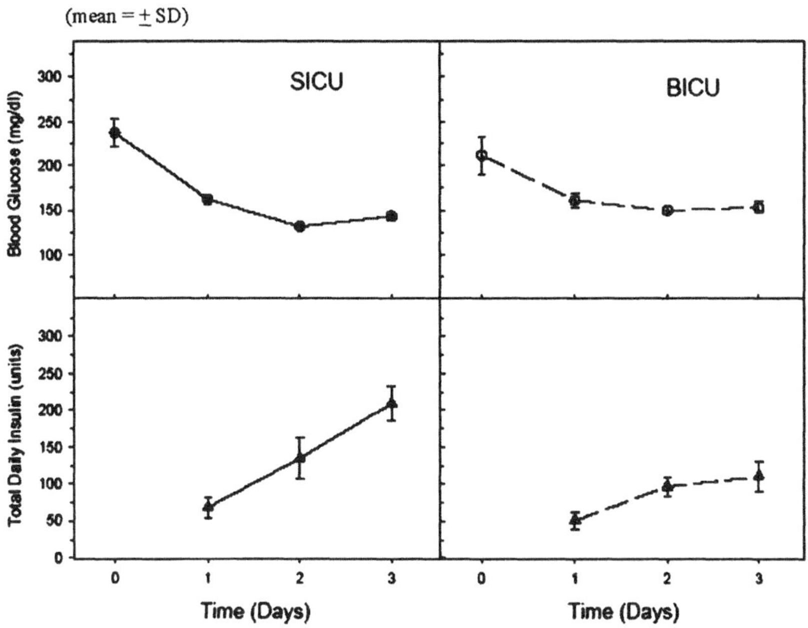

FIGURE 1.—Average glucose levels in the upper panel and the average daily insulin requirements in the lower panel for all patients admitted to the surgical intensive care unit (SICU) (*left panels*) and the burn ICU (BICU) (*right panels*). (Reprinted from Gibson BR, Galiatsatos P, Rabiee A, et al. Intensive insulin therapy confers a similar survival benefit in the burn intensive care unit to the surgical intensive care unit. *Surgery.* 2009;146:922-930, with permission from Elsevier.)

for at least 72 hours. Data were analyzed to determine if tight glycemic control (blood glucose ≤150 mg/dL by day 3) is associated with reduced morbidity and mortality.

Results.—Tight control was better achieved in SICU patients (45%) than in BICU patients (33%). Daily insulin requirements were approximately 2-fold greater in SICU patients compared with BICU patients ($P < .05$). Tight control in both SICU and BICU patients was associated with a decreased incidence of sepsis compared with poor glycemic control (10% vs 58% and 60% vs 70%, respectively) and a decreased mortality rate (0 vs 58% and 20% vs 50%; SICU vs BICU, respectively). The percentage of total body surface area burned in BICU patients was 10% and 45% in the ≤150 and >150 mg/dL groups. Mortality rate in the poor control group was >10-fold greater than that of the tight control group; for patients ≥65 years of age, mortality was nearly double than that of patients <65 years of age. The greatest mortality rate (62%) was seen in patients >65 years of age with poor control.

Conclusion.—Tight control with IIT is associated with an increased survival rate in both BICU and SICU patients. Age is associated with survival, with patients older than 65 years of age having the greatest mortality rate (Fig 1).

▶ Tight glucose control in critically ill patients has substantial positive outcomes. Maintenance of euglycemia with intensive insulin therapy has been associated with reduced mortality, morbidity, and duration of stay in critically ill surgical patients, largely due to a striking reduction in infectious complications.

Currently, the use of intensive insulin therapy to achieve tight glycemic control is becoming a standard practice in many medical facilities. However, achievement of tight glycemic control is extremely difficult and seldom achieved. Other recent studies have failed to confirm this beneficial relationship. It is still not clear whether tight control should be the goal and whether, or to what degree, it is beneficial. In this selection, the authors look at burn and surgical intensive care unit (BICU and SICU) populations specifically.

They demonstrated that tight glycemic control is associated with reduced mortality in both the SICU (0% vs 58%) and the BICU (20% vs 50%) patients receiving intensive insulin therapy. Patient survival in the BICU was associated with tight glycemic control as well as a lower percentage of total body surface area burned and younger age. This preliminary study reveals an association between improved management of blood glucose and beneficial outcomes in adult burn victims, and indicates the need for a larger study to confirm these findings. Also, the data suggest that hyperglycemia may be especially difficult to control in elderly as well as in burn patients, and these patients may be at higher risk for infection and mortality.

Further exploration of the benefit of tight glycemic control in the elderly is warranted.

D. W. Mozingo, MD

Methicillin-Resistant *Staphylococcus aureus* Furunculitis in the Outpatient Burn Setting

Warner P, Neely A, Bailey JK, et al (Shriners Hosps for Children, Cincinnati, OH)

J Burn Care Res 30:657-660, 2009

Methicillin-resistant *Staphylococcus aureus* (MRSA) is becoming more predominant in the community. We have seen increasing cases of furunculitis in our outpatient burn clinic, which appear to develop weeks after the initial burn injury and in patients with limited inpatient stays. We performed a 3-year retrospective review of all outpatient burn patients who developed furunculitis. Data analyzed included length of hospital stay, type of injury sustained, culture and sensitivity results, and treatment provided. A total of 28 patients were identified with MRSA furunculitis, which presented as painful, hard, indurated boils with minimal purulent drainage. Adults had less extensive burn injuries (mean of 12% TBSA adults vs 20% TBSA children) with shorter hospital stays (mean 8 days adults vs 22 days children). Fifty-seven percent of the patients had multiple furuncules, involving both burned and nonburned areas. Patients with furunculitis had a less resistant MRSA strain than those without furunculitis. Of the 22 patients who received systemic antibiotic coverage, 14 (58%) were successfully treated with 1 antibiotic regimen, whereas 8 (33%) required multiple antibiotics. In this study, furunculitis in the outpatient setting was believed to be consistent with community-acquired MRSA. Incision and drainage was not sufficient in patients with multiple furuncles, and systemic antibiotics were administered. Through increased awareness of the prevalence of community-acquired MRSA in the community, appropriate antibiotic treatment can be initiated, and the discomfort and transmission risk associated with this disease can be minimized.

▶ Methicillin-resistant *Staphylococcus aureus* (MRSA) is becoming more prevalent in the community setting. Athletes, prisoners, and military recruits have been identified as high-risk groups for community-acquired MRSA (CA-MRSA). In the United States, CA-MRSA is associated with 2 clones. Its virulent USA400 clone can potentially cause severe and fatal diseases such as necrotizing fasciitis. The less virulent strain, USA300, is associated with localized skin and soft tissue infections. In healthy individuals, CA-MRSA most commonly presents as a furuncle whose management requires incision and drainage and normally does not require antibiotic treatment, though multiple lesions, recurrent lesions, and lesions with significant cellulitis often do.

The authors of this selection have described an increased trend of furunculitis in the outpatient burn population. These infections appear weeks after the initial injury and in patients with limited inpatient stay. Most patients they described had multiple furuncles, requiring incision and drainage with systemic antibiotic treatment (Fig 2 in the original article). In this study, furunculitis in the outpatient setting was felt to be consistent with CA-MRSA, even in patients with hospital stays of more than 48 hours.

Risk factors appeared to be male sex and injury sustained in an outdoor setting. Incision and drainage were not sufficient in patients with multiple furuncles, and antibiotics were used. I have observed a similar increase in CA-MRSA complicating the postburn course as well. Culture and sensitivity testing remains important because not all skin and soft tissue infections in the postburn period are due to MRSA.

D. W. Mozingo, MD

Pruritus in Burns: Review Article

Goutos I, Dziewulski P, Richardson PM (Stoke Mandeville Hosp, Buckinghamshire, UK; Broomfield Hosp, Chelmsford, UK)

J Burn Care Res 30:221-228, 2009

Pruritus represents a common and distressing feature of burn wounds. Over the last decades, significant advances in neuroanatomical and neurophysiological knowledge have resulted in the elucidation of the mediators and pathways involved in the transmission of pruritic impulses. A plethora of therapeutic approaches have been evaluated mostly in small-scale studies involving burns patients targeting both the peripheral and the central components of the neurologic pathway. Antihistamines, doxepin, massage therapy, and transcutaneous electrical nerve stimulation are effective strategies to combat pruritus in burns patients. Recent studies have provided preliminary evidence regarding the effectiveness of gabapentin and ondansetron. The area of burns pruritus is under-researched and large-scale studies are required to reinforce the armamentarium of specialists with evidence-based regimens for the treatment of this highly distressing symptom.

▶ Pruritus is a common and disabling feature of healing and healed burn wounds. The reported incidence of severe itching is as high as 87% in adult and 100% in pediatric patients with burns. Pruritus can complicate the recovery of all types of burn wounds, including those treated conservationally and donor and recipient areas in grafted patients. The authors of this selection have presented a comprehensive review of the subject.

The area of pruritus research is under-researched and as a result many protocols adopted by health care professionals reflect empirical approaches with little evidence-based information. The recent advances in the neuroanatomical and neurophysiological mechanisms of pruritus have spurred interest in exploring new therapeutic avenues. There is good evidence that antihistamines, doxepin, transcutaneous electrical nerve stimulation (TENS), and massage therapy are effective strategies. Recently, gabapentin and ondansetron have shown promising results as agents to ameliorate pruritic symptoms in patients with burns. These agents will require larger scale studies to prove their efficacy in the treatment of patients with burns.

D. W. Mozingo, MD

Recombinant Thrombin: Safety and Immunogenicity in Burn Wound Excision and Grafting

Greenhalgh DG, Gamelli RL, Collins J, et al (Univ of California, Sacramento; Loyola Univ Med Ctr, Maywood, IL; et al)

J Burn Care Res 30:371-379, 2009

This study evaluated the safety, immunogenicity, and hemostatic effect of recombinant human Thrombin (rThrombin), in patients undergoing skin grafting for burns. This was a phase 2 multiple site, single-arm, open-label study in patients receiving partial- or full-thickness autologous grafts. rThrombin was applied using a spray applicator to newly excised wounds of 1 to 4% body surface area at 5 minutes intervals for up to 20 minutes, after point source bleeding was stopped. Adverse events, skin graft survival, and formation of anti-rThrombin antibodies were measured at baseline and Day 29. There were no deaths or study drug discontinuations. Adverse events occurred in 63 of 72 patients (88%), and were typical of sequelae of skin grafting. Hemostasis was achieved within 20 minutes after application of rThrombin in 65 of 71 patients (91.5%). Skin graft failure occurred in 4 patients (6%). At the day 29 evaluation, for those patients who returned, 88.9% had ≥90% graft survival. One patient (1 of 70, 1.4%) had specific, low titer antibodies to rThrombin at baseline, but no increase in titer posttreatment; a second patient (1 of 62, 1.6%), developed antibodies to rThrombin at day 29. None of the antibodies neutralized native human thrombin. In excised burn wounds, hemostasis at 20 minutes was achieved in 91.5% of patients and skin graft survival was excellent. There was a low rate of antibodies to rThrombin at baseline (1.4%) and a low rate of anti-rThrombin antibody formation at day 29 (1.6%). rThrombin was well tolerated when administered with a pump spray.

▶ Surgical hemostasis is particularly important for the success of synchronous burn wound excision and placement of partial-thickness skin grafts. The goal of burn wound excision is to create a graft recipient site with a healthy vascular bed that is free from necrotic tissue, infection, fluid, or blood. Consequently, skin graft recipient site preparation often results in significant bleeding, especially after tangential or sequential excision. Using grafts prepared as sheets of skin as opposed to meshed grafts improves cosmetic outcomes; however, fluid accumulation under such grafts, including hematoma formation, can jeopardize graft take. Most techniques used to prepare a skin graft site include a number of techniques that enhance hemostasis.

One common method of graft bed hemostasis following burn wound excision is the use of topically applied thrombin, typically administered by spray applicator, in addition to surgical hemostasis. Thrombin plays an essential role in hemostasis, directly activating fibrin clot formation, platelets, and other procoagulant cofactors when vascular injury is present. Currently available thrombin-containing products are either plasma-derived or manufactured by recombinant technology.

The use of human plasma-derived thrombin is associated with a number of potential safety risks, including transmission of pathogens associated with plasma-borne infectious diseases, such as viral hepatitis, acquired immunodeficiency syndrome, and transmissible spongiform encephalopathies.

Human exposure to bovine-derived thrombin has been associated with the induction of allergic reactions, including anaphylaxis. The development of anti-bovine thrombin antibodies that cross-react with human coagulation factors II and V has also been described. The risk of developing anti-bovine thrombin product antibodies seems to increase with repeated exposure to bovine thrombin, and in patients with extensive burns, repeated exposure is the norm.

D. W. Mozingo, MD

The Association Between Blood Alcohol Level and Infectious Complications Among Burn Patients

Griffin R, Poe AM, Cross JM, et al (Univ of Alabama at Birmingham)
J Burn Care Res 30:395-399, 2009

Approximately 50% of fatal and 15% of nonfatal burn-injured patients have detectable blood alcohol content (BAC) at the time of admission, and it is hypothesized that alcohol exacerbates burn-related immunosuppression. The purpose of this study was to evaluate the association between BAC and infectious complications in burn patients. The study population consisted of 1161 burn patients admitted to a large academic burn center between January 1998 and June 2007. Patients were categorized into no BAC (0.0 g/100 ml), low/moderate BAC (>0.0 and <0.1 g/100 ml) and high BAC (≥0.1 g/100 ml) groups based on BAC at time of admission. Risk ratios (RRs) and 95% confidence intervals (CIs) were calculated for associations between pneumonia, sepsis, urinary tract infection, line infection, and wound infection and BAC, adjusted for total burn surface area and inhalation injury. Relative to no BAC patients, both low/moderate and high BAC patients had nonsignificantly increased risk

TABLE 3.—Crude and Adjusted Risk Ratios* (RRs) and 95% Confidence Intervals (CIs) for the Association Between Blood Alcohol Levels (in g/100 ml) and Pneumonia Stratified by Presence of Inhalation Injury

	BAC >0.0 and <0.1		BAC ≥0.1	
	Crude	Adjusted†	Crude	Adjusted†
No inhalation injury	1.68 (0.51–5.61)	1.64 (0.49–5.48)	3.29 (1.41–7.67)	2.92 (1.25–6.82)
Inhalation injury	1.61 (0.57–4.51)	1.80 (0.63–5.10)	1.09 (0.35–3.34)	1.20 (0.39–3.71)

BAC, blood alcohol content.
*RRs compared with BAC 0.0 group.
†Analysis is adjusted for total burn surface area.

for most infectious complications. High BAC patients were at significantly increased risk for any infectious complication (RR 2.06, CI 1.25–3.41) and pneumonia (RR 2.06, CI 1.04–4.09) and a nonsignificantly increased risk of urinary tract infection (RR 2.12, CI 0.0.94–4.78). Results suggest that preinjury alcohol consumption places patients at an increased risk for infectious complications, most notably pneumonia. Further studies examining the relationship between alcohol and pneumonia among burn patients will help elucidate the reason for the increased risk observed in the current study and suggest ways to prevent infection for this particular subgroup of burn patients.

▶ Many of the 40 000 individuals hospitalized for burn injuries in the United States have consumed alcohol before their injury. In trauma and burn patients, it has been observed that such patients have a higher risk of developing infectious complications, requiring more surgical procedures, and have a longer hospital stay. There are several mechanisms by which alcohol consumption might increase the risk of infectious complications. Burn injuries are associated with immunosuppression, even in the absence of alcohol consumption. It has been suggested that alcohol produces a synergistic immunosuppressive effect.

Bacterial translocation has been shown to be increased in the presence of both alcohol and burn injury when compared with either insult alone in a rat model. Little is known regarding the association between alcohol intoxication and infections in patients with burns. This study evaluated the association between alcohol and infectious complications in patients with burns admitted to a large urban academic burn center and stratified them with regard to blood alcohol concentration (BAC). Patients with higher BAC levels were more likely to develop pneumonia and other infectious complications (Table 3). Further studies will be required to elucidate this association.

D. W. Mozingo, MD

The Beneficial Effects of Plasma Exchange After Severe Burn Injury

Klein MB, Edwards JA, Kramer CB, et al (Univ of Washington Burn Ctr, Seattle; Univ of Washington, Seattle)

J Burn Care Res 30:243-248, 2009

Severe burn injury results in a systemic inflammatory response that leads to increased capillary permeability and fluid leak into the interstitium. This global systemic capillary leak can be attributed, at least in part, to inflammatory mediators produced as a result of cellular injury. Plasma exchange has been used in the management of a number of illnesses with a significant inflammatory component, and, therefore, may have a role in the early management of burn injury. The purpose of this study was to review our institutional experience using plasma exchange in the management of severe burn injury. We performed a retrospective review of all patients receiving plasma exchange at our burn center between

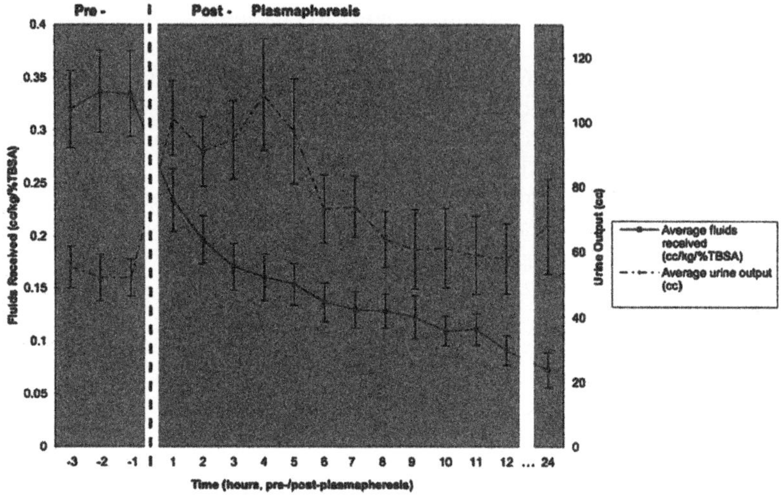

FIGURE 1.—Fluid received and urine output before and after plasma exchange therapy. (Reprinted from Klein MB, Edwards JA, Kramer CB, et al. The beneficial effects of plasma exchange after severe burn injury. *J Burn Care Res.* 2009;30:243-248, with permission from the American Burn Association.)

2001 and 2005. Data collected included the following: burn size, presence of inhalation injury, resuscitation fluid received, urine output, lactate levels, base deficit levels, and hematocrit before and after the exchange procedure. A total of 37 patients underwent plasma exchange during the 5-year study period and seven patients underwent two plasma exchange treatments. Average TBSA burned was 48.6% (range 18–82) and 73% of patients sustained an inhalation injury. After plasma exchange, hourly fluid volume received significantly decreased ($P < .05$) and base deficit, lactate, and hematocrit levels significantly improved. Plasma exchange in the early resuscitation period was associated with decreased fluid administration, as well as increased urine output in the period during and immediately after the procedure. These data suggest that plasma exchange may provide a useful tool in the management of severe burn injury (Fig 1).

▶ There has been increasing concern over the morbidity associated with large fluid volumes that patients receive during burn resuscitation, the so-called fluid creep.

Excessive fluid administration to the burn patient may result in extremity and abdominal compartment syndrome, adult respiratory distress syndrome, and pneumonia.

Many proinflammatory molecules have been implicated as mediators of the postburn response that drives edema formation.

Therapeutic plasma exchange is a technique of extracorporeal blood purification that removes large molecular weight particles, such as inflammatory mediators, from the circulating blood volume. A procedure that could abrogate the effects of the systemic inflammatory response and reduce fluid requirements could benefit the management of the severely burned patient. In this selection, the authors reviewed the effects of plasma exchange on fluid volume received, urinary output, and serum markers of resuscitation efficacy and found a significant beneficial effect on all parameters (Fig 1).

The study suffers from being retrospective in nature, but the differences between groups are quite convincing. Future studies will be required to define the optimal criteria for plasma exchange and to better define the differences in patient outcomes related to this therapy.

D. W. Mozingo, MD

The Effect of Burn Center and Burn Center Volume on the Mortality of Burned Adults—An Analysis of the Data in the National Burn Repository

Light TD, Latenser BA, Kealey GP, et al (Univ of Iowa Carver College of Medicine; et al)

J Burn Care Res 30:776-782, 2009

Regional variations of care, and improved outcomes with larger volumes, have been well described in the medical and surgical literature for a variety of conditions including heart surgery, vascular surgery, and orthopedic surgery. Burn care has not been recently subjected to such an analysis. The National Burn Repository (NBR) contains de-identified patient and burn center data to allow this analysis. The NBR was queried for adult burn patients admitted for an acute thermal burn injury. A multivariable regression analysis to identify risk of death was performed incorporating patient characteristics, de-identified burn center, and burn center volume. Patient characteristics such as age, size of burn, mechanism of burn, inhalation injury, race, and sex determine mortality. There is also a statistically significant difference in death rates when individual,

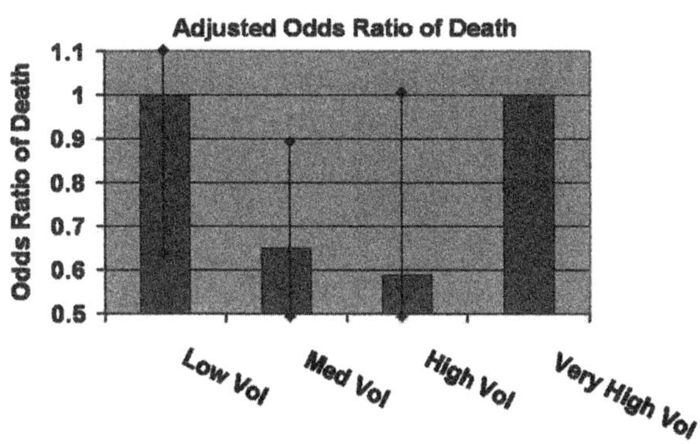

FIGURE 2.—Effect of volume on odds ratio of death when controlled for treating facility and patient characteristics ($P < .017$). Very high volume is standard of comparison for the other volume classifications. Lower is better. (Reprinted from Light TD, Latenser BA, Kealey GP, et al. The effect of burn center and burn center volume on the mortality of burned adults—an analysis of the data in the National Burn Repository. *J Burn Care Res*. 2009;30:776-782, with permission from the American Burn Association.)

de-identified centers are compared. This difference in care persists even when accounting for burn center volume. Analysis of registries like the NBR, insurance claims databases, and statewide hospital discharge databases may help identify opportunities to improve burn care. According to this analysis of data available in the NBR, burn mortality depends not only on patient characteristics but also where the patient is treated. Mortality does not linearly improve with burn center volume and plateaus with increasing burn center size. The optimal burn center size is a complicated and contentious question. Future discussions about burn center size and density should incorporate not only mortality but also the region's ability to absorb surges in volume, and the optimal "staffing" ratios for the multidisciplinary aspects of burn care (Fig 2).

▶ The authors of this selection state that increasing burn center volume does not correlate with improved survival. This finding differs from other types of surgical procedures, such as heart and transplant surgery, where a linear relationship between mortality and operative volume has been described. Although it may seem reasonable that increasing center annual patient volumes would improve outcomes such as mortality, this hypothesis was not supported across all volume categories in this study (Fig 2). Patients treated in low-volume centers had poorer outcomes. Mortality improved at the middle- and high-volume centers (100-200 and 200-300 patients per year); however, the very high-volume centers (greater than 300 burn admissions per year) had the same mortality risk as the lowest volume centers.

One possible explanation for this observation may be that the severity of such patients may not be adequately reflected in the risk-adjustment models. Also, inconsistent classification of mechanism between facilities in different volume categories may introduce bias. The data, however, continue to show the same results when this variable was eliminated from the analysis. It would be interesting to repeat this study using data from other national databases.

D. W. Mozingo, MD

The Effect of Virtual Reality on Pain and Range of Motion in Adults With Burn Injuries

Carrougher GJ, Hoffman HG, Nakamura D, et al (Univ of Washington, Seattle; Wake Forest Univ Baptist Med Ctr, Winston-Salem, NC; et al)

J Burn Care Res 30:785-791, 2009

Few studies have empirically investigated the effects of immersive virtual reality (VR) on postburn physical therapy pain control and range of motion (ROM). We performed a prospective, randomized controlled study of the effects of adding VR to standard therapy in adults receiving active-assisted ROM physical therapy, by assessing pain scores and maximal joint ROM immediately before and after therapy on two consecutive days. Thirty-nine inpatients, aged 21 to 57 years (mean 35 years), with a mean TBSA burn of 18% (range, 3–60%) were studied using a within-subject, crossover design. All patients received their regular pre-therapy pharmacologic analgesia regimen. During physical therapy sessions on two consecutive days (VR one day and no VR the other day; order randomized), each patient participated in active-assisted ROM exercises with an occupational or physical therapist. At the conclusion of each session, patients provided 0 to 100 Graphic Rating Scale measurements of pain after each 10-minute treatment condition. On the day with VR, patients wore a head-position-tracked, medical care environment-excluding VR helmet with stereophonic sound and interacted in a virtual environment conducive to burn care. ROM measurements for each joint exercised were recorded before and after each therapy session. Because of nonsignificant carryover and order effects, the data were analyzed using simple paired *t*-tests. VR reduced all Graphic Rating Scale pain scores (worst pain, time spent thinking about the pain, and pain unpleasantness by 27, 37, and 31% respectively), relative to the no VR condition. Average ROM improvement was slightly greater with the VR condition; however, this difference failed to reach clinical or statistical significance ($P = .243$). Ninety-seven percent of patients reported zero to mild nausea after the VR session. Immersive VR effectively reduced pain and did not impair ROM during postburn physical therapy. VR is easily used in the hospital setting and offers a safe, nonpharmacologic adjunctive analgesic treatment.

▶ Comprehensive rehabilitation therapy is essential for patients with severe burn injuries. Rehabilitation begins shortly after the patient's admission to the hospital and includes therapeutic positioning, splinting, use of physical agents, and therapeutic exercise. Therapeutic exercise plays a key role in the prevention of permanent impairments caused by burn scar and skin graft contractures.

Patients often experience significant procedural pain during postburn physical therapy. The pain experienced often limits the effectiveness of therapy and consequently leads to secondary complications. Since procedural pain often cannot be adequately controlled with pharmacologic agents alone, psychological techniques, such as distraction and hypnosis, have been used. Immersive virtual reality is a new form of cognitive distraction and has been found to be an effective adjunct for analgesic during postburn physical therapy. A particular contribution of this selection is that patients were able to remain in the virtual environment for longer durations of time than have been reported in earlier studies that used this modality, thus enhancing their compliance with rehabilitation therapy.

D. W. Mozingo, MD

The Incidence and Outcome of Extubation Failure in Burn Intensive Care Patients

Smailes ST, Martin RV, McVicar AJ (Broomfield Hosp, Chelmsford, Essex, UK; Anglia Ruskin Univ, Essex, UK)
J Burn Care Res 30:386-392, 2009

To identify the incidence and outcome of extubation failure in patients with burn. Retrospective cohort study in a tertiary burn intensive care unit. A review of the casenotes of 132 consecutive adult patients with burn admitted between 2001 and 2005, and requiring mechanical ventilation for >24 hours, was undertaken. Sixty-seven patients underwent extubation and entered data analyses. Extubation failure was defined as reintubation within 48 hours. The outcomes of interest were incidence and cause of extubation failure, duration of mechanical ventilation (DMV), length of stay (LOS), and mortality. The patients who succeeded and failed extubation were similar in terms of age, sex, burn size ($P = .3$), and incidence of inhalation injury ($P = .1$). Of 67 planned extubations, 20 (30%) failed. DMV (22.5 vs. 4 days; $P < .001$), intensive care LOS (1.20 vs. 0.41 days/% burn; $P < .001$), and hospital LOS (1.90 vs. 1.18 days/% burn; $P < .003$) were significantly longer in reintubated patients when compared with those who extubated successfully. Extubation outcome, burn size, and age provided the best predictive model for patient outcome ($P = .02$), but extubation outcome was the only predictor that operated individually ($P = .05$). The aetiology of extubation failure in 15 (75%) patients was poor pulmonary toilet. The incidence of extubation failure in this homogenous population of patients with burn is higher than general intensive care patients (30% vs. 4–23%). The DMV, lengths of intensive care, and hospital stay are significantly longer in patients who failed extubation. In addition to burn size and age, extubation outcome is an important predictor of intensive care mortality. The indication for reintubation in most patients is poor airway clearance (Table 3).

▶ Pulmonary dysfunction is the most common form of organ failure developing in thermally injured patients. Smoke inhalation injury increases the risk of respiratory failure and the need for prolonged mechanical ventilation. Although the

TABLE 3.—Patient Outcome

	Extubation Failure	Extubation Success	*P*
Duration of mechanical ventilation (d)	22.50 (14.50–30.25)	4.00 (2.00–9.00)	<.001
Intensive care LOS/% burn	1.20 (0.71–1.85)	0.41 (0.26–0.68)	<.001
Hospital LOS/% burn	1.90 (1.38–3.70)	1.18 (0.83–1.70)	<.003
Mortality*	3	1	.08

Data presented as median (interquartile range).
LOS, length of stay.
*Mortality is expressed as numbers of patients.

outcome of patients with smoke inhalation injury has improved significantly in recent years, prolonged need for mechanical ventilation and the determination of the optimal time to extubate mechanically ventilated patients remains a challenge. Unnecessary delay in discontinuing mechanical ventilation increases the incidence of complications such as tracheal injury and stenosis, ventilator-associated pneumonia, volutrauma and barotrauma, and the length of intensive care unit (ICU) stay. Extubation failure, and subsequent reintubation, is associated with adverse outcomes in terms of morbidity and mortality in general medical and surgical intensive care patients. It has been found to carry an 8-fold higher odds ratio for the development of nosocomial pneumonia. In addition, reintubation is a predictor of other pulmonary complications and mortality. The authors categorize extubation failure in patients with burn injury in an effort to distinguish the additional comorbidity of this occurrence (Table 3). This group of patients is difficult to study in this respect because the patients for whom the problem of reintubation often occurs are those with extensive burns and smoke inhalation injury, a population that may require mechanical ventilation for weeks to months after injury.

The weaknesses of this study are associated with its retrospective nature and the relatively small sample size. A prospective study may provide more data regarding the causes for extubation failure, and collaboration with similar units would enable the power to detect the effect of the extent of burn and age on these outcomes.

D. W. Mozingo, MD

4 Critical Care

A Central Venous Line Protocol Decreases Bloodstream Infections and Length of Stay in a Trauma Intensive Care Unit Population

Duane TM, Brown H, Borchers CT, et al (Virginia Commonwealth Univ, Richmond)

Am Surg 75:1166-1170, 2009

We evaluated the benefit of a central venous line (CVL) protocol on bloodstream infections (BSIs) and outcome in a trauma intensive care unit (ICU) population. We prospectively compared three groups: Group 1 (January 2003 to June 2004) preprotocol; Group 2 (July 2004 to June 2005) after the start of the protocol that included minimizing CVL use and strict universal precautions; and Group 3 (July 2005 to December 2006) after the addition of a line supply cart and nursing checklist. There were 1622 trauma patients admitted to the trauma ICU during the study period of whom 542 had a CVL. Group 3 had a higher Injury Severity Score (ISS) compared with both Groups 2 and 1 (28.3 ± 13.0 *vs* 23.5 ± 11.7 *vs* 22.8 ± 12.0, $P = 0.0002$) but had a lower BSI rate/1000 line days (Group 1: 16.5; Group 2: 15.0; Group 3: 7.7). Adjusting for ISS group, three had shorter ICU length of stay (LOS) compared with Group 1 (12.11 ± 1.46 *vs* 18.16 ± 1.51, $P = 0.01$). Logistic regression showed ISS ($P = 0.04$; OR, 1.025; CI, 1.001–1.050) and a lack of CVL protocol ($P = 0.01$; OR, 0.31; CI, 0.13–0.76) to be independent predictors of BSI. CVL protocols decrease both BSI and LOS in trauma

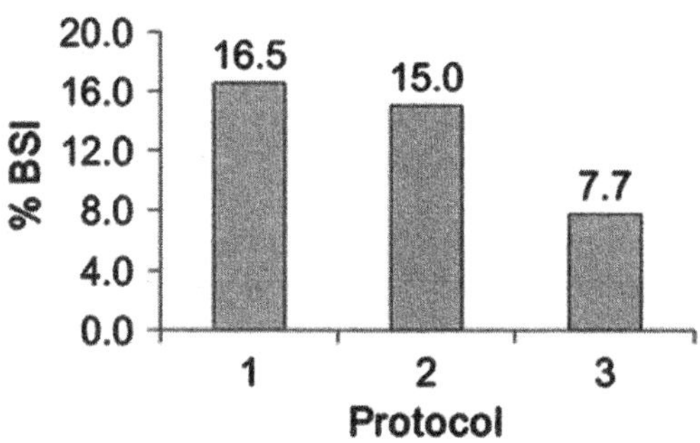

FIGURE 1.—Bloodstream infections (BSIs) per 1000 line days. (Reprinted from Duane TM, Brown H, Borchers CT, et al. A central venous line protocol decreases bloodstream infections and length of stay in a trauma intensive care unit population. *Am Surg.* 2009;75:1166-1170, with permission from Elsevier.)

patients. Strict enforcement by a nurse preserves the integrity of the protocol (Fig 1).

▶ Central venous catheterization is often required in the intensive care unit. It provides valuable access for resuscitation, administration of multiple drugs, monitoring of systemic functioning, and feeding.

Unfortunately, it has often been the source of significant morbidity and mortality. In addition to mechanical and thrombotic complications, central venous line (CVL)-related bloodstream infections (BSIs), as many as 80 000 each year, are another major adverse event. Although recent advances in the types of catheters have reduced the number of central line infections in recent years, mortality rates associated with these infections are still high. Recent changes in government reimbursement guidelines suggest elimination of payment for many hospital-acquired infections, including possibly catheter-related BSIs. The consequent escalation of uncompensated care may strain resources further. The investigators hypothesized that the use of a protocol for the insertion and management of central venous catheters in a trauma ICU would result in a decrease in infectious complications, lengths of stay, and overall charges. They demonstrated that the effectiveness of this approach continued over time (Fig 1).

D. W. Mozingo, MD

Differences in outcome between obese and nonobese patients following severe blunt trauma are not consistent with an early inflammatory genomic response

Winfield RD, Delano MJ, Dixon DJ, et al (Univ of Florida College of Medicine, Gainesville; Washington Univ in St Louis, MO; et al)
Crit Care Med 38:51-58, 2010

Objectives.—Obesity has been demonstrated to alter a number of acute and chronic medical conditions. The effect of obesity on severely injured patients, however, remains incompletely defined. We sought to unravel potential physiologic and genomic alterations induced by obesity in severely injured blunt trauma patients.

Design.—A retrospective review of clinical and genomic information contained in the Inflammation and the Host Response to Injury multicenter trauma-related database examining the relationship between body mass index and the early genomic response from peripheral blood leukocytes to patient outcome following severe blunt trauma was performed.

Setting.—Multicenter collaboration between university-based academic trauma centers.

Patients.—Severely injured blunt trauma patients enrolled in the database.

Interventions.—None.

Measurements and Main Results.—Univariate analysis of 455 severely injured trauma patients using the National Institutes of Health/World Health Organization body mass index classification system revealed significant increases in morbidity, including longer intensive care unit stays and a greater number of ventilator days, cardiac arrests, episodes of acute renal failure, and patients developing multiple organ failure. Regression modeling identified body mass index class as being independently associated with adverse outcomes and increased morbidity but an inverse relationship with mortality in patients who suffered severe blunt traumatic injury. Initial leukocyte genomic expression patterns between 163 patients in the four different body mass index groupings did not differ; however, analysis of gene differences between body mass index classes occurring over time demonstrated significant changes in 513 probe sets with significant pathway differences being related to cellular metabolism.

Conclusions.—Increasing body mass index is associated with increased morbidity following severe blunt trauma. The initial blood leukocyte inflammatory response to blunt trauma does not appear to differ significantly between patients despite increasing body mass index. Resolution of the inflammatory response may differ between patients on the basis

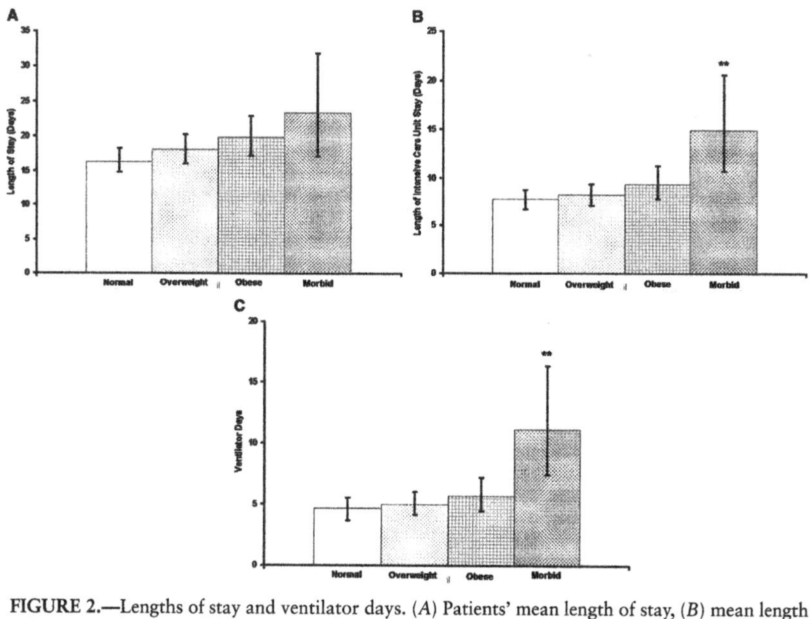

FIGURE 2.—Lengths of stay and ventilator days. (*A*) Patients' mean length of stay, (*B*) mean length of intensive care unit stay, and (*C*) mean number of ventilator days are provided for patients in each body mass index classification. Columns represent mean values, with error bars demonstrating 95% confidence intervals. **Significantly greater number of days for morbidly obese patients compared with patients classified as normal and overweight, $p < .05$. (Courtesy of Winfield RD, Delano MJ, Dixon DJ, et al. Differences in outcome between obese and nonobese patients following severe blunt trauma are not consistent with an early inflammatory genomic response. *Crit Care Med.* 2010;38:51-58.)

of body mass index; however, additional work is needed to clarify the potential causality of this finding.

▶ The relationship between increased body weight and risk for disease continues to be a major national health concern. The National Institutes of Health classifies individuals according to the body mass index to assess the risk for development of obesity-related comorbid diseases. As body mass index increases above 25, the risk of diseases such as hypertension, hyperlipidemia, diabetes mellitus, cancer, obstructive sleep apnea, pulmonary hypertension, right heart failure, fatty liver disease, osteoarthritis, and renal failure increase markedly. The authors of this study confirmed that increased body mass index was associated with the development of complications and poorer outcomes following blunt trauma (Fig 2). They could not predict this based on the initial inflammatory genomic response; however, the time-based series analysis provides insight into temporal inflammatory differences in the obese and morbidly obese trauma patients.

A new set of potential targets was identified in the areas of nutrition and metabolism on which to focus the future research.

D. W. Mozingo, MD

Early Cytokine Production Risk Stratifies Trauma Patients for Multiple Organ Failure

Jastrow KM III, Gonzalez EA, McGuire MF, et al (Univ of Texas Med School at Houston; Univ of Texas School of Health Information Sciences at Houston; et al)

J Am Coll Surg 209:320-331, 2009

Background.—Shock is a prime inciting event for postinjury multiple organ failure (MOF), believed to induce a state of injurious systemic inflammation. In animal models of hemorrhagic shock, early (<24 hours) changes in cytokine production are an index of the systemic inflammatory response syndrome. However, their predictive value in trauma patients remains to be fully elucidated.

Study Design.—In a prospective observational pilot study of > 1 year at an urban Level I trauma center, serial (every 4 hours) serum cytokine levels were determined during a 24-hour period using multiplex suspension immunoassay in patients with major torso trauma (excluding severe brain injury) who met criteria for standardized shock resuscitation. Temporal cytokine expression was assessed during shock resuscitation in severe trauma patients to predict risk for MOF. MOF was assessed with the Denver score.

Results.—Of 48 study patients (mean age 39 ± 3 years, 67% men, 88% blunt mechanism, mean Injury Severity Score 25 ± 2), MOF developed in 11 (23%). MOF patients had a considerably higher mortality (64% versus 3%) and fewer ICU-free days (3.5 ± 2 versus 17.8 ± 1.3 days) compared with non-MOF patients. Traditional predictors of MOF, including age (45 ± 7 versus 38 ± 3 years; $p = 0.21$), Injury Severity Score (26 ± 3 versus 25 ± 2; $p = 0.67$), admission hemoglobin (11.4 ± 0.9 versus 12.1 ± 0.5 g/dL; $p = 0.22$), international normalized ratio (1.6 ± 0.2 versus 1.4 ± 0.06; $p = 0.17$), and base deficit (9.0 ± 2 versus 7.1 ± 0.8; $p = 0.19$), were not significantly different between MOF and non-MOF patients. Statistical analysis identified six candidate predictors of MOF: inducible protein 10, macrophage inflammatory protein-1β, interleukin-10, interleukin-6, interleukin-1Ra, and eotaxin.

Conclusions.—These data provide insight into cytokine expression during traumatic shock that can enable earlier identification of patients at risk for development of MOF.

▶ There are many unanswered questions about acute organ failure syndromes and the pathophysiology that drives organ dysfunction in the setting of major trauma. Evidence is accumulating that suggests cytokines are implicated in the pathogenesis of critical illness.

In this prospective study, 48 critically injured trauma patients received standardized resuscitation and treatment protocols, and a battery of cytokine measurements were made at timed intervals throughout their hospital course.

MOF developed in 11 patients and was associated with a 64% mortality rate. Differences in cytokine concentrations between multiple organ failure and non-multiple organ failure patients were detectable as early as 4 to 8 hours after injury and statistical analysis identified 6 candidate cytokines, which might permit earlier identification of patients at risk for developing multiple organ failure. Early prediction of multiple organ failure risk may enable alternate treatment strategies to be used in these critically ill patients.

D. W. Mozingo, MD

Early Packed Red Blood Cell Transfusion and Acute Respiratory Distress Syndrome after Trauma

Chaiwat O, Lang JD, Vavilala MS, et al (Univ of Washington School of Medicine, Seattle; et al)

Anesthesiology 110:351-360, 2009

Background.—Transfusion of packed red blood cells (PRBCs) is a risk factor for acute respiratory distress syndrome (ARDS) in trauma patients. Yet, there is a paucity of information regarding the risk of ARDS with incremental PRBCs exposure.

Methods.—For this retrospective analysis, eligible patients from National Study on Costs and Outcomes of Trauma were included. Our main exposure was defined as units of PRBCs transfused during the first 24 h after admission. The main outcome was ARDS.

Results.—A total of 521 (4.6%) of 14070 patients developed ARDS, and 331 patients (63.5%) who developed ARDS received PRBCs

TABLE 4.—Effect of the Amount of Transfused PRBCs on ARDS and In-hospital Mortality Adjusted for Significant Confounders

	ARDS, aOR (95% CI)	In-hospital Death, aOR (95% CI)
PRBC units		
1–5	1.88 (0.77–4.62)	1.13 (0.64–2.02)
6–10	2.48 (1.17–5.26)*	1.52 (0.82–2.83)
> 10	2.62 (1.08–6.37)*	0.93 (0.27–3.17)

aOR = adjusted odds ratio; ARDS = acute respiratory distress syndrome; PRBC = packed red blood cell.
*$P < 0.05$; Referent group = 0 PRBC units.

transfusion. Injury severity, thoracic injury, polytrauma, and pneumonia receiving more than 5 units of fresh frozen plasma and 6–10 units of PRBCs were independent predictors of ARDS. Patients receiving more than 5 units of PRBCs had higher risk of developing ARDS (patients who received 6–10 units: adjusted odds ratio 2.5, 95% CI 1.12–5.3; patients who received more than 10 units: odds ratio 2.6, 95% CI 1.1–6.4). Each additional unit of PRBCs transfused conferred a 6% higher risk of ARDS (adjusted odds ratio 1.06; 95% CI 1.03–1.10).

Conclusions.—Early transfusion of PRBCs is an independent predictor of ARDS in adult trauma patients. Conservative transfusion strategies that decrease PRBC exposure by even 1 unit may be warranted to reduce the risk of ARDS in injured patients (Table 4).

▶ Research over the past decade has demonstrated that allogeneic blood transfusion is associated with immunomodulatory effects that are implicated in the development of acute respiratory distress syndrome (ARDS) in trauma patients. Alterations in immunomodulation and proinflammatory mediators are considered the culprits.

Transfusion of packed red blood cells (PRBCs), platelets, and fresh-frozen plasma are all associated with the development of ARDS in trauma patients; however, transfusion of more than 10 units of PRBCs has been identified as a major risk factor for ARDS in trauma patients.

It is still unknown how much of the relationship between blood transfusion and ARDS is a result of the transfusion itself or the result of other confounders, such as injury severity, chest trauma, shock, pneumonia, and long bone fractures. Most previous studies investigating these questions are single center and are statistically underpowered to definitively answer this question. Using the National Study on Cost and Outcomes of Trauma database, the authors of this selection examined the relationship between volume of early PRBC transfusion and ARDS in a sample of over 14 000 trauma patients (Table 4). The investigators determined that each unit of PRBCs transfused increases the risk of ARDS by 6%. This speaks for conservative PRBC transfusion strategies early after trauma and the need for this to be considered in early goal-directed therapy protocols.

D. W. Mozingo, MD

Is the evolving management of intra-abdominal hypertension and abdominal compartment syndrome improving survival?

Cheatham ML, Safcsak K (Orlando Regional Med Ctr, FL)

Crit Care Med 38:402-407, 2010

Objective.—The diagnosis and management of intra-abdominal hypertension and abdominal compartment syndrome have changed significantly over the past decade with improved understanding of the pathophysiology and appropriate treatment of these disease processes. Serial intra-abdominal pressure measurements, nonoperative pressure-reducing interventions, and early abdominal decompression for refractory intra-abdominal hypertension or abdominal compartment syndrome are all key elements of this evolving strategy.

Design.—Prospective, observational study.

Setting.—Tertiary referral/level I trauma center.

Patients.—Four hundred seventy-eight consecutive patients requiring an open abdomen for the management of intra-abdominal hypertension or abdominal compartment syndrome.

Interventions.—Patients were managed by a defined group of surgical intensivists using established definitions and an evidence-based management algorithm. Both univariate and multivariate analyses were performed to identify patient and management factors associated with improved survival.

Measurements and Main Results.—Whereas patient demographics and severity of illness remained unchanged over the 6-yr study period, the use of a continually revised intra-abdominal hypertension/abdominal

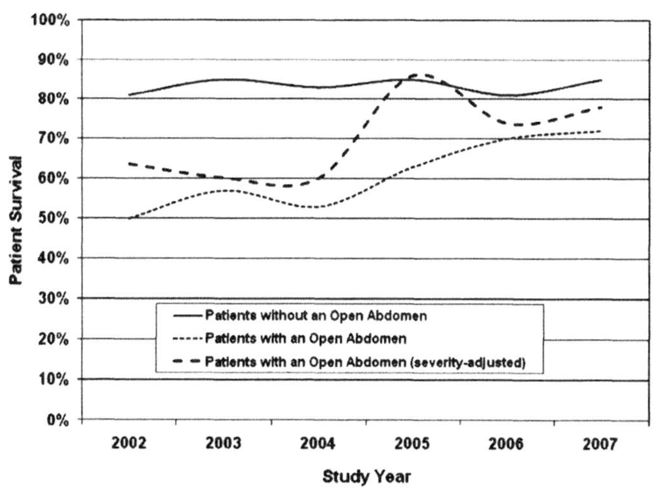

FIGURE 1.—Severity-adjusted patient survival. (Courtesy of Cheatham ML, Safcsak K. Is the evolving management of intra-abdominal hypertension and abdominal compartment syndrome improving survival? *Crit Care Med.* 2010;38:402-407.)

compartment syndrome management algorithm significantly increased patient survival to hospital discharge from 50% to 72% ($p = .015$). Clinically significant decreases in resource utilization and an increase in same-admission primary fascial closure from 59% to 81% were recognized. Development of abdominal compartment syndrome, prophylactic use of an open abdomen to prevent development of intra-abdominal hypertension/abdominal compartment syndrome, and use of a multi-modality surgical/medical management algorithm were identified as independent predictors of survival.

Conclusions.—A comprehensive evidence-based management strategy that includes early use of an open abdomen in patients at risk significantly improves survival from intra-abdominal hypertension/abdominal compartment syndrome. This improvement is not achieved at the cost of increased resource utilization and is associated with an increased rate of primary fascial closure.

▶ The diagnosis and treatment of critically ill patients with intra-abdominal hypertension (IAH) and abdominal compartment syndrome (ACS) have changed significantly over the past 10 years with improved understanding of the pathophysiology and timely and appropriate treatment of these conditions. Serial intra-abdominal pressure (IAP) measurements, nonoperative pressure-reducing interventions, and early abdominal decompression in refractory cases are all important components of this evolving experience. In this selection, the authors explain the evolution of the concepts of IAH and correlate their improving survival over the past 10 years with refinements in diagnosis and technique. Fig 1 depicts these improvements.

The study does have several limitations: Most of the patients did not have IAP measurements recorded before the management of IAH was initiated. Nevertheless, postdecompression IAP measurements in the intensive care unit remain an important part of the algorithm for guiding resuscitation and preventing organ dysfunction attributable to IAH/ACS. Another limitation of the study is that it does not directly include IAH/ACS patients who did not require abdominal decompression.

D. W. Mozingo, MD

Local and Systemic Consequences of Large Retroperitoneal Clot Burdens

Loor G, Bassiouny H, Valentin C, et al (Univ of Chicago, IL; The Univ of Chicago Hosps, IL)

World J Surg 33:1618-1625, 2009

Background.—There is a paucity of data regarding the impact of retroperitoneal hematoma (RPH) volumes, as detected by computed tomography (CT) scanning, on patient morbidity and mortality. Therefore, we wanted to determine the natural history of RPHs and the effect of size on local and systemic outcomes.

Methods.—We performed a volumetric analysis of CT-documented RPHs managed at our institution between 1985 and 2006 along with a retrospective chart review.

Results.—We included 81 cases of RPH in this study. The mean Acute Physiology, Age, and Chronic Health Evaluation II (APACHE II) score was 12.8 ± 0.72 (score ± SE). By univariate analysis, the size of the hematoma showed a significant correlation with the development of local mass effects, delayed mass effects, 6-month mortality, major morbidity, pulmonary complications, fluid overload, and the requirement for operative evacuation ($p < 0.05$). Receiver operating characteristic analysis revealed that a size ≥1600 cm^3 was >80% sensitive and specific for predicting a delayed mass effect or an increase in 6-month mortality. Multivariate analysis controlling for factors such as APACHE II and packed red blood cells transfused showed that the volume of the RPH was an

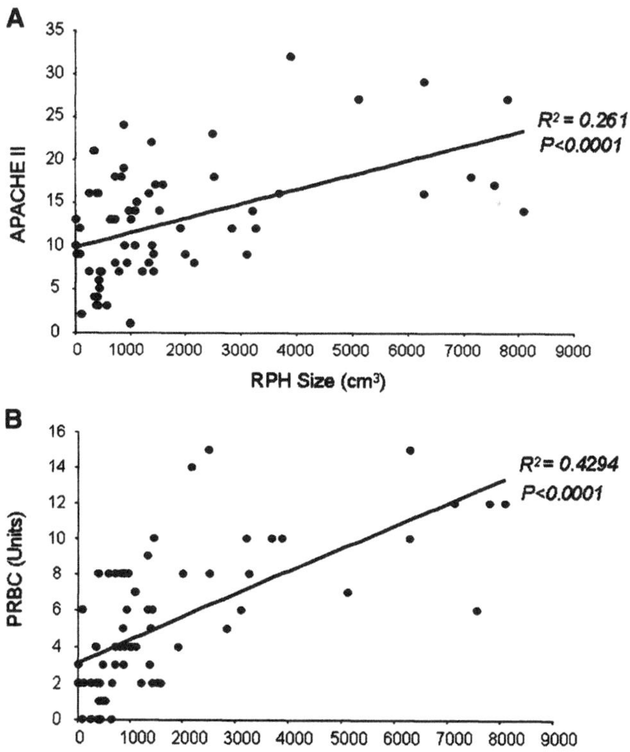

FIGURE 4.—A, Relation between the size of the RPH and the Acute Physiology, Age, and Chronic Health Evaluation II (*APACHE II*) score. B, Relation between size and packed red blood cell (*PRBC*) units transfused. (With kind permission from Springer+Business Media: Loor G, Bassiouny H, Valentin C, et al. Local and systemic consequences of large retroperitoneal clot burdens. *World J Surg.* 2009;33:1618-1625.)

independent predictor for the development of local mass effects, pulmonary insufficiency, and fluid overload.

Conclusions.—Large RPHs are clearly associated with worse patient outcomes. Surgical intervention may be warranted for the treatment of RPHs $\geq$1600 cm^3.

▶ Retroperitoneal hematomas develop spontaneously or as a result of iatrogenic or traumatic causes. These hematomas have been associated with significant morbidity and mortality. General surgeons and vascular surgeons are often consulted to evaluate patients who have developed a retroperitoneal hematoma. Since anticoagulation and endovascular therapies are now commonplace, it is probable that the occurrence of this complication will increase. Although many retroperitoneal hematomas are self-limited and can be treated conservatively, they may also lead to considerable morbidity and systemic manifestations. Reported complications include abscess formation, ileus, and persistent lower abdominal pain and femoral neuropathy. The size of the hematoma may play an important role in determining the development of a mass-associated complication due to the unyielding nature of the retroperitoneal space. Surgical decompression is primarily reserved for cases where such a mass effect has occurred. It is not clear whether there is a benefit from evacuating the hematoma in all cases.

This selection reviews a single institution's experience with retroperitoneal hematomas. It has not been previously determined whether there is a specific hematoma size that dictates intervention. Traditionally, stable and asymptomatic hematomas are managed conservatively, and only a small number of patients undergo operative decompression.

The magnitude of the clot burden was shown to have a major impact on local and systemic outcomes (Fig 4). Patients with hematomas greater than 1600 cm^3 are more likely to develop significant morbidity and mortality. Based on these data, it is possible that evacuating large hematomas may prevent adverse outcomes; however, a prospective study of matched hematomas greater than 1600 cm^3 may be required to show a beneficial effect of surgical evacuation on the outcome.

D. W. Mozingo, MD

Methicillin-Resistant Staphylococcus Aureus in a Surgical Intensive Care Unit

Recinos G, Inaba K, Dubose J, et al (Univ of Southern California Med Ctr, Los Angeles; Wilford Hall Med Ctr, LAFB, TX)
Am Surg 75:1077-1080, 2009

The rate of methicillin-resistant *Staphylococcus aureus* (MRSA) infections has increased significantly over the last years, especially from community-associated MRSA (CA-MRSA) sources. The true prevalence of these multidrug-resistant infections among the trauma patient

TABLE 2.—Outcomes for Patients with MRSA Infection

Outcomes	Patients with MRSA (n = 36)	HA-MRSA (n = 23)	CA-MRSA (n = 13)	P value
Death (%)	11.1% (4/36)	8.7% (2/23)	15.4% (2/13)	0.540
ICU LOS (days), mean ± SD	20.4 ± 14.6	22.9 ± 15.5	18.0 ± 13.9	0.229
HLOS (days), mean ± SD	34.9 ± 41.2	42.7 ± 47.1	25.3 ± 31.1	0.037
HLOS after infection (days), mean ± SD	34.9 ± 41.3	34.3 ± 40.3	15.2 ± 6.4	0.552
Ventilation days, mean ± SD	14.9 ± 16.4	18.0 ± 19.8	9.8 ± 6.4	0.271
Total charges ($), mean ± SD	310,110 ± 305,696	364,231 ± 323,719	242,458 ± 276,630	0.091

The *P* values for categorical variables were derived from χ^2 test or Fisher's exact test; *P* values for continuous variables were derived from Student's *t* test or Mann Whitney test.
SD, standard deviation; ICU LOS, Intensive Care Unit Length of Stay.

population, however, is not well defined. A retrospective review of our surgical intensive care unit (SICU) database from April 2003 to April 2007 was performed to identify all trauma patients surviving 48 hours or more that had a positive culture result during their SICU stay. The results of the cultures were examined. A total of 582 SICU patients with 2,860 cultures were assessed for MRSA infection. Among these, 368 cultures (12.9%) in 36 patients were reported as MRSA positive. Thirteen of these patients fulfilled the criteria for a CA-MRSA infection. When outcomes were analyzed, no significant difference in mortality (8.7% *vs* 15.4%, $P = 0.540$) or hospital related charges ($364,231 ± 323,719 *vs* $242,458 ± 276,630, $P = 0.091$) was noted. Patients with a hospital-acquired MRSA infection, however, had longer hospital lengths of stay (42.7 ± 47.1 *vs* 25.3 ± 31.1, $P = 0.037$) than their community-associated counterparts. MRSA constitutes an important source of infection among critically ill trauma patients. CA-MRSA organisms may play an increasing pathogenic role in this population (Table 2).

▶ Infectious complications remain a significant cause of morbidity and mortality among patients admitted to hospitals, particularly among those who are critically ill. Increasing rates of infection caused by resistant gram-positive organisms, mostly methicillin-resistant *Staphylococcus aureus* (MRSA), represent an ongoing concern in the intensive care unit (ICU) setting. MRSA was once characteristically considered a hospital-acquired source of infection, but community-acquired MRSA is emerging as an additional source of these drug-resistant organisms.

Some have suggested that trauma patients may be at an increased risk for the development of MRSA-related infections from community-acquired sources. Although the impact of community-acquired MRSA infection on morbidity and mortality following trauma is not well known, it is likely that the burden of a multidrug-resistant infection places trauma patients at a higher risk for adverse outcomes.

The objective of this retrospective review was to determine the prevalence of hospital-associated MRSA and community-acquired MRSA among a population of critically ill trauma patients. The authors also sought to identify the potential impact of community-acquired MRSA on patient outcomes after trauma. The differences in outcomes attributed to the source of MRSA are reviewed in Table 2, included in this selection. The study was retrospective in nature and not powered sufficiently to identify differences in mortality between groups. A larger, perhaps multi-institutional, prospective data collection is indicated.

D. W. Mozingo, MD

Personalized Medicine: Genetic Variation and Loss of Physiologic Complexity Are Associated With Mortality in 644 Trauma Patients

Norris PR, Canter JA, Jenkins JM, et al (Vanderbilt Univ, Nashville, TN; et al)
Ann Surg 250:524-530, 2009

Objective.—Personalized medicine merges genetics, physiology, and patient outcome. Loss of physiologic complexity (heart rate [HR] variability) is a bedside biomarker for autonomic nervous system (ANS) dysfunction. We hypothesized that variability in ANS receptor proteins (genetics) and loss of complexity (physiology) are independently associated with mortality in critical illness.

Summary Background Data.—Decreased HR complexity has been associated with increased mortality and morbidity in trauma and other critically ill populations. Genetic variations in alpha-1A and beta-2 adrenergic receptors (ADRA1A, ADRB2) have been associated with changes in smooth muscle tone in various tissues, and implicated in bronchial hyper-responsiveness, metabolic syndrome, and other disorders.

Methods.—A cohort of 644 trauma intensive care unit (ICU) admissions had complexity data and genetic samples. Two ANS receptor polymorphisms (rs1048101, Alpha ADRA1A and rs1042714, Beta ADRB2) were genotyped. Physiologic complexity at various points in the ICU stay was measured using previously-studied integer HR multiscale entropy (MSE) over 6-hour intervals (~21,600 HR data points/interval/patient). Logistic regression assessed the concurrent relationship of genotypes, complexity, and probability of survival, an acuity score incorporating age, injury mechanism/severity, and admission vitals, to risk of death.

Results.—Of total, 96 patients (15%) died. Nonsurvivors had lower complexity at early, middle, and late portions of ICU stay (median MSE at least 25% less in nonsurvivors, $P < 0.001$) and lower incidence of the GG ADRB2 genotype (7.5% vs. 18.3%, $P < 0.001$). In multivariable logistic regression, the GG ADRB2 genotype carried ~3-fold decrease in mortality odds (odd ratio [OR] = 0.33, $P = 0.01$), independent of significant effects in HR MSE (OR = 0.93, $P < 0.001$), and probability of survival (OR = 0.22, $P < 0.001$).

Conclusions.—This first study to simultaneously examine ANS genetics, the biomarker complexity, and mortality concludes: (1) ANS genetics and physiologic complexity are independently related to mortality;

(2) Genetics and complexity add information over traditional acuity scoring (probability of survival); and (3) Simultaneous assessment of ANS physiology and genetics may yield novel research, diagnostic, and therapeutic opportunities in critical illness.

▶ This study is the first to report genetic and physiologic indicators related to the autonomic nervous system in a large population of critically ill patients. The authors also were able to define how these factors simultaneously contribute to the risk of death. The single nucleotide polymorphisms coding for adrenergic receptors α_{1A} and β_2 were examined together with heart rate complexity measurements. This group of researchers has previously reported associations of these genotypes and early heart rate complexity with trauma patient risk. In this study, the authors expanded the duration of heart rate complexity measurements beyond the first 24 hours to include time periods throughout the intensive care unit stay. They hypothesized that adrenergic receptor genotypes and heart rate complexity would provide independent information regarding acuity-adjusted risk of mortality.

This type of work is just beginning to define important and previously unrecognized variation in genetic and physiological variables. The scope of how this will affect future monitoring, diagnostic, and prognostic capabilities is unknown, but the possibilities are intriguing.

D. W. Mozingo, MD

Pulmonary Embolism After Injury: More Common Than We Think?

Menaker J, Stein DM, Scalea TM (Univ of Maryland Med Ctr, Baltimore)

J Trauma 67:1244-1249, 2009

Background.—We have previously demonstrated that pulmonary embolism (PE) can occur early and explain hypoxia immediately after injury. We hypothesized that an increased awareness of early PE would result in an increased incidence, an earlier diagnosis, and a decreased mortality of PE after injury.

Methods.—The trauma registry identified patients diagnosed with a PE between time period (TP) 1 (June 1999 and December 2004) and TP 2 (January 2005 and December 2006). Demographics, injury specific data, time from injury to diagnosis, diagnostic modality, and mortality were compared with a *t* test for the two TPs.

Results.—There were 35,424 and 15,022 patients, respectively, treated in our trauma center during the two study periods. During TP1, 94 (0.27%) patients were diagnosed with PE. Mean age was 45 years (±18.5) and mean Injury Severity Score (ISS) was 23 (±11.4); 81.9% were men and 91.6% sustained blunt trauma. Eighty-three (0.55%) patients in TP2 were identified with a PE. Mean age was 43 years (±17.4) and mean ISS was 23 (±13.0); 78.3% were men and 86.7% sustained blunt trauma. In TP1, the diagnosis was confirmed by a computed

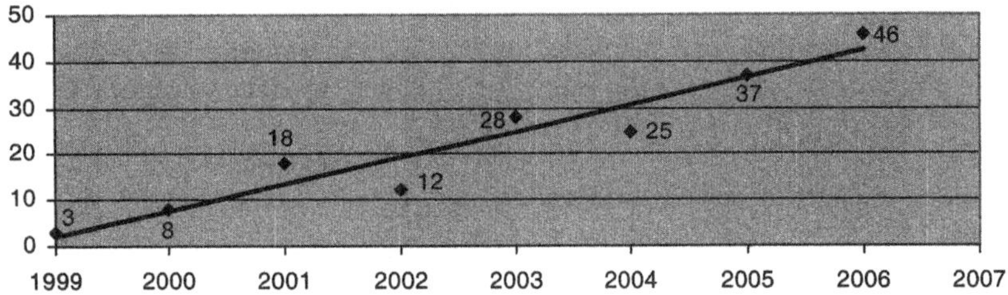

FIGURE 5.—Pulmonary embolism trend over 6 years. (Courtesy of Menaker J, Stein DM, Scalea TM. Pulmonary embolism after injury: more common than we think? *J Trauma.* 2009;67:1244-1249.)

tomography (CT) in 76 of 94 (80.9%) patients. In TP2, the CT scan diagnosed 80 of 83 (96.4%) patients. Time to diagnosis was postinjury day 11.8 (±14) in TP1 and 9.2 (±11.5) in TP2. Mortality in patients diagnosed with PE was 10.6% in TP1 and 9.6% in TP2.

Conclusion.—Our incidence of PE has doubled from 0.27% to 0.55% in a 6-year TP when mean ISS and thromboembolic prophylaxis protocols have remained the same. We attribute this increase in incidence to heightened awareness through recent publications, as well as 24 hour availability of multiple multidetector-row spiral CT scanners and not necessarily an increase in prevalence of PE.

▶ Pulmonary embolism (PE) continues to be a known complication after trauma. Although previously thought to have a low incidence after trauma, this may no longer be the case.

This retrospective review performed at the R Adams Cowley Shock Trauma Center demonstrates that the incidence of PE has doubled from 0.27% to 0.55% in a 6-year time period when mean injury severity and thromboembolic prophylaxis protocols have not changed (Fig 5). Heightened clinical awareness is needed with this, and other recent publications demonstrate that PE may be underdiagnosed in trauma patients. Probably all diagnosed pulmonary emboli warrant treatment; however, the clinical significance and the need for definitive treatment of peripheral and small clots are unknown, and further research is needed.

D. W. Mozingo, MD

The relationship between nutritional intake and clinical outcomes in critically ill patients: results of an international multicenter observational study

Alberda C, Gramlich L, Jones N, et al (Alberta Health Services Edmonton, Canada; Kingston General Hosp, Ontario, Canada)
Intensive Care Med 35:1728-1737, 2009

Purpose.—The objective of this study was to examine the relationship between the amount of energy and protein administered and clinical outcomes, and the extent to which pre-morbid nutritional status influenced this relationship.

Methods.—We conducted an observational cohort study of nutrition practices in 167 intensive care units (ICUs) across 37 countries. Patient demographics were collected, and the type and amount of nutrition received were recorded daily for a maximum of 12 days. Patients were followed prospectively to determine 60-day mortality and ventilator-free days (VFDs). We used body mass index (BMI, kg/m^2) as a marker of nutritional status prior to ICU admission. Regression models were developed to evaluate the relationship between nutrition received and 60-day mortality and VFDs, and to examine how BMI modifies this relationship.

Results.—Data were collected on 2,772 mechanically ventilated patients who received an average of 1,034 kcal/day and 47 g protein/day. An increase of 1,000 cal per day was associated with reduced mortality [odds ratio for 60-day mortality 0.76; 95% confidence intervals (CI) 0.61–0.95, $p = 0.014$] and an increased number of VFDs (3.5 VFD, 95% CI 1.2–5.9, $p = 0.003$). The effect of increased calories associated with lower mortality was observed in patients with a BMI <25 and ≥35 with no benefit for patients with a BMI 25 to <35. Similar results were observed when comparing increasing protein intake and its effect on mortality.

Conclusions.—Increased intakes of energy and protein appear to be associated with improved clinical outcomes in critically ill patients, particularly when BMI is <25 or ≥35.

▶ The optimal amount of calories and protein required by critically ill patients to reduce morbidity and mortality remains controversial. In some observational studies, a cumulative energy deficit or caloric debt is associated with adverse clinical outcomes in critically ill patients, while another observational study suggests that feeding fewer-than-goal calories, between 33% and 66% of estimated energy needs, resulted in improved clinical outcomes compared with patients who received closer to 100% of goal intake. This study identified that pre-illness body weight and nutritional status were major determinants of the outcome, and that those patients with a relatively low body mass index (BMI) seemed to benefit the most from aggressive nutritional intervention.

Randomized trials where delivery of goal calories is optimized in critically ill patients at the extremes of BMI are necessary to test this further. Future randomized trials need to consider the pre-intensive care unit (ICU) nutritional status in their design.

D. W. Mozingo, MD

Transfusion and Pneumonia in the Trauma Intensive Care Unit: An Examination of the Temporal Relationship

Vandromme MJ, McGwin G Jr, Marques MB, et al (Univ of Alabama at Birmingham)

J Trauma 67:97-101, 2009

Background.—Transfusion has been demonstrated to be associated with pneumonia in injured patients, and blood of older storage age may potentiate this morbidity. It remains unclear, however, whether this association is causal, as prior studies have not accounted for prepneumonia versus postpneumonia transfusion. We sought to evaluate the temporal relationship between transfusion and pneumonia and the influence of blood age on this relationship.

Methods.—Admissions to a Level I trauma center between July 2004 and October 2007 with the following characteristics were selected for inclusion: overall length of stay of ≥4 days; intensive care unit length of stay of ≥1 day; and ≥1 ventilator days. Date(s) of transfusion and blood storage age defined as "old" ≥14 days and "young" <14 days were obtained. Pneumonia was diagnosed by bronchoalveolar lavage ($>10^5$ colonies/mL). Risk ratios (RR) and 95% confidence intervals (CIs) were calculated for the association between pneumonia and both date (in relation to pneumonia) and age of blood transfused, adjusted for age, gender, injury severity, mechanism of injury, ventilator days, and transfusion volume.

Results.—A total of 1,615 patients met study criteria. Adjusted RR (CI) for the association between pneumonia and receipt of blood at any time was 1.99 (1.39–2.86). However, when postpneumonia transfusions were disregarded, no association was observed (RR 1.33; CI 0.98–1.80). Analysis by blood age, however, demonstrated that prepneumonia transfusion of exclusively older blood was significantly associated with an increased risk of pneumoinia (adjusted RR 1.42; CI 1.01–2.02), whereas transfusion of exclusively younger units (adjusted RR 1.02; CI 0.62–1.67) or mixed units (adjusted RR 1.35; CI 0.98–1.87) were not.

Conclusions.—Prior reports of an association between transfusion and pneumonia may reflect transfusions received after pneumonia rather than etiologically relevant transfusions received before the onset of pneumonia. Transfusion of exclusively older blood, however, increased the risk of pneumonia, further suggesting the importance of blood age with respect to outcomes in trauma patients.

▶ Ventilator-associated pneumonia is a nosocomial infection associated with increased morbidity and mortality and is encountered in trauma patients with considerable frequency.

The Centers for Disease Control and Prevention report a median incidence of 11.4 cases of ventilator-associated pneumonia per thousand ventilator days observed in trauma intensive care units compared with a median incidence of 3.7 cases per thousand ventilator days observed in medical intensive care units.

Previous reports have speculated a causal relationship between transfusion and pneumonia. This conclusion may be erroneous, reflecting transfusions received as a consequence of pneumonia and critical illness rather than relevant transfusions received before the onset of pneumonia.

After accounting for the temporal relationship between transfusion and pneumonia, the authors of this selection concluded that stratification of patients according to transfusion storage age demonstrated increased risk of pneumonia on receipt of old blood, whereas the transfusion of young blood and mixed units did not.

This result draws further attention to the potential consequences of transfusing relatively older blood to injured patients.

Prospective validation of the deleterious effects of transfusion of older blood is warranted before consideration of any changes in blood banking practice.

D. W. Mozingo, MD

Transfusion of Aged Packed Red Blood Cells Results in Decreased Tissue Oxygenation in Critically Injured Trauma Patients

Kiraly LN, Underwood S, Differding JA, et al (Oregon Health and Science Univ, Portland)

J Trauma 67:29-32, 2009

Background.—Blood transfusion is a common event in the treatment of injured patients. The effect of red blood cell transfusion on tissue oxygenation is unclear. The transfusion of older blood has been shown to be detrimental in retrospective studies. This study aims to study the effect of the age of the blood transfused on the tissue oxygenation using near infrared spectroscopy.

Methods.—Thirty-two critically injured trauma patients for whom a blood transfusion had been ordered were recruited. Each patient had a transcutaneous probe placed on the thenar eminence. The probe was placed 1 hour before the transfusion and left in place until 4 hours after transfusion. Tissue oxygen saturation (Sto_2) was recorded every 2 minutes. The Sto_2 area under the curve (AUC) over time periods was calculated. A control group ($n = 16$), not transfused, was recruited. The transfusion group was divided into two groups by blood age. One group received blood less than 21 days old, (new blood, $n = 15$) and the other received blood 21 days old or greater (old blood, $n = 17$). The data were analyzed for significance with Kendall's W and Wilcoxon's signed rank test ($p < 0.05$).

Results.—Baseline characteristics were not significantly different between groups. The baseline AUC did not differ between groups. The old blood group demonstrated a significant decline in Sto_2 comparing its baseline period to its transfusion period ($p < 0.05$). There was no similar decline in the control group or the new blood group. The posttransfusion period AUC for the old blood group was also lower versus baseline

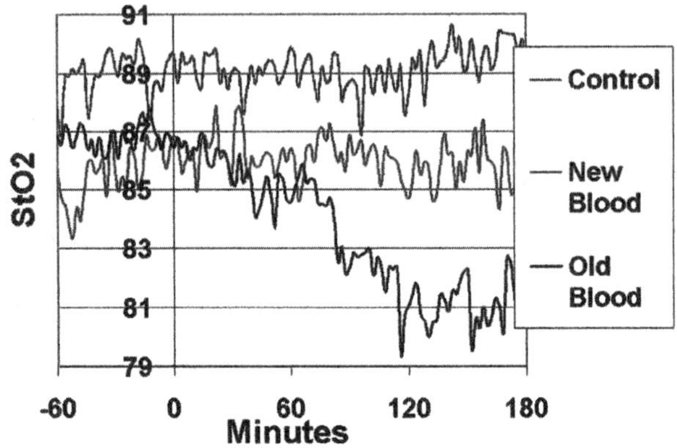

FIGURE 2.—Tissue oxygenation versus time. Time 0 is defined as the start of transfusion. (Courtesy of Kiraly LN, Underwood S, Differding JA, et al. Transfusion of aged packed red blood cells results in decreased tissue oxygenation in critically injured trauma patients. *J Trauma*. 2009;67:29-32.)

($p = 0.06$). There was a moderate correlation between increasing age of blood and decrease in oxygenation ($r = 0.5$).

Conclusions.—There was a decrease in peripheral tissue oxygenation in patients receiving older red blood cells. There was no oxygenation decrease in patients receiving blood less than 21 days. This indicates that factors in stored blood may influence the peripheral vasculature and oxygen delivery.

▶ This selection was chosen, as it clearly demonstrated a decrease in tissue oxygenation associated with the transfusion of red blood cells more than 21 days old (Fig 2). This decrease was measured as a trend even after the blood transfusion had been completed. This finding is in distinct contrast to the true goals of red blood cell transfusion.

This study does have several limitations. The number of patients in each group is relatively small. Additional observations with larger numbers will be necessary to confirm the findings of this study. These results show that the transfusion of older red blood cells fails to produce the desired effects on tissue oxygenation and may actually be harmful. Further study is warranted to investigate the mechanism that produces this effect and the negative outcomes that have been reported.

D. W. Mozingo, MD

Protein C depletion early after trauma increases the risk of ventilator-associated pneumonia

Cohen MJ, Bir N, Rahn P, et al (Univ of California, San Francisco)
J Trauma 67:1176-1181, 2009

Introduction.—Mechanically ventilated trauma patients have a high risk for the development of ventilator-associated pneumonia (VAP). We have recently reported that reduced plasma protein C (PC) levels early after trauma/shock are associated with coagulopathy and mortality. Furthermore, trauma patients with tissue injury and shock are at higher risk for the development of VAP.

Objective.—We hypothesized that low PC levels early after trauma are associated with an increased susceptibility to VAP in trauma patients.

Methods.—Fifty-nine acutely injured, intubated trauma patients were admitted to the critical care unit. Serial blood samples were drawn and coagulation factors were measured. VAP was diagnosed by presence of bacteria on bronchial alveolar lavage specimen, bilateral infiltrates on chest roentgenogram, and fever or elevated white blood cell count.

Results.—There were no differences in demographic or injury characteristics between patients who developed VAP and those who did not. As expected, patients who developed VAP had more ventilator days, hospital days, intensive care unit days, and greater mortality (all $p < 0.05$). Patients in both groups had lower mean PC levels at 6 hours compared with baseline. Noninfected patients' PC subsequently returned to near baseline levels, whereas those patients who eventually acquired VAP had significantly lower PC levels at both 12 and 24 hours (12 hours: 79 vs. 96%, $p = 0.05$; 24 hours: 75 vs. 97% $p = 0.02$). Soluble endothelial PC receptor (sEPCR) levels were also lower at 24 hours (82 vs. 99% in the noninfected group, $p = 0.04$).

Discussion.—The activation of PC pathway early after trauma may protect the vascular endothelium by both its anticoagulant and cytoprotective effects. However, trauma patients who later developed VAP have significantly lower plasma levels of PC within 24 hours after injury, suggesting a possible consumption of this vitamin K-dependent protein and an inhibition of its activation by inflammatory mediators. EPCR is involved in the activation of PC and is also a mediator of its cytoprotective effects.

Conclusion.—Critically ill trauma patients have an early activation of the PC pathway, associated with a rapid decrease in the plasma levels of this protein and increase in EPCR. Plasma levels of PC return to normal levels within 24 hours in most patients. However, patients who go on to acquire VAP have persistently low plasma levels of PC in the immediate period after trauma. Whether PC could play a mechanistic role in the host response against nosocomial lung infection warrants further study.

► Ventilator-associated pneumonia is the most common nosocomial infection in trauma patients and is associated with an increase in ventilator days, intensive care unit and hospital stay, other infectious complications, and mortality. This selection presents evidence of a relationship between protein C depletion early after trauma and the later development of ventilator-associated pneumonia (Fig 2 in the original article). This has been described in nontrauma sepsis patient populations; however, this study provides the first data indicating that there is a depletion of protein C that begins early after trauma and that this depletion is associated with the later development of ventilator-associated pneumonia. This same research group has previously shown that there is a profound activation of protein C that occurs immediately after trauma and shock in severely injured patients. Protein C is a serine protease that is activated through a thrombin dependent reaction with thrombomodulin and the endothelial protein C receptor. Once activated, activated protein C binds irreversibly to and deactivates factors Va and VIIIa. The importance of the anticoagulant and cytoprotective effects of protein C on the development of nosocomial infection and end-organ damage remains uncertain. There are several clinical implications of their preliminary findings. Recombinant activated protein C is the only approved drug for the treatment of septic shock. Even so, its use has been limited by the perception that it is too expensive and often given too late. Because protein C activation and depletion can occur as early as 6 hours after trauma, this might warrant the consideration of early monitoring and correction of plasma levels of activated protein C if a true causative relationship with ventilator-associated pneumonia could be defined.

D. W. Mozingo, MD

Validation of the Riboleukogram to Detect Ventilator-Associated Pneumonia After Severe Injury

Cobb JP, Moore EE, Hayden DL, et al (Washington Univ in St Louis, MO; Massachusetts General Hosp, Boston)

Ann Surg 250:531-538, 2009

Objective.—We hypothesized that circulating leukocyte RNA profiles or "riboleukograms" detect ventilator-associated pneumonia after blunt trauma.

Summary Background Data.—A pilot microarray study of 11 ventilator-associated pneumonia (VAP) patients suggested that 85 leukocyte genes can be used to diagnose VAP. Validation of this gene set to detect VAP was tested using data from an independent patient cohort.

Methods.—A total of 158 intubated blunt trauma patients were enrolled at 5 centers, where 57 (36%) developed VAP. Patient age was 34.2 ± 11.1 years; 65% were male. Circulating leukocyte GeneChip U133 2.0 expression values were measured at time 0.5, 1, 4, 7, 14, 21, and 28 days after injury. DChip normalized leukocyte transcriptional profiles were analyzed using repeated measures logistic regression. A compound covariate model based on leukocyte gene transcriptional profiles in a training subset of patients was tested to determine predictive accuracy for VAP 4 days prior to clinical diagnosis in the test subset.

Results.—Using gene expression values measured on each study day at an FDR <0.05, 27 (32%) of the 85 genes were associated with the diagnosis of VAP 1 to 4 days before diagnosis. However, the compound covariate model based on these 85 genes did not predict VAP in the test cohort better than chance ($P = 0.27$). In contrast, a compound covariate model based upon de novo transcriptional analysis of the 158 patients predicted VAP better than chance 4 days before diagnosis with a sensitivity of 57% and a specificity of 69%.

Conclusion.—Our results validate those described in a pilot study, confirming that riboleukograms are associated with the development of VAP days prior to clinical diagnosis. Similarly, a riboleukogram predictive model tested on a larger cohort of 158 patients was better than chance at predicting VAP days prior to clinical diagnosis.

▶ Ventilator-associated pneumonia is the most common nosocomial infection in the critically ill, occurring in up to 20% of the patients receiving mechanical ventilation. The rate of ventilator-associated pneumonia is highest in trauma patients and is associated with a higher mortality rate in those who are less severely injured. Because ventilator-associated pneumonia also increases ventilator and intensive care unit (ICU) days, the resulting increase in associated costs is substantial. The significant increase in morbidity, mortality, and cost associated with ventilator-associated pneumonia makes it an obvious target for quality care initiatives.

Preventative strategies have been effective in significantly decreasing the rates of ventilator-associated pneumonia; however, improvements in the diagnosis and treatment of ventilator-associated pneumonia have not been forthcoming. The diagnostic criteria for ventilator-associated pneumonia remain controversial. It is difficult to distinguish pneumonia from tracheal colonization in patients with other forms of lung injury. There is a tendency for clinicians to overdiagnose this condition because of the serious consequences of untreated pneumonia.

Advances in molecular diagnostics, thus, hold great promise for ventilator-associated pneumonia, especially if these tests could determine the causative organism earlier.

D. W. Mozingo, MD

5 Transplantation

Introduction

Transplantation in 2009 underwent changes in resources and reimbursement, oversight, research interests, and patient problems that resulted in an array of publications. The selection of manuscripts is representative of much of the dialogue that has occurred within the organ transplantation community. What follows is a brief discussion of the articles that I reviewed this year.

One of the significant oversight issues that recently occurred within the practice of organ transplantation was the stipulation by the Centers for Medicare and Medicaid (CMS) that individual transplant programs demonstrate specific institutional resources, processes, and performance requirements as necessary components for participation in the national Medicare reimbursement program. To the degree that a specific program is found to be lacking in a specific area, the consequence could lead to lack of payment for transplant care for patients with Medicare funding. The ASTS[1] responded to the CMS organ-specific conditions of participation with an analysis of existing centers that reached threshold performances to remove federal funding, the time required to return to compliance and mitigating factors that are not included within the risk-adjusted performance metric. While many other facets of the multilayered oversight of transplantation can be further discussed, the Society responded with many cogent issues. Without a doubt, the dialogue will continue with significant ramifications for other facets of surgery where outcome-driven reimbursement is important.

The numbers of people awaiting organ transplants in the US is now more than 100 000, yet the annual number of deceased donors has been static at about 8000. This disparity exists despite the fact that the numbers of people with end-stage kidney failure (the driver of the wait list) continues to increase much faster than the numbers of organs available. The numbers of people that would potentially benefit from extrarenal organ transplantation is not presently known, so the shortfall is conjecture. The Transplant Growth and Management Collaborative (TGMC) resulted in a 3-year increase in the availability of organ donors; however, the numbers of donors have plateaued and the organ shortage persists. An analysis of the information provided to the Organ Procurement and Transplant Network (OPTN) was analyzed.[2] The authors found that the demographics of deceased donors is changing: 1) there continues to be a decline in the numbers of young, standard donors declared dead by neurologic criteria (the ideal organ donor); 2) there is an increase in older donors, largely associated with vascular disease in the brain; and 3) the use of organs from donors declared dead by circulatory criteria is becoming a significant component of the nation's organ supply. Probably as a consequence of obtaining organs from non-traditional donors, the total numbers of organs retrieved from the nation's donor pool has not significantly changed, but to the transplant surgeon, the quality of the organs offered for transplantation has shifted. The consistent decline in live organ donors has been of significant import. This trend began in 2004 and has continually persisted. The authors highlight many of the factors associated with the changing scope of organ donation and utilization. They speculate about the impact of factors ranging from increased CMS oversight, the TGMC effect, and electronic notification for organ availability. Regardless of the reasons, the availability of high-quality organs for transplantation has not kept pace with the numbers of people that would benefit from organ transplantation.

Surprisingly, there has been little clinical research performed to improve the quality of organs after donation. While retrospective and laboratory experience has suggested that adrenergic agents given to organ donors would lead to improved outcomes, no clinical research had confirmed the hypotheses. To test the hypotheses, a randomized clinical trial[3] was performed through the auspices of Eurotransplant, in which donors were randomized to either conventional management of circulatory support or given a routine infusion of low-dose dopamine (4 μg/kg/min). The outcome of the kidneys retrieved from the donors was assessed. While the long-term functional outcome was the same despite how the kidney donors were managed, the probability of a kidney recipient being dialysis free immediately after transplantation was significantly increased by receiving a kidney from a donor in the dopamine pre-treatment group. The average duration of therapy before organ removal was short, the median duration being only 344 minutes. While there are shortcomings associated with this study, the results suggest that minor changes in donor management strategies may greatly impact upon the outcomes for the recipients.

To date, the recipient of a kidney from a live donor receives a substantially longer freedom from dialysis and death than does a recipient of a deceased donor kidney; however, the consequence(s) of kidney donation for the live donor has not been well studied. While there had been anecdotal reports of dire consequences, a population study had been lacking. The Minnesota group assessed their single center experience[4] of 3698 kidney donors who donated between 1963 and 2007. The observed kidney donor survival was compared to matched controls from the Human Mortality Database. The rate of development of ESRD within the donors was less than that observed within the general population (180 vs 268 cases/million persons/year). Analysis of other variables did not demonstrate any significant detrimental differences from the general population.

Most donors had preserved GFR, normal albumin excretion and an excellent quality of life. While results may be different with significantly altered donor characteristics, the existing paradigm suggests that the opportunity to donate a kidney does not have a significant detrimental impact upon the average kidney donor.

The hallmark of live donation has been the opportunity to donate directly to someone whom the donor knows. Initially it was thought that receiving a kidney from a family member (with similar genetic material) would be particularly advantageous; however, it is now recognized that other than an identical haplotype match, the important variable for excellent long-term kidney function is receiving a kidney from a live donor. This recognition has led to a different form of sharing when an incompatible donor-recipient pair (DP 1) occurs. Under these circumstances, it is sometimes possible to find a suitable recipient from another incompatible donor pair (DP 2) that could accept the kidney from the donor of DP1. This would free the donor from DP2 to donate to either the recipient of DP1 or another incompatible pair. As long as the recipient of DP1 eventually receives a live donor kidney, the result of moving the donation away from an incompatible group into a larger pool potentially increases the numbers of donors willing to donate kidneys. The impact that this form of donation would have on transplantation is currently unknown. The enthusiasm was manifested in the illustrative report published in the.[5] The process has the potential of having a significant impact upon the ability to have more recipients receive kidneys from live donors. This would result in significant benefit to the subset of the wait list. There are some pitfalls such as skewing the wait list away from O recipients, how to choose a recipient when more than one acceptable person is available and adjudication of the inevitable conflicts that will occur when the process does not go as anticipated.

One of the major concerns over the past several years has been the increasing recognition that the recipient of an organ transplant can get a disease through the graft that they had not wanted. Biovigilance is an issue not only for the transplant community, but also for the tissue and blood communities. Recognition and response to potential agents recognized to be in the donor organ can be a logistical tour de force. The difficulty of identification of which organs are at risk and with what certainty is problematic. In 1994, the Public Health Service released a list of behaviors/tests that putatively identified a subset of the population at "high risk" for blood-borne viral pathogens (HIV in particular, but also HBV and HCV). An analysis of the OPTN database[6] revealed that recipients of organs from "high risk" kidneys had similar graft and patient survival as the recipients of kidneys from donors not identified to have any of the risk factors. There have been multiple high-profile reports of disease transmission through organ transplantation that will likely influence the various oversight agencies to attempt new techniques to make the nation's organ supply safer.

A topic that has become an important issue for the kidney transplant community is treating people with antibodies directed against the histocompatibility antigens on the donor kidney. As the presence of these sorts of antibodies had previously been associated with hyperacute rejection and loss of grafts, they were thought to be a contraindication to transplantation. Several events have led to changing of those thoughts. First, technology has changed. Where in previous times, antibodies directed against donor alloantigens were identified by complement fixation and lysis, current techniques allow for FACS analysis of the cells and also the use of beads labeled with human HLA to identify antibody. Needless to say, the numbers of people with antibody directed against other human HLA have increased. In a study of 165 patients with donor-specific antibody (DSA) and a negative complement-fixation, outcomes were assessed.[7] It was found that only antibody to Class I MHC was associated with a worsened outcome (with a negative complement dependent crossmatch). Ability to predict clinical outcomes with the use of laboratory techniques is undergoing significant transformation. In the event that DSA is found in association with rejection, several therapeutic approaches have been described. The use of IVIG was first popularized and then the combination of plasmapheresis, IVIG and anti-CD20 was proposed. A comparison of the 2 therapies was performed.[8] It was suggested that IVIG alone resulted in inferior results compared with plasmapheresis, IVIG and anti-CD20. A more recent approach has been to treat recipients with DSA with a proteasome inhibitor, such as bortezomib, to disrupt antibody production. This is a potent therapy that is beginning to find a place in the management of the sensitized kidney recipient.[9]

The recent Institute of Medicine analysis of the organ donation process within the US concluded that organs from donors declared dead through circulatory criteria should be a major solution to the national organ shortage. This has proven to have mixed benefits. Long-term kidney function in recipients of organs from such donors has proven to be satisfactory. Liver recipients have had contradictory results, although there has been a growing sentiment that the increased proportion of bile duct complications and need for re-transplantation make these very inferior grafts. A US and UK article highlight the same issues from two sides of the Atlantic. In the US report,[10] the livers from donors with circulatory death had an inferior survival and the recipients had an increased rate of re-listing and re-transplantation, despite a mean recorded warm ischemia time of only 15.8 minutes. The UK experience is remarkably similar[11] with inferior graft survival and increased rates of ischemic cholangiopathy. Combined, these two papers reinforce the clinical perception that there is great heterogeneity in the quality and outcomes from transplanted DCD livers. Donor management and organ preservation strategies must be designed to maximize organ function and minimize arterial and biliary complications after transplantation if these organs are to achieve routine use.

Other than the availability of organs for the pediatric population, the numbers of people on the wait list for the other transplanted organs (pancreas, lung, heart, and intestine) is less than the numbers of donors. Diabetes is a common disease in the renal failure population and the role of beta cell replacement therapies through transplantation has remained somewhat undetermined. In several centers, extensive experience has been gained with whole organ pancreas transplantation along with kidney transplantation. The U Wisconsin group reported their experience with 1000 simultaneous pancreas-kidney transplants.[12] Despite changes in management of the exocrine function, immunosuppression, donor selection, and preservation over a protracted time period, the survival of the diabetic patient with renal failure is significantly improved when beta cell replacement occurs concomitantly with kidney transplantation. Transplantation of the intestine is emerging as an appropriate therapy for many individuals with an inability to maintain nutritional balance through enteral means; however, intestinal transplantation has been complicated by the highest rate of post transplant lymphoproliferative disease of any organ transplants. The U Pittsburgh reported the evolution of PTLD in their experience[13] demonstrating that as immunosuppressive and antiviral regimens changed, so did the outcomes. Concomitant with changes in drug regimens, improvements in patient and graft survival occurred. These gains have been important to increasing acceptance of intestinal transplantation as a major therapy in people with intestinal failure. Lung transplantation has been limited to a certain extent by the frequency of lung-associated pathology in the donor population. Expansion of organ availability through the use of retrieval of lungs from donors after declaration of death from circulatory criteria has been addressed.[14] There is a growing consensus that such lungs can be transplanted with reasonable success. The newest form of organ transplant has been the composite vascular allograft (VCA). While hand transplants have been evolving over the past decade, interest in replacement of the severely disfigured face has captured the imagination of the reconstructive surgeons. The various aspects and planning that went into the near-total face transplant at the Cleveland Clinic is discussed.[15] To the extent that the issues of VCA differ from those of organ transplantation, reconciliation of allocation and process with organs will need to occur.

The possibility that one could use organs from animals in human therapy has been sought for years. The barriers have been significant and include hyperacute rejection and more conventional immunoresponsiveness. The creation of a composite graft of thymus and kidney from an α1,3-galactosyltransferase knockout animal has been designed as yet another step towards the clinical reality of xenotransplantation.[16] More steps will need to be taken if xenotransplantation is to be actualized.

Cell transplantation has been proposed as an adjunct therapy for either cure or a manner to reestablish compensated organ failure. Most investigations have sought to isolate differentiated cells from organs (ie, islet transplantation for diabetes or hepatocytes for liver decompensation); however, the prospect of forcing autologous cells to differentiate into cells capable of function is appealing. It has been shown that peripheral blood mononuclear cells can be forced to differentiate into cells that have many characteristics of liver cells (NeoHeps). An experimental murine model of acute liver failure demonstrated improved animal survival being treated by either isolated hepatocytes or NeoHeps.[17] Development of therapies that use autologous cells may prove to be of significant benefit as the variable of immune response to the cells will be minimized.

A holy grail of organ transplantation has been the search for tolerance generation to alloantigens. Recognition of the role of regulatory T cells and attenuating or countering the proinflammatory is starting to develop,[18] which many think will facilitate this goal; however, T cells compartmentalize and circulate differently in the transplant population. In a study of lung transplant recipients, Tregs were followed in peripheral circulation and BAL fluid found in protocol bronchoscopy.

There was a disparity between what was observed in the peripheral circulation as compared to cells retrieved from the airway.[19] It is likely that immunologic monitoring may not be a simple task in the complex world of allograft transplants.

The issues and problems associated with transplantation have taken on extreme issues relating to social parameters of resource availability and varying quality of organs as well as a fundamental need to better understand the immunologic adaptations that occur after transplantation.

Timothy L. Pruett, MD

References

1. Abecassis MM, Burke R, Klintmalm GB, et al. American Society of Transplant Surgeons transplant center outcomes requirements—a threat to innovation. *Am J Transplant.* 2009;9:1279-1286.
2. Tuttle-Newhall JE, Krishnan SM, Levy MF, McBride V, Orlowski JP, Sung RS. Organ donation and utilization in the United States: 1998-2007. *Am J Transplant.* 2009;9:879-893.
3. Schnuelle P, Gottmann U, Hoeger S, et al. Effects of donor pretreatment with dopamine on graft function after kidney transplantation: a randomized controlled trial. *JAMA.* 2009;302:1067-1075.
4. Ibrahim HN, Foley R, Tan L, et al. Long-term consequences of kidney donation. *N Engl J Med.* 2009;360:459-469.
5. Rees MA, Kopke JE, Pelletier RP, et al. A nonsimultaneous, extended, altruistic-donor chain. *N Engl J Med.* 2009;360:1096-1101.
6. Reese PP, Feldman HI, Asch DA, et al. Transplantation of kidneys from donors at increased risk for blood-borne viral infection: recipient outcomes and patterns of organ use. *Am J Transplant.* 2009;9:2338-2345.
7. Billen EV, Christiaans MH, van den Berg-Loonen EM. Clinical relevance of Luminex donor-specific crossmatches: data from 165 renal transplants. *Tissue Antigens.* 2009;74:205-212.
8. Lefaucheur C, Nochy D, Andrade J, et al. Comparison of combination Plasmapheresis/IVIg/anti-CD20 versus high-dose IVIg in the treatment of antibody-mediated rejection. *Am J Transplant.* 2009;9:1099-1107.
9. Trivedi HL, Terasaki PI, Feroz A, et al. Abrogation of anti-HLA antibodies via proteasome inhibition. *Transplantation.* 2009;87:1555-1561.

10. Skaro AI, Jay CL, Baker TB, et al. The impact of ischemic cholangiopathy in liver transplantation using donors after cardiac death: the untold story. *Surgery.* 2009; 146:543-552.
11. Pine JK, Aldouri A, Young AL, et al. Liver transplantation following donation after cardiac death: an analysis using matched pairs. *Liver Transpl.* 2009;15: 1072-1082.
12. Sollinger HW, Odorico JS, Becker YT, D'Alessandro AM, Pirsch JD. One thousand simultaneous pancreas-kidney transplants at a single center with 22-year follow-up. *Ann Surg.* 2009;250:618-630.
13. Abu-Elmagd KM, Mazariegos G, Costa G, et al. Lymphoproliferative disorders and de novo malignancies in intestinal and multivisceral recipients: improved outcomes with new outlooks. *Transplantation.* 2009;88:926-934.
14. Puri V, Scavuzzo M, Guthrie T, et al. Lung transplantation and donation after cardiac death: a single center experience. *Ann Thorac Surg.* 2009;88:1609-1614.
15. Siemionow M, Papay F, Alam D, et al. Near-total human face transplantation for a severely disfigured patient in the USA. *Lancet.* 2009;374:203-209.
16. Griesemer AD, Hirakata A, Shimizu A, et al. Results of gal-knockout porcine thymokidney xenografts. *Am J Transplant.* 2009;9:2669-2678.
17. Glanemann M, Gaebelein G, Nussler N, et al. Transplantation of monocyte-derived hepatocyte-like cells (NeoHeps) improves survival in a model of acute liver failure. *Ann Surg.* 2009;249:149-154.
18. Boros P, Bromberg JS. Human FOXP3+ regulatory T cells in transplantation. *Am J Transplant.* 2009;9:1719-1724.
19. Neujahr DC, Cardona AC, Ulukpo O, et al. Dynamics of human regulatory T cells in lung lavages of lung transplant recipients. *Transplantation.* 2009;88: 521-527.

American Society of Transplant Surgeons transplant center outcomes requirements–a threat to innovation

Abecassis MM, Burke R, Klintmalm GB, et al (Northwestern Univ, Chicago, IL)
Am J Transplant 9:1279-1286, 2009

The transplant center regulations recently published by the Centers for Medicare and Medicaid (CMS) mandate that observed program-specific survival outcomes to fall within expected risk-adjusted outcomes. Meeting these outcomes is essential to continued participation in the Medicare program. Both donor and recipient variables not considered in current risk adjustment models can result in inferior outcomes and therefore may cause an overestimation of transplant center expected performance, precluding participation in the federally funded Medicare program. We reviewed the most recent four reporting periods published by the Scientific Registry for Transplant Recipients on their public website. We identified kidney, liver and heart transplant programs that were flagged for having outcomes statistically lower than expected as well as those that failed to meet CMS criteria. We also analyzed whether center volumes correlated with outcomes in these centers. We highlight the need for mitigating factors that could justify inferior outcomes under specific circumstances. Failure to reach consensus on such a mechanism for appeal may result in risk-averse behavior by transplant centers with respect to innovation and therefore hamper the ability to advance the field of transplantation. We propose a methodology that may address this emerging dilemma.

▶ Organ transplantation has been in the midst of changing social oversight and economics. The advent of the conditions of participation to receive Medicare payments has had a profound impact upon transplant programs throughout the country. For a field that has been so heavily dependent upon innovation to achieve improvements in care, these changes have had great effect. The American Society of Transplant Surgeons' response is important in defining some of the areas of concern from the transplant community. The need to continue the dialog with those charged with oversight of the community will continue to be important.

T. Pruett, MD

Organ donation and utilization in the United States: 1998-2007

Tuttle-Newhall JE, Krishnan SM, Levy MF, et al (Duke Univ Health System, Durham, NC)

Am J Transplant 9:879-893, 2009

Organ transplantation remains the only life-saving therapy for many patients with organ failure. Despite the work of the Organ Donation and Transplant Collaboratives, and the marked increases in deceased donors early in the effort, deceased donors only rose by 67 from 2006 and the number of living donors declined during the same time period. There continue to be increases in the use of organs from donors after cardiac death (DCD) and expanded criteria donors (ECD). This year has seen a major change in the way organs are offered with increased patient safety measures in those organ offers made by OPOs using DonorNet. Unfortunately, the goals of 75% conversion rates, 3.75 organs transplanted per donor, 10% of all donors from DCD sources and 20% growth of transplant center volume have yet to be reached across all donation service areas (DSAs) and transplant centers; however, there are DSAs that have not only met, but exceeded, these goals. Changes in organ preservation techniques took place this year, partly due to expanding organ acceptance criteria and increasing numbers of ECDs and DCDs. Finally, the national transplant environment has changed in response to increased regulatory oversight and new requirements for donation and transplant provider organizations.

▶ One of the major changes that occurred over the past decade has been in the quality and quantity of organs available to be transplanted. While the number of people waiting for organs has increased, the number of organs available for them has not kept up with the increase. The number of organs from older donors and donors declared dead through circulatory criteria has increased, and the number of the younger (standard) donors has diminished. Additionally, the number of living donors has also decreased. While the reasons for these changes have been the source of considerable conjecture, what should not be questioned is that the United States is not meeting the needs of those who would benefit from organ transplantation. A discipline needs to be applied to the donation community as it is to the transplant community to discern observed versus expected performance to obtain organs for the people of the country. This article is descriptive of many of the pressures on and methods used by the donation community to increase the number of available organs.

T. Pruett, MD

Effects of Donor Pretreatment With Dopamine on Graft Function After Kidney Transplantation: A Randomized Controlled Trial

Schnuelle P, Gottmann U, Hoeger S, et al (Univ Med Centre Mannheim, Germany; et al)

JAMA 302:1067-1075, 2009

Context.—Kidney graft function after transplantation can be improved through pharmacological donor pretreatment to limit organ injury from cold preservation.

Objective.—To determine whether pretreatment of brain-dead donors with low-dose dopamine improves early graft function in human renal transplant recipients.

Design, Setting, and Patients.—Randomized, open-label, multicenter, parallel-group trial of 264 deceased heart-beating donors and 487 subsequent renal transplants performed at 60 European centers between March 2004 and August 2007 (final follow-up, December 31, 2008). Eligible donors were stable under low-dose norepinephrine with a normal serum creatinine concentration on admission.

Interventions.—Donors were randomized to receive low-dose dopamine (4 μg/kg/min).

Main Outcome Measures.—Dialysis requirement during first week after transplantation.

Results.—Dopamine was infused for a median of 344 minutes (IQR, 215 minutes). Dialysis was significantly reduced in recipients of a dopamine-treated graft. Fewer recipients in the treatment group needed multiple dialyses (56/227; 24.7%; 95% CI, 19.0%-30.3%; vs 92/260; 35.4%; 95% CI, 29.5%-41.2%; $P = .01$). The need for multiple dialyses posttransplant was associated with allograft failure after 3 years (HR, 3.61; 95% CI, 2.39-5.45; $P < .001$), whereas a single dialysis was not (HR, 0.67; 95% CI, 0.21-2.18; $P = .51$). Besides donor dopamine (OR, 0.54; 95% CI, 0.35-0.83; $P = .005$), cold ischemic time (OR, 1.07; 95% CI, 1.02-1.11 per hour; $P = .001$), donor age (OR, 1.03; 95% CI, 1.01-1.05 per year; $P < .001$), and recipient body weight (OR, 1.02; 95% CI, 1.01-1.04 per kg; $P = .009$) were independent explanatory variables in a multiple logistic regression model. Dopamine resulted in significant but clinically meaningless increases in the donor's systolic blood pressure (3.8 mm Hg; 95% CI, 0.7-6.9 mm Hg; $P = .02$) and urine production before surgical recovery of the kidneys (29 mL; 95% CI, 7-51 mL; $P = .009$) but had no influence on outcome.

Conclusion.—Donor pretreatment with low-dose dopamine reduces the need for dialysis after kidney transplantation.

Trial Registration.—clinicaltrials.gov Identifier: NCT00115115.

▶ Clinical studies to discern differences in the management of the deceased organ donor have been very uncommon. This study through Eurotransplant database demonstrated that treatment of the heart-beating organ donor with low-dose dopamine (4 μg/kg/min for a median of 344 minutes) yielded kidneys with an improved immediate function rate. While the ultimate outcome of the kidneys was not affected in this study, the benefits and cost savings from avoiding dialysis for the recipients are considerable. The impact of the low-dose dopamine on other organs was not assessed. This type of study needs further repetition to discern therapeutic management strategies for other donated organs.

T. Pruett, MD

Long-Term Consequences of Kidney Donation

Ibrahim HN, Foley R, Tan L, et al (Univ of Minnesota, Minneapolis; Chronic Disease Res Group, Minneapolis, MN)

N Engl J Med 360:459-469, 2009

Background.—The long-term renal consequences of kidney donation by a living donor are attracting increased appropriate interest. The overall evidence suggests that living kidney donors have survival similar to that of nondonors and that their risk of end-stage renal disease (ESRD) is not increased. Previous studies have included relatively small numbers of donors and a brief follow-up period.

Methods.—We ascertained the vital status and lifetime risk of ESRD in 3698 kidney donors who donated kidneys during the period from 1963 through 2007; from 2003 through 2007, we also measured the glomerular filtration rate (GFR) and urinary albumin excretion and assessed the prevalence of hypertension, general health status, and quality of life in 255 donors.

Results.—The survival of kidney donors was similar to that of controls who were matched for age, sex, and race or ethnic group. ESRD developed in 11 donors, a rate of 180 cases per million persons per year, as compared with a rate of 268 per million per year in the general population. At a mean ($\pm$SD) of 12.2 ± 9.2 years after donation, 85.5% of the subgroup of 255 donors had a GFR of 60 ml per minute per 1.73 m^2 of body-surface area or higher, 32.1% had hypertension, and 12.7% had albuminuria. Older age and higher body-mass index, but not a longer time since donation, were associated with both a GFR that was lower than 60 ml per minute per 1.73 m^2 and hypertension. A longer time since donation, however, was independently associated with albuminuria. Most donors had quality-of-life scores that were better than population norms, and the prevalence of coexisting conditions was similar to that among controls from the National Health and Nutrition Examination Survey (NHANES) who were matched for age, sex, race or ethnic group, and body-mass index.

Conclusions.—Survival and the risk of ESRD in carefully screened kidney donors appear to be similar to those in the general population. Most donors who were studied had a preserved GFR, normal albumin excretion, and an excellent quality of life.

▶ Results of kidney transplantation from a live donor are on average superior to any kidney from a deceased donor. There has been a persistent debate from within the community relating to the subsequent long-term health risks to a kidney donor. To a certain extent, the safety of kidney donation has been reaffirmed by the findings of this article. The survival curves of controls and donors are virtually superimposable. However, as with the changing profile of deceased donors, so live kidney donors have changed. It is not clear whether the adverse effects will occur in the older, nonwhite kidney donors with well-controlled hypertension. This article speaks to the need for continued surveillance of this population. While the results certainly speak to the general safety of the procedure, there are more than enough uncertainties to lead us to continue to understand the uninephric condition.

T. Pruett, MD

A Nonsimultaneous, Extended, Altruistic-Donor Chain

Rees MA, Kopke JE, Pelletier RP, et al (Univ of Toledo Med Ctr, OH; Univ of Cincinnati, OH; Alliance for Paired Donation, Maumee, OH; et al)

N Engl J Med 360:1096-1101, 2009

We report a chain of 10 kidney transplantations, initiated in July 2007 by a single altruistic donor (i.e., a donor without a designated recipient) and coordinated over a period of 8 months by two large paired-donation registries. These transplantations involved six transplantation centers in five states. In the case of five of the transplantations, the donors and their coregistered recipients underwent surgery simultaneously. In the other five cases, "bridge donors" continued the chain as many as 5 months after the coregistered recipients in their own pairs had received transplants. This report of a chain of paired kidney donations, in which the transplantations were not necessarily performed simultaneously, illustrates the potential of this strategy.

▶ A significant amount of media attention has been generated when a live donor donates a kidney to someone other than the intended recipient, only to have that person receive a kidney from a different, but compatible donor. The extended, nonsimultaneous altruistic-donor chain has been demonstrated to be possible. To the extent that the chain results in more patients being transplanted, such a tactic will prove extraordinarily valuable. However, it is still not clear what criteria should be applied to identify which potential recipient should be chosen to receive when more than 1 waitlisted person is identified as compatible. Does this form of matching constitute kidney allocation, and, if so, what criteria should be applied to the matching algorithms? There are many issues that will need to be addressed before this type of transplantation becomes routine.

T. Pruett, MD

Transplantation of Kidneys from Donors at Increased Risk for Blood-Borne Viral Infection: Recipient Outcomes and Patterns of Organ Use

Reese PP, Feldman HI, Asch DA, et al (Univ of Pennsylvania, Philadelphia)
Am J Transplant 9:2338-2345, 2009

Kidney transplantation from deceased donors classified as increased risk for viral infection by the Centers for Disease Control (CDC) is controversial. Analyses of Organ Procurement and Transplantation Network (OPTN) data from 7/1/2004 to 7/1/2006 were performed. The primary cohort included 48 054 adults added to the kidney transplant wait list. Compared to receiving a standard criteria donor (SCD) kidney or remaining wait-listed, CDC recipients (HR 0.80, $p = 0.18$) had no significant difference in mortality. In a secondary cohort of 19 872 kidney recipients at 180 centers, SCD (reference) and CDC (HR 0.91, $p = 0.16$) recipients had no difference in the combined endpoint of allograft failure or death. Among centers performing >10 kidney transplants during the study period, the median proportion of CDC transplants/total transplants was 7.2% (range 1.1–35.6%). Higher volume transplant centers were more likely to use CDC kidneys compared to low and intermediate volume centers ($p < 0.01$). An analysis of procured kidneys revealed that 6.8% of SCD versus 7.8% of CDC ($p = 0.13$) kidneys were discarded. In summary, center use of CDC kidneys varied widely, and recipients had good short-term outcomes. OPTN should collect detailed data about long-term outcomes and recipient viral testing so the potential risks of CDC kidneys can be fully evaluated.

► One of the clear risks after organ transplantation is the possibility of acquiring an infectious or malignant disease through the organ. When HIV and HCV were transmitted through organ transplantation in 2007, a flurry of regulatory activity was generated around types of testing that should be performed on the organ donor, what type of information/informed consent should be given and obtained from the recipient, and how the donation community should characterize the organ donor for reporting and allocation purposes. The knowledge database relating to the risk of disease transmission is not complete. From a patient and graft survival perspective, recipients of organs from PHS/CDC defined as high-risk donors fare as well as recipients from standard organ donors. The unfortunate fact is that organs are discarded from these donors, often with little evidence that a recipient is at higher risk of acquiring a disease. The current reporting system does little to provide complete risk information regarding organs available for transplant in the United States. Because of the safety drumbeat, there is an increasing effort to develop a biovigilance system within the United States.

T. Pruett, MD

Clinical relevance of Luminex donor-specific crossmatches: data from 165 renal transplants

Billen EV, Christiaans MH, van den Berg-Loonen EM (Univ Hosp Maastricht, The Netherlands)

Tissue Antigens 74:205-212, 2009

The clinical significance of the presence of donor-specific anti-human leucocyte antigen (HLA) antibodies (DSA) prior to renal transplantation detected solely by solid-phase techniques remains unclear. This study was designed to determine the clinical relevance of the recently introduced bead-based Luminex donor-specific crossmatch (LumXm). A group of 165 patients transplanted between 1997 and 2001 were tested. Of 165 recipients transplanted with a negative complement-dependent cytotoxicity crossmatch, 32 proved to have a positive Luminex crossmatch. Sixteen were positive for class I, 15 were positive for class II, 1 was both class I and II positive and 133 recipients were negative. Acute rejection (AR)-free survival for all recipients was 77%, and there was no difference in AR-free survival between LumXm-positive and LumXm-negative recipients. Overall graft survival after a median follow-up time of 8 years was 56%. Recipients with a positive class I LumXm had worse long-term graft survival ($P = 0.006$). In recipients with a positive class I LumXm, 5-year graft survival was 41% vs 70% in negative patients and 10-year graft survival was 27% vs 56%. Positivity for class II LumXm was not a significant risk factor for graft failure ($P = 0.7$). In conclusion, pretransplant DSA detected by the LumXm had no impact on AR episodes. Class II LumXm positivity proved no significant risk factor for graft failure, but the value of the class II LumXm is questionable. A positive class I LumXm resulted in worse long-term graft survival compared with a negative one.

► Identification of patients with preformed antibodies to antigens that are expressed on a donor organ has been a technique to exclude transplantation because of the risk for rapid rejection. The historical laboratory technique to identify such antibodies has been cell based, that is, antibody binding to cells with known antigens were used to discern antigen specificity. Technology has changed and the use of beads coated with recombinant human antigen is now available to characterize antibodies for those on the waiting list. This has raised innumerable questions regarding the translation of old knowledge in the light of new techniques. This article is representative of the community's efforts to understand the outcomes associated with the new tests. In these patients with negative pretransplant testing using the old tests, 32 patients were found to have donor-specific antibodies using the solid phase testing. Episodes of acute rejection were not different between those with and without donor-specific antibody. There appeared to be earlier graft dysfunction in recipients with class II antibodies, but 5-year graft survival was not different from those without antibodies. However, in recipients with antibodies against the class I antigens, 5-year graft survival was associated with inferior results. Other studies have demonstrated somewhat different results, but this article is representative of the efforts that the community is making to understand the effects of changing technology on the likelihood that kidney transplantation will be successful.

T. Pruett, MD

Comparison of Combination Plasmapheresis/IVIg/Anti-CD20 Versus High-Dose IVIg in the Treatment of Antibody-Mediated Rejection

Lefaucheur C, Nochy D, Andrade J, et al (Saint-Louis Hosp, Paris, France; Georges Pompidou European Hosp, Paris, France)

Am J Transplant 9:1099-1107, 2009

Different strategies appear to improve the success in treatment of antibody-mediated rejection (AMR), although no one best method has yet emerged. The objective of this study was to compare the efficacy of the combination of Plasmapheresis/intravenous immunoglobulin (IVIg)/anti-CD20-based regimes versus high-dose IVIg alone in the treatment of AMR. Group A (12 patients) was treated with high-dose IVIg between January 2000 and December 2003; group B (12 patients) was treated by Plasmapheresis/IVIg/anti-CD20 between January 2004 and December 2005. Graft survival at 36 months was 91.7% in group B versus 50% in group A ($p = 0.02$). Donor-specific human leukocyte antigens (DSA) levels detected by Luminex single antigen (Luminex SA) and ELISA, 3 months postrejection are significantly lower in group B than in group A: DSA ELISA class 2 score 6–8 ($p = 0.02$), DSA mean intensity of fluorescence (MFI) max ($p = 0.009$) and DSA mean MFI ($p = 0.0004$). The persistence of elevated DSA levels posttreatment is more frequent in patients with graft loss as compared to those with preserved renal function: score 6–8 on ELISA ($p = 0.04$); mean MFI ($p = 0.00009$) and MFImax ($p = 0.018$). We conclude that: (1) high dose IVIg alone is inferior to Plasmapheresis/IVIg/anti-CD20 as therapy for AMR and (2)DSA postrejection can be quantified using solid phase assays, showing that 3 months after AMR, DSA levels are higher in patients with graft loss.

► With the increased recognition of donor-specific antibody, techniques to modify the detection (and hopefully the outcomes) have grown. The use of intravenous immunoglobulin (IVIg) with or without the addition of anti-CD20 (CD20 is a protein on B cells but not plasma cells) has become quite popular as a technique to diminish antibody levels in the recipient serum. This article is representative of the literature, with a small group of study patients (12 patients in each study arm) to compare therapies for antibody-mediated rejection. In this article, anti-CD20 was associated with improved outcomes compared with the 12 patients that did not receive the antibody. However, what is not discussed are the goals of the therapy. Both groups received plasmapheresis: what was the goal of therapy? Was it met and in what percentage of patients? Should there be different goals of therapy in patients with different stimuli to produce donor-specific antibody? Does the person sensitized from a prior transplant differ from one who has a different stimulation through pregnancy or transfusion? There is still much to be learned about this problem.

T. Pruett, MD

Abrogation of Anti-HLA Antibodies via Proteasome Inhibition

Trivedi HL, Terasaki PI, Feroz A, et al (Inst of Kidney Diseases and Res Centre [IKDRC]-Inst of Transplantation Sciences [ITS], Ahmedabad, Gujarat, India; Terasaki Foundation Laboratory, Los Angeles, CA; et al)

Transplantation 87:1555-1561, 2009

Background.—Current treatments for autoantibody-mediated diseases (i.e., systemic lupus erythematosus) and alloantibodies (in transplant) are minimally effective. Although they deplete naïve B cells, plasmablasts, and transiently reduce antibody concentrations, they are minimally effective against long-lived, antibody-producing plasma cells. In transplantation, plasma cells produce antibodies directed against human leukocyte antigen (HLA) antigens causing poor allograft survival. We report the first clinical experience with a plasma cell depleting therapy, bortezomib, to abrogate anti-HLA antibodies in transplantation (outside of rejection) in an attempt to improve long-term allograft survival.

Methods.—Eleven patients with anti-HLA alloantibodies were treated with bortezomib. All patients underwent plasmapheresis to aid in removal of antibodies and to determine the effect of bortezomib. Serial measurements of anti-HLA antibody levels were conducted weekly by single antigen bead on Luminex platform.

Results.—Bortezomib treatment elicited substantial reduction in both donor-specific antibody (DSA) and non-DSA levels. Antibodies were directed against DSA in 8 of 11 cases. Mean time to antibody appearance was 2 months posttransplant. Within 22 days (median) from treatment initiation, 9 of 11 patients' antibody levels dropped to less than 1000 mean fluorescence intensity. Of two patients without successful depletion, all had peak mean fluorescence intensity more than 10,000. At a mean follow-up of approximately 4 months posttreatment, all patients have stable graft function. Minimal transient side effects were noticed with bortezomib in the form of gastrointestinal toxicity, thrombocytopenia, and paresthesias.

Conclusions.—Bortezomib therapy effectively abrogates anti-HLA antibodies. Hence, removal of antibodies, by proteasome inhibition, represents a new treatment strategy for transplantation and may have benefit in autoimmune-related disease.

▶ Bortezomib, a proteasomal inhibitor, is a drug developed for the treatment of multiple myeloma. It has been found to deplete plasma cells through a variety of mechanisms. It has had some success in the treatment of acute rejection but may also have a role in abrogating antibodies directed against alloantigens. This article describes the effect of bortezomib but is hampered by the small number of patients and the peculiar use of a clonal stimulation and depletion protocol of donor-specific leukocyte transfusion, cyclophosphamide, irradiation, and thymoglobulin. No calcineurin inhibitors, mammalian target of rapamycin inhibitors, or antiproliferative agents (MMF) were used. In patients with donor-specific antibody, bortezomib was used. It is virtually impossible to ascertain the relative effects of the conditioning treatments from the therapeutic treatments. The confounding variables make application to the usual world of transplant recipients very difficult.

T. Pruett, MD

The impact of ischemic cholangiopathy in liver transplantation using donors after cardiac death: The untold story

Skaro AI, Jay CL, Baker TB, et al (Northwestern Univ, Chicago, IL)
Surgery 146:543-553, 2009

Background.—Liver transplantation (LT) from donation after cardiac death (DCD) donors is increasingly being used to address organ shortages. Despite encouraging reports, standard survival metrics have overestimated the effectiveness of DCD livers. We examined the mode, kinetics, and predictors of organ failure and resource utilization to more fully characterize outcomes after DCD LT.

Methods.—We reviewed the outcomes for 32 DCD and 237 donation after brain death (DBD) LT recipients at our institution.

Results.—Recipients of DCD livers had a 2.1 times greater risk of graft failure, a 2.5 times greater risk of relisting, and a 3.2 times greater risk of retransplantation compared with DBD recipients. DCD recipients had a 31.6% higher incidence of biliary complications and a 35.8% higher incidence of ischemic cholangiopathy. Ischemic cholangiography was primarily implicated in the higher risk of graft failure observed after DCD LT. DCD recipients with ischemic cholangiography experienced more frequent rehospitalizations, longer hospital stays, and required more invasive biliary procedures.

Conclusion.—Related to higher complication rates, DCD recipients necessitated greater resource utilization. This more granular data should be considered in the decision to promote DCD LT. Modification of liver allocation policy is necessary to address those disadvantaged by a failing DCD graft.

▶ Livers from donors declared dead through circulatory criteria are used for transplantation. As time progresses, it becomes more certain that these organs do not offer the same outcomes to recipients as those from heart-beating donors. This single-center report stresses many of the problems with graft failure and the need for relisting but especially stresses the biliary complications. Whether the bile duct complications can be addressed through technical and donor management methods or is an inevitable consequence of that form of death is uncertain. One would prefer that livers from this type of donor would have similar and predictable outcomes as those from donors with neurologic death.

T. Pruett, MD

Liver Transplantation Following Donation After Cardiac Death: An Analysis Using Matched Pairs

Pine JK, Aldouri A, Young AL, et al (St James's Univ Hosp, UK)

Liver Transpl 15:1072-1082, 2009

Grafts from donation after cardiac death (DCD) donors are used to increase the number of organs available for liver transplantation. There is concern that warm ischemia may impair graft function. We compared our DCD recipients with a case-matched group of donation after brain death (DBD) recipients. Between January 2002 and April 2008, 39 DCD grafts were transplanted. These were matched with 39 DBD recipients on the basis of identified variables that had a significant impact on mortality. These were used to individually match DCD and DBD patients with similar predictive mortality. We compared patient/graft survival, primary non-function (PNF), and rates of complications. Of all liver transplants, 6.1% were DCD grafts. PNF occurred twice in the DCD group. The incidence of nonanastomotic biliary strictures (NABS; 20.5% versus 0%, $P = 0.005$) and hepatic artery stenosis (HAS; 12.8% versus 0%, $P = 0.027$) in the DCD group was higher. One-year (79.5% versus 97.4%, $P = 0.029$) and 3-year (63.6% versus 97.4%, $P = 0.001$) graft survival was lower in the DCD group. Three-year patient survival was also lower (68.2% versus 100%, $P < 0.0001$). Our study is the first to use case-matched patients and compare groups with similar predictive mortality. There was a higher incidence of NABS and HAS in the DCD group. NABS were likely a result of warm ischemia. HAS may have been due to ischemia or arterial injury during retrieval. The DCD group had significantly poorer outcomes, but DCD grafts remain a valuable resource. With careful donor/recipient selection, minimization of ischemia, and good postoperative care, acceptable results can be achieved.

▶ Experience from this European center confirms that livers from donation after cardiac death (DCD) donors do not behave in a similar fashion as those from neurologically declared dead donors. The near universal experience that these organs are inferior grafts cannot be dismissed. The issue will be whether enough understanding can be gained that will permit acceptable outcomes with routine use.

T. Pruett, MD

One Thousand Simultaneous Pancreas-Kidney Transplants at a Single Center With 22-Year Follow-Up

Sollinger HW, Odorico JS, Becker YT, et al (Univ of Wisconsin, Madison)
Ann Surg 250:618-630, 2009

Objective.—Simultaneous pancreas-kidney transplantation (SPK) is a procedure which frees the diabetic patient with end-stage nephropathy from dialysis and daily insulin injections. The purpose of this study is to report long-term outcomes of this procedure, and describe surgical and medical complications.

Methods.—The analysis includes 1000 consecutive SPKs performed between 1985 and 2007. Bladder drainage was used in 390 patients and enteric drainage in 610 patients. In 362 patients, SPK transplantation was performed before initiation of dialysis.

Results.—Patient survival at 1, 10, and 20 years is 97%, 80%, and 58%; kidney survival is 91%, 63%, and 38%; and pancreas survival is 88%, 63%, and 36%, respectively. There was no difference ($P > 0.19$) for patient, kidney, and pancreas survival between bladder and enteric drainage. Major surgical complications for bladder-drained patients were anastomotic leaks, urological complications, and infections. For enteric-drained patients, major surgical complications were infection, bleeding, and enzyme leak. Principal causes of death were myocardial infarction (n = 23), cerebrovascular accident (n = 18), and renal failure (n = 15). Graft failure for the kidney was due to acute rejection (n = 48), chronic rejection (n = 146), and death with a functioning graft (n = 99). Graft failure for the pancreas was caused by chronic graft loss (n = 44), thrombosis (n = 31), rejection (n = 80), and death with a functioning graft (n = 125). A total of 113 patients were retransplanted with either living related or unrelated donor kidneys (n = 64) or deceased donor kidneys (n = 42). Survival for retransplanted kidneys is 84% at 1 year and 68%

at 5 years. Surviving bladder-drained patients underwent enteric conversion (>50%) for severe recalcitrant metabolic or urologic complications, most commonly enzyme leaks, hematuria, and recurrent urinary tract infection.

Conclusions.—Diabetic patients with end-stage renal failure have a poor prognosis without transplantation. Transplantation with SPK provides a marked extension of the patient's life and freedom from insulin injections. Enteric drainage is currently the surgical technique of choice. SPK transplantation should be considered the treatment of choice in this patient population.

▶ Pancreas transplantation at the same time as a kidney transplantation has become a major therapy for type I diabetic patients with kidney failure. As this patient population's outcomes are so poor with dialysis, it has been questioned whether the benefits of glycemic control associated with pancreas transplantation offset the other morbidities associated with the added procedure. Experience from centers with a significant commitment to the application of pancreas transplantation to the population has shown many evolutions of therapy. The experience reported in this article describes only that with simultaneous pancreas-kidney transplant but discusses the evolution from bladder drainage to enteric drainage and current ideas relating to immunosuppression. Type I diabetes and associated renal failure is a disastrous disease that can be effectively treated by organ transplantation. The variables associated with good outcomes are considerable and require significant experience to achieve consistent good results.

T. Pruett, MD

Lymphoproliferative Disorders and De Novo Malignancies in Intestinal and Multivisceral Recipients: Improved Outcomes With New Outlooks

Abu-Elmagd KM, Mazariegos G, Costa G, et al (Univ of Pittsburgh, PA)

Transplantation 88:926-934, 2009

Background.—Early experience with intestinal and multivisceral transplantation was plagued with high risk of rejection and posttransplant lymphoproliferative disorders (PTLD). To improve outcome, innovative management and immunosuppressant strategies were sequentially evolved.

Methods.—With initiation of the program in 1990, serial monitoring of Epstein-Barr-Viral load was introduced in 1994 with adoption of preemptive antiviral therapy. In 1995, cyclophosphamide or daclizumab induction was added to the tacrolimus-steroid-based multiple drug immunosuppressions. Such a conventional approach was replaced in 2001 with a novel immunosuppressive protocol consisting of recipient pretreatment with a single dose of rabbit antithymocyte globulin or alemtuzumab and posttransplant tacrolimus monotherapy.

Results.—With a total of 395 consecutive primary recipients, de novo malignancy(s) developed in 61 (15%) patients, with PTLD in 52 (13%), and nonlymphoid cancer (NLC) in 13 (3.2%). Malignancy was donor driven in 3 (4.6%) recipients and associated with graft-versus-host disease in 7 (11.4%). Children were at a significantly higher risk ($P < 0.001$) of PTLD, and adults were more vulnerable ($P = 0.01$) to NLC. With multivariate analyses, type of immunosuppression, recipient age, splenectomy, and treatment of rejection were significant PTLD risk factors.

Conclusions.—Despite pretransplant lymphoid depletion, preemptive antiviral therapy and minimization of posttransplant immunosuppression significantly reduced PTLD morbidity ($P = 0.0001$) and mortality ($P = 0.001$) with no impact on NLC. Patient survival was also improved ($P = 0.0001$) with 91% at 1 year and 75% at 5 years.

▶ One of the significant limitations for recipients of intestinal and multivisceral transplantation has been the development of lymphomas after the procedure. Many monitoring, prophylactic therapies and immunosuppression have changed since the introduction of intestinal transplantation and associated with the change has been a significant reduction in post-transplant lymphoproliferative disorder morbidity and mortality. Whether the benefit is the consequence of experience and numbers or whether it is from the heightened monitoring and changes in drug therapies is not clear. As the incidence of nonlymphoid cancers did not change, the presumption is that changes in immunosuppressive and viral monitoring strategies are most likely associated.

T. Pruett, MD

Lung Transplantation and Donation After Cardiac Death: A Single Center Experience

Puri V, Scavuzzo M, Guthrie T, et al (Washington Univ, St Louis, MO)
Ann Thorac Surg 88:1609-1615, 2009

Background.—Lung donation after cardiac death (DCD) can enlarge the donor pool. Single-center reports have shown comparable outcomes after lung transplantation using conventional donors versus DCD in small numbers of patients.

Methods.—We performed a retrospective review of DCD experience at a single lung transplant program using a prospective database.

Results.—Between January 2003 and April 2008, 293 lung transplantations were performed, including 11 bilateral transplantations (3.7%) using DCD lungs. Similar criteria were used to assess donor quality. The hospital mortality for DCD recipients was 2 of 11 (18%) and overall mortality was 4 of 11 (36%) by 18 months of follow-up. Seven DCD patients (64%) are alive with a median follow-up of 32 months. The DCD group was comparable to the control group in age and ischemic times. The 4 deaths, when compared with 7 DCD survivors, had longer ischemic time (293 minutes versus 232 minutes) and a higher incidence of nonlocal donors (3 of 4 versus 1 of 7).

Conclusions.—At our center, early outcomes after DCD lung transplantations are somewhat inferior to those of series from other centers but approach national averages for conventional lung transplantation. Thus, DCD lung transplantation has the potential to increase the donor pool but must be offered cautiously.

▶ Like the liver, there have been considerable efforts to increase the utilization of organs from nontraditional donors. The outcomes of transplants of lungs from donors declared dead through circulatory criteria (donation after cardiac death [DCD]) are satisfactory but have still not been thoroughly evaluated. This report demonstrates that although the results are satisfactory, these lungs may not tolerate cold ischemia. The numbers are still too small, and there is a need for better stratification of data, if the use of these lungs is to become commonplace.

T. Pruett, MD

Near-total human face transplantation for a severely disfigured patient in the USA

Siemionow M, Papay F, Alam D, et al (Cleveland Clinic, OH)

Lancet 374:203-209, 2009

Background.—Multiple reconstructive procedures are common for the reconstruction of complex facial deformities of skin, soft tissues, bony structures, and functional subunits, such as the nose, lips, and eyelids. However, the results have been unsatisfactory. An innovative approach entailing a single surgical procedure of face allograft transplantation is a viable alternative and gives improved results.

Methods.—On Dec 9, 2008, a 45-year-old woman with a history of severe midface trauma underwent near-total face transplantation in which 80% of her face was replaced with a tailored composite tissue allograft. We addressed issues of immunosuppressive therapy, psychological and ethical outcomes, and re-integration of the patient into society.

Findings.—After the operation, the patient did well physically and psychologically, and tolerated immunosuppression without any major complication. Routine biopsy on day 47 after transplantation showed rejection of graft mucosa; however, a single bolus of corticosteroids reversed rejection. During the first 3 weeks after transplantation, the patient accepted her new face; 6 months after surgery, the functional outcome has been excellent. In contrast to her status before transplantation, the patient can now breathe through her nose, smell, taste, speak intelligibly, eat solid foods, and drink from a cup.

Interpretation.—We show the feasibility of reconstruction of severely disfigured patients in a single surgical procedure using composite face allotransplantation. Therefore, this should be taken in consideration as an early option for severely disfigured patients.

► Vascularized composite allografts are becoming of age. Extremity and face transplants are increasingly being offered to people with severe debility but not necessarily organ failure. The transplant center entering into this form of therapy has new issues to consider. This report discusses many of the issues that were confronted with the planning and execution of a face transplant. As the therapy becomes more commonplace, it will be necessary to adjust the retrieval, allocation, and monitoring of donors and recipients.

T. Pruett, MD

Results of Gal-Knockout Porcine Thymokidney Xenografts

Griesemer AD, Hirakata A, Shimizu A, et al (Massachusetts General Hosp, Boston)

Am J Transplant 9:2669-2678, 2009

Clinical transplantation for the treatment of end-stage organ disease is limited by a shortage of donor organs. Successful xenotransplantation could immediately overcome this limitation. The development of homozygous α 1,3-galactosyltransferase knockout (GalT-KO) pigs removed hyperacute rejection as the major immunologic hurdle to xenotransplantation. Nevertheless, GalT-KO organs stimulate robust immunologic responses that are not prevented by immunosuppressive drugs. Murine studies show that recipient thymopoiesis in thymic xenografts induces xenotolerance. We transplanted life-supporting composite thymokidneys (composite thymus and kidneys) prepared in GalT-KO miniature swine to baboons in an attempt to induce tolerance in a preclinical xenotransplant model. Here, we report the results of seven xenogenic thymokidney transplants using a steroid-free immunosuppressive regimen that eliminated whole-body irradiation in all but one recipient. The regimen resulted in average recipient survival of over 50 days. This was associated with donor-specific unresponsiveness *in vitro* and early baboon thymopoiesis in the porcine thymus tissue of these grafts, suggesting the development of T-cell tolerance. The kidney grafts had no signs of cellular infiltration or deposition of IgG, and no grafts were lost due to rejection. These results show that xenogeneic thymus transplantation can support early primate thymopoiesis, which in turn may induce T-cell tolerance to solid organ xenografts.

► Hurdles to xenotransplantation have been significant. The existence of natural antibodies against the terminal saccharide epitope (galactose-α 1,3-galactose) and the consequence of early graft thrombosis were major hurdles to overcome. With the development of knockout animals without the enzyme to make epitope, xenotransplantation was thought to be eminent. However, kidneys from α 1,3-galactosyltransferase knockout (GalT-KO) pigs still had significant rejection episodes due to strong xenogeneic T-cell immunity. The protective modulating role of the thymus has been recognized for some time. These authors demonstrated that concomitant transplantation of a graft with combined pig GalT-KO thymus and kidney allows for significant long-term function and improved results when transplanted into a baboon. This finally provides some hope that xenotransplantation may become a clinical reality.

T. Pruett, MD

Transplantation of monocyte-derived hepatocyte-like cells (NeoHeps) improves survival in a model of acute liver failure

Glanemann M, Gaebelein G, Nussler N, et al (Universitätsmedizin Berlin, Germany)

Ann Surg 249:149-154, 2009

Objective.—Investigation of the efficacy of implantation of monocyte-derived hepatocyte-like cells (NeoHeps) in acute liver failure.

Summary Background Data.—Extended liver resection or split liver transplantation is still associated with high morbidity and mortality because of postoperative liver insufficiency. In view of liver support systems, implantation of isolated hepatocytes or hepatocyte-like cells such as NeoHeps is increasingly under discussion.

Methods.—Twenty-four hours before subtotal hepatectomy, cells of different origin [A: human mononuclear cells (24 × 10(6)); B: NeoHeps (16 × 10(6)); C: NeoHeps (24 × 10(6)); D: rat hepatocytes (24 × 10(6))] were injected into the spleen of Wistar rats. After an observation period of 5 days, animal survival, postoperative weight, and signs of encephalopathy were recorded. At the end of the observation period, blood was collected for laboratory analysis.

Results.—Transplantation of both rat hepatocytes and NeoHeps significantly improved animal survival when compared with control animals (group A: 21%), reaching 72% in group D ($P = 0.001$), 50% in group C ($P = 0.04$), and 36% in group B ($P = 0.22$). Moreover, animals in these groups postoperatively experienced less frequently signs of encephalopathy, as well as earlier weight increase when compared with group A.

Discussion.—Hepatocyte transplantation is a practicable and successful treatment option in case of liver insufficiency because implantation of NeoHeps or primary rat hepatocytes had an improving effect on survival. The promising data of the present study warrants further analysis to elucidate the role of NeoHeps in treatment of acute postoperative liver failure to a greater extent.

► In some diseases, cell transplantation should be as effective as organ transplantation. If successful transplantation of autogeneic cells were possible, the need for immunosuppression would be avoided. While stem cell transplants have captured most attention, the observation that other cells can assume various phenotypes could potentially be another source of organs. Demonstration that manipulation and infusion of peripheral blood mononuclear cells resulted in improved survival of mice with acute liver failure is an exciting proof of concept.

T. Pruett, MD

Dynamics of human regulatory T cells in lung lavages of lung transplant recipients

Neujahr DC, Cardona AC, Ulukpo O, et al (Emory Univ School of Medicine, Atlanta, GA)

Transplantation 88:521-527, 2009

Background.—Despite advances in the field of lung transplantation, the median survival after lung transplant remains below 5 years. Early rejection is a risk factor for the development of chronic rejection. In animal models of transplant tolerance, regulatory T cells (Tregs) can prevent the establishment of rejection.

Methods.—This study was designed to explore the dynamics of Tregs focally and systemically in lung transplant recipients. Sequential surveillance bronchoscopy results were available in 51 patients with at least four sequential samples recovered from each patient at defined times posttransplant. In 36 individuals, a complete year of follow-up data for BAL was analyzed. In 33 of these individuals had a complete year of follow-up data for peripheral blood monocyte cell specimens were also analyzed. Lung lavage cells were recovered from each bronchoscopy and corresponding blood draw and subjected to polychromatic flow cytometry. The percentage of CD4 lymphocytes, which expressed the intracellular transcription factor FoxP3 was recorded at each point. At each time point, lung biopsy specimens were scored for rejection.

Results.—Lung Treg frequency was significantly more variable than blood Treg frequency. Treg frequency in the lung was increased in the aftermath of acute rejection. In contrast, lung Treg frequency declined sequentially in patients demonstrating continued quiescence. Mean BAL Treg level integrated over the first transplant year correlated inversely with the degree of acute cellular rejection. In contrast, blood Treg levels demonstrated no correlation with lung pathology.

Conclusions.—Lung Tregs increase in the setting of acute cellular rejection, whereas declining levels of BAL Tregs correlates with immunologic quiescence.

▶ One would hope that the circulating cells in the blood would be representative of what is happening at a distal site. Unfortunately, when one examines the cells within the peripheral blood and organs, the populations of cells do not appear to be of the same composition. Understanding cell trafficking and homing signals will help better design cell therapies for clinical application.

T. Pruett, MD

6 Surgical Infection

Introduction

Infection continues to be a significant component of the surgeon's practice. Often, a surgeon's skills are necessary for resolution of an infection and occasionally an infection is produced in the wound that a surgeon makes. In either case, the morbidity for the person with the infection is at best troublesome. Prevention of surgical site infections (SSI) has been a goal since surgery began. The identification of techniques that can minimize risk is continually being refined and expanded. What follows is a brief discussion of the articles that I reviewed this year.

It has repetitively been demonstrated that SSIs are not only an unwanted outcome for the patient, but also is more expensive in terms of health care. This finding was again reaffirmed by assessing outcomes from over 25 000 selected colorectal cases.[1] Several observations were made. First, current rates of SSI were low—3.7%; however, people with higher SENIC scores (sicker) and those procedures with significant potential for contamination (stoma formation) were significantly more likely to develop SSI than those with lower scores. It is not surprising that costs associated with providing care for people with SSI is higher than in those without infection. Because of the greater resource expenditure associated with SSI, hospital epidemiologists are continually looking for methods to estimate rates. Most assessments are made through chart review and documentation. An automated approach assessing patient antibiotic utilization linked with ICD-9 codes during either the hospitalization of the procedure or a readmission was effective in identifying patients with SSI, but more importantly found that the rates were nearly double that identified through conventional practice.[2] Consistent identification of SSI is an important portion of hospital epidemiology and this tool may be useful.

Many process elements have been associated with reduction in frequency of SSI, such as eliminating preop skin shaves, timely administration of antimicrobial administration immediately prior to incision, etc. Assessment of operative techniques and risk of wound complications has long been taught as influencing SSI, but a recent randomized study comparing "wide" fascial closure techniques to "short" and frequent closure led to the striking finding that shorter, more frequent sutures were associated with fewer SSI and a lower rate of dehiscence.[3] OR technique has long been predicated upon maintenance of aseptic practice. A review of the surgical outcomes demonstrated that holes in surgical gloves were associated with a two-fold increase in SSI over baseline.[4] The use of wound protectors that are designed to minimize contamination of the subcutaneous tissues while performing procedures in an infected field has been debated. A randomized study of use of a wound protector in people undergoing open appendectomy demonstrated a reduction of SSI from 14.6% to 1.6% by the utilization of a wound protector.[5] While many criticisms can be made of these studies, the message that surgical techniques have influence on SSI is irrefutable and the careful surgical technique and minimization of wound contamination will influence outcomes. Adjuncts in the perioperative time period have generated significant debate. Supplemental oxygen administered to the surgical patient has been the subject of numerous studies, with ambiguous results. A meta-analysis of randomized, double-blind studies comparing supplemental oxygen delivery in the peri-operative period[6] demonstrated a beneficial effect. The use of allogenic/blood bank transfusions has repetitively been demonstrated to increase the risk for post operative infections (SSI and others). A recent report of outcomes after cardiac and orthopedic surgery reconfirmed that people receiving transfusions were more likely to develop infections.[7] In this era of shortened hospitalizations, the observation that almost 50% of the infections occurred outside of the hospital is an important observation. The shifting delivery style of health care will change the observed set of adverse events. Not all surgical wounds have the same predisposition for infection. Surgical procedures in areas with poor blood supply and significant endogenous contamination are particularly susceptible. While clean procedures should typically have an SSI rate of less than 5%, peripheral vascular procedures in the infrainguinal region have traditionally been much higher. Despite knowledge of the variety of factors associated with reduction of SSI, the current rate of 9.4% still emphasizes the importance of variables associated with external bacterial contamination and the capacity for host immunity and healing.[8]

The organisms that cause surgical infections have traditionally been part of either the patient flora or, in the truly ill, the hospital flora. The community and hospital bacterial flora is becoming increasingly resistant to conventional antimicrobial agents. When this trend is associated with a decreasing pipeline of new agents, it has been the cause for concern. The Infectious Diseases Society of America has continued its clarion alarm that the adaptation of bacteria within our environment to antimicrobial agents is becoming an increasing problem within our community.[9] The practicing surgeon needs to be aware of the changes in his or her locale as the therapies for common organisms may not be constant. One of the major issues has been whether in vitro sensitivities that describe "appropriate" therapies for bacteria isolated from surgical wounds significantly influence outcomes. A retrospective analysis of treatment of SSI was performed with a comparator of appropriate or inappropriate spectrum of antibacterial agents[10] to the isolated organisms. Although it was found that inappropriate therapy was associated with longer length of stay and cost, the variables were considerable. Unfortunately, the presence of bacteria and other organisms that have become resistant to whole classes of antimicrobial agents is probably here to stay. The multiple drug-resistant gram-negative bacteria (MDRGNB) represents a serious problem for the hospitalized patient. These organisms often colonize the GI tract and are very slow to clear.[11] In following patients colonized with MDRGNB, it was noticed that persistence of colonization did not require antibiotic administration and *Proteus* MDRGNB appeared to persist in the GI flora for a protracted period of time. To the extent that such organisms are present with the fecal contamination of an operative wound or fistula, they are involved with surgical infections. Such infections can be very complicated and have marginal response to antimicrobial treatments. Methicillin-resistant *Staphylococcus aureus* is a bacterium that poses an increasing problem for the person who requires surgical interventions. As the organism increasingly penetrates the community, the epidemiology community is searching for ways to assess for outbreaks from either virulent organisms or breaches in protocol to minimize patient-to-patient transmission. In this regard, the application of PCR analysis of the coagulase gene (that protein that is thought to define *Staph aureus*) has been done.[12] This appears to be a practical and reasonably reliable process and will likely be used within surgical areas to assess the adequacy of techniques that minimize cross-colonization. In this study, the patterns of coagulase in methicillin-sensitive and -resistant bacteria appeared to be similar, although there were clear differences in bacteria. Such techniques have been used to assess other types of bacterial infections, such as *C. difficile*.[13] It is important to recognize that the bacterial flora that cause infections are not static and indeed even when the specific infection appears to be caused by a constant organism, there are often significant strain differences. This shift in microbial flora is even further witnessed in a survey of sternal SSI that demonstrated the recent and evolving role of *Candida sp* after cardiac surgery. They demonstrated in heart patients the same phenomena observed in general surgery patients: that a population afflicted by yeast tends to be sicker on the ventilator and in the hospital a longer period of time than those with more conventional infection. The striking variable of this study was the absence of *Candida* with surgical wounds for the first 3 years of observation and then its appearance. This timeline is suggestive of a change in hospital flora that had significant changes impacting outcomes.

Some diseases that were traditionally treated by surgical therapies have had a change in approach. Mycotic vascular infections were traditionally treated with resection of the involved vessel and extra-anatomic bypass. The advent of endovascular stenting has often led to the placement of an intralumenal device and subsequent treatment with antimicrobials. The experience of 11 patients treated with a combination of luminal therapy, antibiotics, and percutaneous drainage as needed demonstrated early excellent results,[14] but a real risk for progression and appearance in other sites of mycotic infection. While such therapy is a valuable adjunct, durability of treatment must be balanced with comorbidities of the patient. Colonic diverticular disease is another entity that has seen significant changes in recommended therapies. While there has been a marked reduction in colonic resections for chronic disease and abscess, the surgical procedures for perforation has remained reasonably stable.[15] The trends support the observation and contention that fewer colonic resections for diverticular diseases has not led to an increase in emergency surgical procedures for perforation, obstruction, or complicated disease.

Despite the tendency to delay or minimize treatments for many diseases traditionally managed through radical surgery, optimal management of certain infections is still best defined by the thoughtful surgeon. Surgical debridement of the phlegmon associated with necrotizing pancreatitis remains the mainstay of treatment. While morbidities associated with this disease remain high and recovery is protracted, survival after surgical management of this malady has become much lower than in the past.[16] With widespread migration of peoples from around the world, it is important to recognize those infectious diseases in which surgical therapy plays a major role. Hydatid disease is one such disease where, despite anti-parasitic therapies, disease persistence and spread can still occur. A variety of surgical techniques have been devised to provide effective eradication of the disease and reduce the risk of anaphylaxis associated with spillage of cyst contents.[17]

Surgeons live in a hazardous environment. Not only is the patient at risk for exposure and development of infection, the surgeon is as well. HIV is one of many infectious pathogens with which the practicing surgeon is likely to come in contact. In an era of multiple drug-resistant viruses, the question of how quick, how long, and with what should the exposed surgeon be treated? While much of the information is conjecture, current advice states that early treatment is better than late and that a course of no fewer than 28 days is optimal.[18] Treatment is associated with about an 80% reduction in risk of contracting HIV, but follow-up is required.

Infection continues to be a major component of surgical practice. The prevention of infection in the perioperative period is associated with improved patient outcomes and lower costs. Both are highly desirable in the era of outcomes and cost awareness. Besides prevention of surgical associated infections, recognition that surgical interventions are often necessary for optimal outcomes of some infections should not be lost. In the era of minimally invasive surgery and interventional radiologic treatments, the optimal use of open, operative intervention is often underestimated. While one should attempt to minimize deforming procedures, infection/source control is usually necessary for successful therapy of surgical infection. Despite the prophet's observation that that "there is nothing new under the sun," applications continue to evolve such that therapies are adapted to changing variables.

Timothy L. Pruett, MD

References

1. Mahmoud NN, Turpin RS, Yang G, Saunders WB. Impact of surgical site infections on length of stay and costs in selected colorectal procedures. *Surg Infect (Larchmt).* 2009;10:539-544.
2. Bolon MK, Hooper D, Stevenson KB, et al. Improved surveillance for surgical site infections after orthopedic implantation procedures: extending applications for automated data. *Clin Infect Dis.* 2009;48:1223-1229.
3. Millbourn D, Cengiz Y, Israelsson LA. Effect of stitch length on wound complications after closure of midline incisions: a randomized controlled trial. *Arch Surg.* 2009;144:1056-1059.
4. Misteli H, Weber WP, Reck S, et al. Surgical glove perforation and the risk of surgical site infection. *Arch Surg.* 2009;144:553-558.
5. Lee P, Waxman K, Taylor B, Yim S. Use of wound-protection system and postoperative wound-infection rates in open appendectomy: a randomized prospective trial. *Arch Surg.* 2009;144:872-875.
6. Qadan M, Akça O, Mahid SS, Hornung CA, Polk HC Jr. Perioperative supplemental oxygen therapy and surgical site infection: a meta-analysis of randomized controlled trials. *Arch Surg.* 2009;144:359-366.
7. Shander A, Spence RK, Adams D, Shore-Lesserson L, Walawander CA. Timing and incidence of postoperative infections associated with blood transfusion: analysis of 1,489 orthopedic and cardiac surgery patients. *Surg Infect (Larchmt).* 2009;10:277-283.
8. LaMuraglia GM, Conrad MF, Chung T, Hutter M, Watkins MT, Cambria RP. Significant perioperative morbidity accompanies contemporary infrainguinal bypass surgery: an NSQIP report. *J Vasc Surg.* 2009;50:299-304.
9. Boucher HW, Talbot GH, Bradley JS, et al. Bad bugs, no drugs: no ESKAPE! An update from the Infectious Diseases Society of America. *Clin Infect Dis.* 2009;48: 1-12.
10. Eagye KJ, Kim A, Laohavaleeson S, Kuti JL, Nicolau DP. Surgical site infections: does inadequate antibiotic therapy affect patient outcomes? *Surg Infect (Larchmt).* 2009;10:323-331.
11. O'Fallon E, Gautam S, D'Agata EM. Colonization with multidrug-resistant gram-negative bacteria: prolonged duration and frequent cocolonization. *Clin Infect Dis.* 2009;48:1375-1381.
12. Himabindu M, Muthamilselvan DS, Bishi DK, et al. Molecular analysis of coagulase gene polymorphism in clinical isolates of methicilin resistant *Staphylococcus aureus* by restriction fragment length polymorphism based genotyping. *Am J Infect Dis.* 2009;5:163-169.
13. Belmares J, Johnson S, Parada JP, et al. Molecular epidemiology of Clostridium difficile over the course of 10 years in a tertiary care hospital. *Clin Infect Dis.* 2009;49:1141-1147.
14. Sörelius K, Mani K, Björck M, Nyman R, Wanhainen A. Endovascular repair of mycotic aortic aneurysms. *J Vasc Surg.* 2009;50:269-274.
15. Ricciardi R, Baxter NN, Read TE, Marcello PW, Hall J, Roberts PL. Is the decline in the surgical treatment for diverticulitis associated with an increase in complicated diverticulitis? *Dis Colon Rectum.* 2009;52:1558-1563.
16. Parikh PY, Pitt HA, Kilbane M, et al. Pancreatic necrosectomy: North American mortality is much lower than expected. *J Am Coll Surg.* 2009;209:712-719.
17. Jamshidi R, Hill A, Harris H. Anaphylaxis caused by recurrent hydatid disease. *Surg Infect (Larchmt).* 2009;10:155-157.
18. Landovitz RJ, Currier JS. Clinical practice. Postexposure prophylaxis for HIV infection. *N Engl J Med.* 2009;361:1768-1775.

Impact of surgical site infections on length of stay and costs in selected colorectal procedures

Mahmoud NN, Turpin RS, Yang G, et al (Hosp of the Univ of Pennsylvania, Philadelphia)

Surg Infect (Larchmt) 10:539-544, 2009

Background.—Length of stay (LOS) and inpatient costs for open-abdomen colorectal procedures have not been examined recently. The aim of this study was to determine LOS and costs for several colorectal procedures in the context of factors potentially associated with surgical site infection (SSI).

Methods.—We used a large U.S. hospital database to identify the variables associated with longer LOS and higher costs for colorectal procedures from January 1, 2005, through June 30, 2006. The study population consisted of all patients >18 years, identified via International Classification of Disease, Ninth Revision, procedural codes for elective colorectal surgery. Patient demographics, surgical procedure, and a modified Study of the Efficacy of Nosocomial Infection Control (SENIC) infection risk score were examined using logistic regression as predictors of LOS ≥1 week and cost ≥$15,000. Patients given cefotetan as surgical prophylaxis were compared with patients given cefazolin/metronidazole. Superficial and deep SSIs were considered; intra-abdominal infection was not.

Results.—The 25,825 patients were of average age 63 years, with 53% being female and 75% being Caucasian. The overall infection rate was 3.7%. The mean LOS was 7.25 days, and the mean ± standard deviation total cost per patient $13,746 ± $13,330. Rates of infection, LOS, and mean hospital costs were all greater for patients with a high SENIC score and increasing disease acuity. Values for these outcome variables were highest for procedures involving stoma formation, followed by operations on the small bowel and large bowel. Variables independently predictive of longer LOS were SSI (odds ratio [OR] 11.74; 95% confidence interval [CI] 9.67, 14.26), age ≥65 years (OR 1.90; 95% CI 1.81, 2.01), and high SENIC score (OR 1.79; 95% CI 1.67, 1.92), whereas Caucasian race (OR 0.86; 95% CI 0.81, 0.91) was predictive of a shorter LOS. Cefazolin/metronidazole was not predictive of a shorter LOS compared with cefotetan (OR 1.06; 95% CI 0.96, 1.17) but was associated with significantly more hospitalizations with costs ≥$15,000 (OR 1.39; 95% CI 1.23, 1.56).

Conclusions.—Length of stay and cost rise proportionally with SENIC score, disease acuity, and patient characteristics such as age. Surgical site infections are significantly and independently associated with LOS and cost and contribute to inpatient morbidity and expense. Cefotetan has limited availability, and substitutions are utilized increasingly. Although equally efficacious in elective colon procedures, cefotetan used as surgical prophylaxis was associated with lower hospitalization costs than cefazolin plus metronidazole.

▶ The occurrence of surgical site infection (SSI) has a significant impact on cost for the United States health care system. Understanding the variables operative during the changing delivery patterns in the United States is important for the practicing surgeon. An 18-month review of 25 825 people undergoing bowel surgery revealed interesting observations. Problems with interpretation of the conclusions from this sort of review reside with the assumptions that are necessary to evaluate the data. The overall infection rate in this study is quite low—below 4%. The definition of SSI was standard, but the authors did not mention where the SSIs were identified. As the data came from a hospital system, it is likely that only infections identified during a hospitalization were captured and those found as an outpatient were not mentioned, and the cost of caring for these people was also probably missed. The authors demonstrated that individuals with significant comorbidities and SSI contribute to higher costs. Hardly shocking, but these data emphasize that it can be expensive to care for those people who are sick.

T. Pruett, MD

Improved surveillance for surgical site infections after orthopedic implantation procedures: extending applications for automated data

Bolon MK, Centers for Disease Control and Prevention Epicenters Program (Northwestern Univ Feinberg School of Medicine, Chicago, IL)

Clin Infect Dis 48:1223-1229, 2009

Background.—Screening methods that use automated data may streamline surgical site infection (SSI) surveillance and improve the accuracy and comparability of data on SSIs. We evaluated the use of automated inpatient diagnosis codes and pharmacy data to identify SSIs after arthroplasty.

Methods.—This retrospective cohort study at 8 hospitals involved weighted, random samples of medical records from 2128 total hip arthroplasty (THA) procedures performed from 1 July 2002 through 30 June 2004, and 4194 total knee arthroplasty (TKA) procedures performed from 1 July 2003 through 30 June 2005. We compared routine surveillance with screening of inpatient pharmacy data and diagnoses codes followed by medical record review to confirm SSI status.

Results.—Records from 696 THA and 1009 TKA procedures were reviewed. The SSI rates were nearly double those determined by routine surveillance (1.32% [95% confidence interval, 0.83%-1.81%] vs. 0.75% for THA; 1.83% [95% confidence interval, 1.43%-2.23%] vs. 0.71% for TKA). An inpatient diagnosis code for infection within a year after the operation had substantially higher sensitivity (THA, 89%; TKA, 81%), compared with routine surveillance (THA, 56%; TKA, 39%). Adding antimicrobial exposure of 7 days after the procedure increased the sensitivity (THA, 93%; TKA, 86%). Record review confirmed SSIs after 51% of THAs and 55% of TKAs that met diagnosis code criteria and after 25% of THAs and 39% of TKAs that met antimicrobial exposure and/or diagnosis code criteria.

Conclusions.—Focused surveillance among a subset of patients who met diagnosis code screening criteria with or without the addition of antimicrobial exposure-based screening was more sensitive than routine surveillance for detecting SSIs after arthroplasty and could be an efficient and readily standardized adjunct to traditional methods.

▶ Reliable surveillance for surgical site infection (SSI) has proven to be vexing. Direct observation of the surgical wound by an independent observer is the most reliable but most expensive. Many other surrogates have been used with moderate to significant discord rates of infection identification. The method described in this article is proposed as an adjunct to decrease the miss rate of certain infections. Using an automated linkage of ICD codes and antibiotic usage through the pharmacy, SSI rates associated with orthopedic implantation procedures were found to be nearly double than identified with conventional infection control measures. One of the reasons is that conventional diagnosis is quite dependent upon microbiology, whereas the technique described in this report tracks physician-prescribing behavior and clinical reaction to a situation. By linking different databases, this approach represents one of many that will potentially deliver a more representative analysis of the incidence of clinically relevant SSI in the surgical population.

T. Pruett, MD

Effect of Stitch Length on Wound Complications After Closure of Midline Incisions: A Randomized Controlled Trial

Millbourn D, Cengiz Y, Israelsson LA (Sundsvall Hosp, Sweden; Umeå Univ, Sweden)

Arch Surg 144:1056-1059, 2009

Hypothesis.—In midline incisions closed with a single-layer running suture, the rate of wound complications is lower when a suture length to wound length ratio of at least 4 is accomplished with a short stitch length rather than with a long one.

Design.—Prospective randomized controlled trial.

Setting.—Surgical department.

Patients.—Patients operated on through a midline incision.

Intervention.—Wound closure with a short stitch length (ie, placing stitches <10 mm from the wound edge) or a long stitch length.

Main Outcome Measures.—Wound dehiscence, surgical site infection, and incisional hernia.

Results.—In all, 737 patients were randomized: 381 were allocated to a long stitch length and 356, to a short stitch length. Wound dehiscence occurred in 1 patient whose wound was closed with a long stitch length. Surgical site infection occurred in 35 of 343 patients (10.2%) in the long stitch group and in 17 of 326 (5.2%) in the short stitch group ($P = .02$). Incisional hernia was present in 49 of 272 patients (18.0%) in the long stitch group and in 14 of 250 (5.6%) in the short stitch group ($P < .001$). In multivariate analysis, a long stitch length was an independent risk factor for both surgical site infection and incisional hernia.

Conclusion.—In midline incisions closed with a running suture and having a suture length to wound length ratio of at least 4, current recommendations of placing stitches at least 10 mm from the wound edge should be changed to avoid patient suffering and costly wound complications.

Trial Registration.—clinicaltrials.gov Identifier: NCT00508053.

▶ Technique has always been an important facet of avoiding complications. This study re-emphasizes that such is still true today. While mass closure is often considered the closure of choice, this study questions the claim and gives alternative rationale for more precision in wound closure without the creation of necrotic tissue. Running suture closure of wounds is now mainstay, but the recommendation that placement of a short interval between stitches (suture length:wound length > 4) has not had solid data. This randomized study gives new rationale to reconsider the practice. Surgical site infection (SSI) was reduced from 10% to 5%, and incisional hernia formation was reduced from 18% to 6%. While there was a slightly lower frequency of dirty wounds in the short suture group, it was not statistically significant and the patient characteristics were otherwise quite comparable. This is a provocative study that should be discussed by all residents in training.

T. Pruett, MD

Surgical glove perforation and the risk of surgical site infection

Misteli H, Weber WP, Reck S, et al (Univ Hosp Basel, Switzerland)

Arch Surg 144:553-558, 2009

Hypothesis.—Clinically apparent surgical glove perforation increases the risk of surgical site infection (SSI).

Design.—Prospective observational cohort study.

Setting.—University Hospital Basel, with an average of 28,000 surgical interventions per year.

Participants.—Consecutive series of 4147 surgical procedures performed in the Visceral Surgery, Vascular Surgery, and Traumatology divisions of the Department of General Surgery.

Main Outcome Measures.—The outcome of interest was SSI occurrence as assessed pursuant to the Centers of Disease Control and Prevention standards. The primary predictor variable was compromised asepsis due to glove perforation.

Results.—The overall SSI rate was 4.5% (188 of 4147 procedures). Univariate logistic regression analysis showed a higher likelihood of SSI in procedures in which gloves were perforated compared with interventions with maintained asepsis (odds ratio [OR], 2.0; 95% confidence interval [CI], 1.4-2.8; $P < .001$). However, multivariate logistic regression analyses showed that the increase in SSI risk with perforated gloves was different for procedures with vs those without surgical antimicrobial prophylaxis (test for effect modification, $P = .005$). Without antimicrobial prophylaxis, glove perforation entailed significantly higher odds of SSI compared with the reference group with no breach of asepsis (adjusted OR, 4.2; 95% CI, 1.7-10.8; $P = .003$). On the contrary, when surgical antimicrobial prophylaxis was applied, the likelihood of SSI was not significantly higher for operations in which gloves were punctured (adjusted OR, 1.3; 95% CI, 0.9-1.9; $P = .26$).

Conclusion.—Without surgical antimicrobial prophylaxis, glove perforation increases the risk of SSI.

▶ Part of the ritual of SSI avoidance has been the maintenance of asepsis during the operative procedure. This study from Basel demonstrated what many had surmised: while a hole in the surgical glove increases the likelihood of wound infection, the risk can be negated with antimicrobial prophylaxis. This was a particularly labor-intensive study with multiple reminders and intraoperative observations. While the risk for SSI increases with identified breaches in aseptic technique, the impact of the common United States practice of double gloving was not evaluated. Despite the limitations of the study, it highlights the importance of maintaining asepsis during periods when the patient's skin is open and the introduction of bacterial contamination significantly increases the risk for SSI.

T. Pruett, MD

Use of Wound-Protection System and Postoperative Wound-Infection Rates in Open Appendectomy: A Randomized Prospective Trial

Lee P, Waxman K, Taylor B, et al (Santa Barbara Cottage Hosp, CA)

Arch Surg 144:872-875, 2009

Objective.—To determine if use of a wound-protection system in open appendectomy decreases the rate of wound infection.

Design.—A randomized prospective trial.

Setting.—A community hospital.

Patients.—One hundred nine patients undergoing open appendectomy.

Intervention.—Randomly assigned conventional retraction or retraction with the wound-protection system. Patients were blinded to the study arm in which they were enrolled. All patients were given standardized preoperative antibiotics. Demographics including age, sex, body mass index, history of diabetes, and tobacco use were recorded. The severity of appendicitis as determined by the attending surgeon at the time of operation was also noted.

Main Outcome Measures.—Incidence of wound infection at 21 days postoperatively.

Results.—Of the 48 patients enrolled in the traditional retraction arm, there were 7 (14.6%) documented wound infections. Of the 61 patients enrolled in the wound-protection device arm, there was 1 (1.6%) wound infection. The severity of appendicitis between the 2 groups was matched. The decrease in incidence of wound infection observed with the wound-protection system was significant ($P = .02$).

Conclusion.—Use of a wound-protection system reduces the incidence of surgical wound infection in open appendectomy.

Trial Registration.—clinicaltrials.gov Identifier: NCT00323453.

▶ Wound protectors have been part of the surgical armamentarium for years but have failed to gain uniform acceptance. The premise is reasonably simple—put a barrier between operative contamination and the soft tissue in order to reduce the risk of residual bacteria at the time of wound closure. The randomized study presented here demonstrates the feasibility of reducing SSI for open appendectomies. While the premise may be right, changing technology limits the applicability of the open approach. Additionally, the efficacy of maintaining an appropriate barrier in other procedures with variable time durations and significant contamination remains questionable. While the idea of wound protection through bacterial barriers is sound, its penetration into clinical practice remains erratic because of the variables.

T. Pruett, MD

Perioperative Supplemental Oxygen Therapy and Surgical Site Infection: A Meta-analysis of Randomized Controlled Trials

Qadan M, Akça O, Mahid SS, et al (Univ of Louisville School of Medicine, KY)

Arch Surg 144:359-366, 2009

Objective.—To conduct a meta-analysis of randomized controlled trials in which high inspired oxygen concentrations were compared with standard concentrations to assess the effect on the development of surgical site infections (SSIs).

Data Sources.—A systematic literature search was conducted using the MEDLINE, EMBASE, and Cochrane databases and included a manual search of references of original articles, poster presentations, and abstracts from major meetings ("gray" literature).

Study Selection.—Twenty-one of 2167 articles met the inclusion criteria. Of these, 5 randomized controlled trials (3001 patients) assessed the effect of perioperative supplemental oxygen use on the SSI rate. Studies used a treatment- inspired oxygen concentration of 80%. Maximum follow-up was 30 days.

Data Extraction.—Data were abstracted by 3 independent reviewers using a standardized data collection form. Relative risks were reported using a fixed-effects model. Results were subjected to publication bias testing and sensitivity analyses.

Data Synthesis.—Infection rates were 12.0% in the control group and 9.0% in the hyperoxic group, with relative risk reduction of 25.3% (95% confidence interval [CI], 8.1%-40.1%) and absolute risk reduction of 3.0% (1.1%-5.3%). The overall risk ratio was 0.742 (95% CI, 0.599-0.919; $P = .006$). The benefit from increasing oxygen concentration was greater in colorectal-specific procedures, with a risk ratio of 0.556 (95% CI, 0.383-0.808; $P = .002$).

Conclusions.—Perioperative supplemental oxygen therapy exerts a significant beneficial effect in the prevention of SSIs. We recommend its use along with maintenance of normothermia, meticulous glycemic control, and preservation of intravascular volume perioperatively in the prevention of SSIs.

▶ Supplemental perioperative oxygen therapy remains one of the simplest conceptual ways to reduce surgical site infections (SSI). The studies performed to assess its efficacy have yielded conflicting results. A meta-analysis of the relevant literature revealed a winnowing of articles. The systematic search of the medical literature using inclusion criteria revealed 2167 articles of which 21 met the inclusion criteria. Of these, only 5 articles (3001 patients) reported the results of randomized trials to assess the effect of perioperative supplemental oxygen on SSI rates and as the invited critique points out, inconsistencies persist even within these articles. However, the evidence still suggests that a reduction of SSI by about 25% is likely associated with supplemental perioperative oxygen (2-6 hours after wound closure), making this a simple, relatively cheap adjunct.

T. Pruett, MD

Timing and incidence of postoperative infections associated with blood transfusion: analysis of 1,489 orthopedic and cardiac surgery patients

Shander A, Spence RK, Adams D, et al (Englewood Hosp and Med Ctr, NJ)

Surg Infect (Larchmt) 10:277-283, 2009

Background.—Transfusion rates remain high in cardiac and orthopedic surgery and differ widely across physician practices in spite of growing knowledge that allogeneic blood transfusion (ABT) is associated with a risk of postoperative infection.

Methods.—This prospective observational study compared the timing and incidence of ABT-associated postoperative infections (PIs) in 1,489 orthopedic or cardiac surgery patients at nine hospitals.

Results.—Of 455 cardiovascular and 1,034 orthopedic surgery patients, 415 (55.6% of the cardiovascular patients and 15.7% of the orthopedic patients) were given ABT. The overall rate of PI during hospitalization was 5.8%. The relative risk of PI was 3.6-fold greater after ABT (50 patients; 12.1%) than in patients not having ABT (36 patients; 3.4%; 95% confidence interval 2.4, 5.4; $p = 0.001$). Postoperative infections appeared both during hospitalization ($n = 86$) and within four weeks after discharge ($n = 81$).

Conclusions.—Patients should be followed for as long as four weeks after discharge to determine the true incidence and risk of ABT-associated PI.

▶ Transfusion has long been associated with increased risk for surgical site infection (SSI). The causes have been many but are typically thought to be associated with changes in perfusion and identification of a sicker population by the skeptics and by immunologic changes in infection susceptibility by those asserting a more direct association. The association persists in this report, and the causality as to why there is a higher rate in those receiving transfusions is not clarified. The study demonstrates that differences in threshold for transfusion exists within different systems. It also demonstrated that a univariate analysis of administration of transfusion was associated with SSI, but whether this risk can be overcome with temperature control, oxygen, and prophylactic antibiotics was not addressed. It remains to be seen how much increased risk of infection through transfusion can be overcome by other techniques.

T. Pruett, MD

Significant perioperative morbidity accompanies contemporary infrainguinal bypass surgery: an NSQIP report

LaMuraglia GM, Conrad MF, Chung T, et al (Massachusetts General Hosp and Harvard Med School, Boston)

J Vasc Surg 50:299-304, 304.e1-4, 2009

Objectives.—A variety of clinical and anatomic factors influence the choice between infrainguinal bypass surgery (BPG) and percutaneous endovascular procedures (PTA) to treat lower extremity vascular disease. The decision, in part, is dependant on periprocedural morbidity. The goal of this study was to document the contemporary morbidity and mortality of infrainguinal BPG, utilizing the previously validated National Surgical Quality Improvement Program (NSQIP) database.

Methods.—Data from the private sector NSQIP, a prospectively validated systematic-sample database, using Current Procedural Terminology (CPT) codes for all infrainguinal BPG performed between January 1, 2005, and December 31, 2006, were analyzed. Study endpoints included 30-day death and NSQIP-defined major complications, including graft failure, differentiated between systemic vs operative-site related complications. Potentially associated clinical variables were assessed by univariate methods to create the multivariate models of factors associated with study endpoints.

Results.—There were 2404 infrainguinal BPG (infrapopliteal distal anastomosis 42%, prosthetic 29%) performed in the study interval with patient variables: age 67 ± 12, male 66%, diabetes 44%, limb salvage indications 48%. The 30-day composite mortality/major morbidity was 19.5%. The overall mortality was 2.7% and correlated with (P value, odds ratio [OR]): patient age (<.001, 1.056), low body weight (.007, 0.988), significant preoperative dyspnea (.03, 1.97), dialysis (.003, 5.26), history transient ischemic attack (.03, 2.43), and bleeding disorder (.02, 2.01). Major complications occurred in 18.7% patients, including 7.4% graft thromboses, and 9.4% wound infections. Major systemic complications occurred in 5.9% and correlated with: age (.001, 1.03), history myocardial infarction (.02, 2.37), dialysis (<.001, 2.52), impaired sensorium (.005, 2.93), and general (vs regional) anesthesia (.04, 1.9). Major operative site-related complications occurred in 15.1% and correlated with: history chronic obstructive pulmonary disease (.04, 1.40), limb salvage indication (<.001, 1.71), impaired sensorium (.01, 2.26), non-independent preoperative functional status (.03, 1.37), and operative time (<.001, 1.002). The combination of dialysis and age >80 was identified as the most powerful high-risk composite for death (13.3-fold) and major complications (2.2-fold).

Conclusion.—Infrainguinal BPG is accompanied by significant major morbidity and mortality in contemporary practice. These results reinforce the precept that stringent indications for BPG should be maintained, when considering the method of lower extremity revascularization.

▶ The desire to decrease surgical site infection (SSI) must be tempered by the reality of conditions in the surgical site. Peripheral vascular surgery is typically performed in an area of reduced perfusion and hence an increased risk for SSI. Additionally, these people have other morbidities that lead to more difficult recovery. While often the practicing surgeon finds SSI to be a price of business, the finding of this report was that the 30-day cardiac complication was low, 1%. While not 1 factor could be identified to explain the outcome, the wound complication rate was around 10%, similar to the prior VA wound infection rate of 12%. Certainly there continues to be a need for better application of techniques to minimize SSI in this high-risk population. It is discouraging after all the studies using prophylactic antimicrobial therapies, aseptic techniques, glucose control, supplemental oxygen delivery, skin protection, etc that the wound infection rate in this population remains persistently high. Perhaps this speaks more to the definitions found in large databases and the confounding clinical variables than it does to some of the technique variables. However, the goals should be to demonstrate techniques that allow for improvements in clinical care.

T. Pruett, MD

Bad bugs, no drugs: no ESKAPE! An update from the Infectious Diseases Society of America

Boucher HW, Talbot GH, Bradley JS, et al (Tufts Univ and Tufts Med Ctr, Boston, MA)

Clin Infect Dis 48:1-12, 2009

The Infectious Diseases Society of America (IDSA) continues to view with concern the lean pipeline for novel therapeutics to treat drug-resistant infections, especially those caused by gram-negative pathogens. Infections now occur that are resistant to all current antibacterial options. Although the IDSA is encouraged by the prospect of success for some agents currently in preclinical development, there is an urgent, immediate need for new agents with activity against these panresistant organisms. There is no evidence that this need will be met in the foreseeable future. Furthermore, we remain concerned that the infrastructure for discovering and developing new antibacterials continues to stagnate, thereby risking the future pipeline of antibacterial drugs. The IDSA proposed solutions in its 2004 policy report, "Bad Bugs, No Drugs: As Antibiotic R&D Stagnates, a Public Health Crisis Brews," and recently issued a "Call to Action" to provide an update on the scope of the problem and the proposed solutions. A primary objective of these periodic reports is to encourage a community and legislative response to establish greater financial parity between the antimicrobial development and the development of other drugs. Although recent actions of the Food and Drug Administration and the 110th US Congress present a glimmer of hope, significant uncertainly remains. Now, more than ever, it is essential to create a robust and sustainable antibacterial research and development infrastructure—one that can respond to current antibacterial resistance now and anticipate evolving resistance. This challenge requires that industry, academia, the National Institutes of Health, the Food and Drug Administration, the Centers for Disease Control and Prevention, the US Department of Defense, and the new Biomedical Advanced Research and Development Authority at the Department of Health and Human Services work productively together. This report provides an update on potentially effective antibacterial drugs in the late-stage development pipeline, in the hope of encouraging such collaborative action.

▶ A mainstay of therapy for surgical patients has been the administration of antibiotics to either kill the offending bacteria or prevent their growth. Recent emergence of bacteria that are resistant to a wide range of antimicrobial agents has been the cause for concern. The Infectious Diseases Society of America (IDSA) has become increasingly concerned about the dearth of agents in the development pipeline and the potential impact on future care. The list of organisms for which the advisory group notes gaps in drug development are common pathogens in the contemporary surgical unit. VRE, MRSA, KPC, and ESBL-GNR are commonly found in surgical wounds of patients. *Acinetobacter baumannii* is becoming a common burn and ventilator-associated organism. Contemporary surgery may be rapidly moving toward a time when the use of effective prophylactic and therapeutic agents to prevent and treat surgical infections is compromised. We should also have the concerns of the IDSA regarding the well-being of our patients.

T. Pruett, MD

Surgical site infections: does inadequate antibiotic therapy affect patient outcomes?

Eagye KJ, Kim A, Laohavaleeson S, et al (Hartford Hosp, CT)
Surg Infect (Larchmt) 10:323-331, 2009

Background.—Complicated skin/skin structure infections involve deeper soft tissues and include surgical site infections (SSIs). Inadequate antibiotic therapy (IAT) has been associated with adverse outcomes in respiratory and blood stream infections, but is seldom evaluated in SSIs. This study assessed the impact of IAT on primary outcomes of length of stay (LOS) and costs in complicated SSIs; identifying risk factors associated with receiving IAT was a secondary objective.

Methods.—This retrospective cohort study of discharges from our 810-bed urban teaching hospital from Quarter 4/2004-Quarter 1/2006 identified 130 patients with complicated SSI among 298 patients with postoperative infections. Superficial infections and infections not involving the skin/skin structures were excluded. Patient characteristics, culture data, and antibiotic history were collected from charts. Inadequate antibiotic therapy was said to have occurred when a drug active against the organism cultured was not given within 24 h of culture. Multiple regression identified variables associated with LOS and increase hospital accounting costs.

Results.—A total of 39 subjects (30%) received IAT; patient characteristics did not differ from those receiving adequate therapy, except that prior antibiotic use was more likely in IAT subjects ($p = 0.053$). Staphylococcus aureus (45% methicillin-resistant) was the most common pathogen (39%). More than one-half (60%) of the subjects received empiric vancomycin. The IAT patients experienced longer post-infection LOS and higher costs (median [25%, 75%]): 10 [6, 21] days vs. 7 [4, 11] days; $p = 0.007$ and $11,746 [$6,652, $28,442] vs. $7,116 [$5,210, $16,443]; $p = 0.04$). Longer LOS was associated significantly with Acute Physiology and Chronic Health Evaluation score, IAT, Pseudomonas infection, and sternal incisions, as were higher costs, excepting Pseudomonas infection. Inadequate antibiotic therapy was more likely in polymicrobial infections ($p < 0.001$), pseudomonal ($p < 0.001$) or enterococcal ($p = 0.002$) infections, and infected abdominal incisions ($p < 0.001$). Methicillin-resistant S. aureus was not associated with adverse outcomes, possibly because empiric therapy frequently included vancomycin.

Conclusions.—Inadequate antibiotic therapy is associated with longer LOS and higher costs in complicated SSIs. Risk factors for IAT include prior antibiotic therapy, polymicrobial infection, infection with P. aeruginosa or Enterococcus spp., and abdominal incisions.

▶ The cost associated with inadequate antibiotic therapy for SSIs was assessed. The data should cause some concerns. Thirty percent of patients with SSI received inadequate antimicrobial therapies. This is especially concerning, as the study time was from 2004-2006, and problems associated with bacterial resistance have not diminished. Those receiving suboptimal therapies had longer hospital stays and costs. Not surprisingly, failure in therapy was more common in polymicrobial, pseudomonal, enterococcal, and intra-abdominal infections. Fortunately, mortality was similar in this small population, but duration of hospitalization and cost of therapy were significantly increased in the population in which inadequate therapy was assessed. Interestingly, MRSA was not a significant pathogen, but as described in this article, vancomycin had become the commonly prescribed drug. This observation demonstrates the commonality of resistant organisms within the hospital setting.

T. Pruett, MD

Colonization with multidrug-resistant gram-negative bacteria: prolonged duration and frequent cocolonization

O'Fallon E, Gautam S, D'Agata EM (Beth Israel Deaconess Med Ctr, Boston, MA)

Clin Infect Dis 48:1375-1381, 2009

Background.—The characteristics of colonization with multidrug-resistant gram-negative bacteria (MDRGNB) in the gastrointestinal tract have not been well defined. Characterizing the duration of colonization, clearance of colonization, and frequency of cocolonization would provide important information for the development of interventions targeting the prevention of MDRGNB spread.

Methods.—From 31 October 2006 through 22 October 2007, serial rectal cultures were obtained every 3-4 weeks from residents of a long-term care facility. Clearance of colonization was defined as ≥ 2 consecutive cultures from which MDRGNB were not recovered. Factors associated with clearance of colonization were analyzed using time-to-event methods.

Results.—Thirty-three patients colonized with 57 MDRGNB isolates were followed up for a median of 211 days (range, 63-356 days). Twenty (61%) of the patients were colonized with ≥ 1 different MDRGNB species (median, 2 strains; range, 1-4 strains). The median duration of MDRGNB colonization was 144 days (range, 41-349 days). Clearance of colonization with all MDRGNB strains occurred in 3 patients (9%). Clearance of MDRGNB colonization, calculated by colonizing strain, occurred in 22 (39%) of 57 MDRGNB colonization episodes, with a rate of colonization clearance of 2.6 episodes per 1000 days. Clearance of multidrug-resistant Proteus mirabilis colonization occurred in 1 (6.7%) of

15 episodes, compared with clearance of 21 (50%) of 42 colonization episodes due to other MDRGNB species (hazard ratio, 0.1; 95% confidence interval, 0.01-0.78; P =.03).

Conclusions.—Patient colonization with MDRGNB is prolonged, and a substantial proportion of patients are colonized with multiple MDRGNB species. Multidrug-resistant P. mirabilis may have a survival advantage in the gastrointestinal tract, compared with other MDRGNB species.

▶ Oftentimes we are under the impression that the antibiotic-resistant organisms are dependent upon the environmental pressure within the hospital system in order to persist. The question of duration of colonization was addressed in this study of patients of a long-term care facility who were colonized with multidrug-resistant gram-negative bacteria (MDRGNB). It was surprising to note that the median duration of colonization was 144 days. A differential strain clearance was also noted, with *Proteus* cleared only once, but other strains of MDRGNB cleared in about 50% of cases. This should stress that the flora of people is likely changing, and previous exposures can result in long-term consequences. There are limitations in the application of the results of this study. There was no mention within the article of whether the subjects were readmitted to a hospital or had a close roommate with frequent readmissions. Additionally, it is likely that non-institutionalized persons will have a different kinetics of gut repopulation than those within a facility. However, despite the limitations of the population and some vagaries of the concomitant care, it should impress the practitioner that MDRGNB can persist for months in the gut flora, and this represents a serious transformation of potential pathogens in the surgical patient.

T. Pruett, MD

Molecular Analysis of Coagulase Gene Polymorphism in Clinical Isolates of Methicilin Resistant *Staphylococcus aureus* by Restriction Fragment Length of Polymorphism Based Genotyping

Himabindu M, Sugapriya Muthamilselvan D, Bishi DK, et al (Indian Inst of Technology Madras, Chennai, Tamil Nadu, India)

Am J Infect Dis 5:170-176, 2009

Problem Statement.—To investigate coagulase gene variants through Restriction Fragment Length Polymorphism (RFLP) amongst clinical isolates of Methicillin-Resistant *Staphylococcus Aureus* (MRSA) collected from Chennai based hospitals.

Approach.—A total of 85 MRSA clinical isolates collected from various clinical sources were studied for the molecular typing purpose. To perform coagulase gene typing, the repeated units encoding hypervariable regions of the *Staphylococcus aureus* coagulase gene were amplified by the PCR followed by AluI and HaeIII restriction enzyme digestion of the PCR product and analyzed for RFLP.

Results.—Cluster analysis performed with Un-weighted Pair Grouping Using Arithmetic Mean Analysis (UPGMA) at >80% similarity level classified all strains into 31 and 21 genotypes based upon AluI and HaeIII RFLP patterns respectively. AluI RFLP patterns gave a high discriminatory index and proved to be better than that of HaeIII in typing of MRSA strains.

Conclusion.—Method investigated in this study, proved to be quick, reliable and useful for typing large number of MRSA strains from various clinical isolates with high fidelity. Grouping of strains based on RFLP patterns of both enzymes, improved the discriminatory index. Finally, using this methodology group of epidemiological strains can be typed reliably and effectively using both enzymes. Significance and impact of the study: This efficient and reliable typing procedure is beneficial to develop efficient infection control measures in hospitals for staphylococcal infection. This typing procedure could be used to analyze large number of strains with in a short period of time and thus useful for epidemiological investigations.

▶ As organisms change within the environment, one should not extrapolate conclusions. The advent of Methicillin-Resistant *Staphylococcus aureus* (MRSA) within the community has received a great deal of lay coverage. It, therefore, becomes important to discern the differences between organisms coming into the hospital from the outside and those that are spread from within the hospital dynamics. Restriction fragment length polymorphism (RFLP) is a technique that can be used to assess variables in the hypervariable regions of the *S aureus* coagulase gene through polymerase chain reaction (PCR) techniques to unravel some of the vagaries around the MRSA organism. The report discusses the relative benefit of different regions of the coagulase gene but in the end describes a technique that will allow for more rational infection control. The PCR tests are not cheap and have some degree of operator dependency. It is important that reliable and simple tests become available so that appropriate infection control can be organized within the care delivery system. Control of what should and can be controlled is an important element of an effective infection control system.

T. Pruett, MD

Molecular epidemiology of Clostridium difficile over the course of 10 years in a tertiary care hospital

Belmares J, Johnson S, Parada JP, et al (Loyola Univ Chicago Med Ctr, Maywood)

Clin Infect Dis 49:1141-1147, 2009

Background.—The molecular epidemiology of endemic and outbreak Clostridium difficile strains across time is not well known.

Methods.—HindIII restriction endonuclease analysis (REA) typing was performed on available clinical C. difficile isolates from 1982 to 1991.

Results.—The annual incidence of C. difficile infection (CDI) ranged from 3.2 to 9.9 cases per 1000 discharges and was significantly higher in 1982, 1983, 1985, and 1991 (high-incidence years) than in other years (mean standard deviation number of cases for the high- vs the low-incidence years, 121.8 ± 20.4 and 70.0 ± 15.0; P = 002). A total of 696 (76.6%) of 908 C. difficile isolates were available for REA typing over the 10-year period. Large clusters (≥10 CDI cases in consecutive months) were caused by REA types B1 and B2 in 1982 and 1983, F2 and B1 in 1985, and K1 in 1991 (high-incidence years). Small clusters of 4-9 CDI cases in consecutive months were caused by REA types G1 (1984), Y4 and Y6 (1987), Y2 (1988), L1 (1989), Y1 (1990), and K1 (1991). Current epidemic REA group BI (unrelated to type B1) was isolated 6 times, twice in 1984, 1988, and 1990.

Conclusions.—Years with a high incidence of CDI were associated with large clusters of specific REA types that changed yearly. The molecular epidemiology of CDI in this hospital was characterized by a wide diversity of C. difficile types and an ever-changing dominance of specific C. difficile types over time. The current epidemic BI group was found sporadically on 6 occasions. A changing CDI molecular epidemiology should be expected in the future.

▶ A 10-year experience in a large facility demonstrated that *Clostridium difficile* infection outbreaks were caused by specific strains but only for finite periods of time. With the passing years, the significant epidemics were found to be associated with different strains. *C difficile* will continue to be associated with hospital-acquired diarrhea. This study demonstrates that the microbial population in the hospital environment is far from static, and vigilance will be required to understand the evolution of nosocomial pathogens.

T. Pruett, MD

Emerging role of Candida in deep sternal wound infection

Modrau IS, Ejlertsen T, Rasmussen BS (Aarhus Univ Hosp Skejby, Denmark)

Ann Thorac Surg 88:1905-1909, 2009

Background.—This study evaluated the overall incidence, prognosis, and risk factors for microbiologically documented Candida deep sternal wound infection (DSWI) after cardiac operations.

Methods.—A retrospective observational study was performed at Aalborg Hospital, Aarhus University Hospital, Denmark, from January 1999 through November 2006. Included were all 83 of 4222 cardiac surgical patients with microbiologically documented DSWI requiring surgical revision. Various potential risk factors in patients with Candida DSWI were compared with those of patients with non-Candida DSWI.

We compared markers of morbidity, in-hospital mortality, and 1-year mortality to evaluate the prognosis of the disease.

Results.—DSWI developed in 2% of all patients, of whom, 17 (20.5%) had Candida DSWI, and 66 (79.5%) had non-Candida etiology. Candida was the primary causative organism in 11 of 17 Candida DSWI cases. No Candida DSWI was found during the first 3 years of the study. In-hospital and 1-year mortality were doubled in patients with Candida DSWI compared with patients with non-Candida DSWI. Candida DSWI was associated with significantly longer stay in the intensive care unit and need of prolonged mechanical ventilation. Risk factors for Candida etiology were Candida colonization in tracheal secretions or urine and reoperation before diagnosis of DSWI.

Conclusions.—Candida was a frequent causative agent of DSWI in our series and was associated with a very high morbidity and mortality. Cardiothoracic patients on mechanical ventilation when colonized with Candida were identified as a high-risk population for subsequent development of Candida DSWI.

▶ *Candida* is another of the hospital pathogens that is associated with significant surgical infections. Its occurrence in surgical wounds is thought to be the consequence of either transient candidemia after the procedure or direct inoculation during the procedure. In this report, almost 2% of cardiac procedures led to the development of deep sternal infections involving *Candida*, and these infections were found to commonly occur in patients who had yeast cultured from tracheal aspirates. Often the infection was associated with multiple organisms, with skin organisms being common. This leads to the hypothesis that a low-grade infection occurs in which yeast can easily also infect. Because yeast prophylaxis is not routine, special concern needs to be given to perioperative patients with colonization and ventilator dependence.

T. Pruett, MD

Endovascular report of mycotic aortic aneurysms

Sörelius K, Mani K, Björck M, et al (Uppsala Univ Hosp, Sweden)

J Vasc Surg 50:269-274, 2009

Purpose.—We report our single-center experience of early and midterm outcome after endovascular repair of mycotic aortic aneurysms (MAA).

Methods.—Case records were retrospectively reviewed of 11 patients who underwent endovascular repair of 13 MAAs between 2000 and 2007. The aneurysms were localized in the aortic arch in 1 patient, descending thoracic aorta in 4, suprarenal abdominal aorta in 3, and infrarenal abdominal aorta in 5.

Results.—Mean follow-up was 27 months. A bleeding aortoesophageal fistula resulted in one in-hospital death ≤30 days. Three patients died later: one each of sepsis, stent migration that caused intestinal ischemia, and an unknown cause. Two patients had recurrent sepsis postoperatively but no vascular complications, two had elevated inflammatory markers during follow-up but were asymptomatic, and three patients had an uneventful follow-up.

Conclusions.—Endovascular treatment for MAA was feasible, with acceptable perioperative mortality and midterm outcome in this single-center case series. Recurrent sepsis and late relapse with a second MAA occurred, indicating the need of long-term antibiotic therapy and follow-up, as well as the possible need for secondary open repair in selected cases. Further research is warranted to evaluate long-term outcome.

▶ Treatment of mycotic aneurysm has traditionally included resection of the infected site with or without extra-anatomic bypass. This time-honored treatment is fraught with morbidity. The advent of endovascular treatment has offered the prospect of a new option. This approach violates the traditional surgical principles stressing that foreign bodies should not be placed in a contaminated field. The interesting component of this report is that not all patients experienced major problems. There was no limb loss from distal emboli and uncontrolled infection. There was 1 death from an aortoesophageal fistula and several persistent infections/new mycotic aneurysms, but with continued antibiotic suppression a surprising stabilization occurred. While clearly not curative, this form of therapy will give more time to plan definitive therapies or accept the option of continued suppression.

T. Pruett, MD

Is the Decline in the Surgical Treatment for Diverticulitis Associated with an Increase in Complicated Diverticulitis?

Ricciardi R, Baxter NN, Read TE, et al (Lahey Clinic, Burlington, MA; Univ of Toronto, Ontario, Canada)

Dis Colon Rectum 52:1558-1563, 2009

Purpose.—Indications for operative intervention in the treatment of diverticulitis have become unclear. We hypothesized that surgical treatment for diverticulitis has decreased resulting in proportionately more complicated diverticulitis cases (free perforation and/or abscess).

Methods.—We conducted a retrospective analysis of patients with diverticular disease in the Nationwide Inpatient Sample from 1991 through 2005. We used diagnostic codes to identify all patient discharges with diverticular disease and then determined the proportion of discharges with diverticulitis, perforated disease, diverticular abscess, and surgical treatment.

Results.—During the study period, 685,390 diverticulitis discharges were recorded. The ratio of diverticulitis discharges increased from 5.1 cases per 1,000 inpatients in 1991 to 7.6 cases per 1,000 inpatients in

2005 ($P < 0.0001$). The proportion of patients who underwent colectomy for uncomplicated diverticulitis declined from 17.9% in 1991 to 13.7% in 2005 ($P <$ 0.0.0001). During the same period, the proportion of free diverticular perforations as a fraction of all diverticulitis cases remained unchanged (1.5%). The proportion of diverticular abscess discharges as a fraction of all diverticulitis cases increased from 5.9% in 1991 to 9.6% in 2005 ($P < 0.0001$). Last, we noted a decrease in diverticular perforations and/or abscess treated with colectomy, 71.0% in 1991 to 55.5% in 2005 ($P < 0.0001$).

Conclusions.—Despite a significant decline in surgical treatment for diverticulitis, there has been no change in the proportion of patients discharged for free diverticular perforation. There was an increase in diverticular abscess discharges, but this finding was not associated with an increase in same stay surgical treatment.

▶ Like the article by Sorelius et al,[1] this article describes the consequences associated with a higher percentage of cases managed through a less invasive treatment that was often thought to be best managed through surgical interventions. While resection of the colon had been the mainstay of diverticular disease, its use has significantly decreased over the past decade. This study uses information from 685 000 discharge diagnoses for diverticular disease. While the diagnoses of diverticulitis increased over the study period, the use of surgical management for the disease decreased. The authors suggest that the absence of perforations and other emergency procedures justifies the reduction in surgical procedures. While this may be true, the lack of granularity of the database does not make this an ironclad conclusion. While emergency surgical therapy for diverticular disease may have been avoided, the authors did not address the less urgent complication of stricture or obstruction. The complete spectrum of disease evolution needs to be assessed when assessing optimal management strategies.

T. Pruett, MD

Reference

1. Sörelius K, Mani K, Björck M, Nyman R, Wanhainen A. Endovascular report of mycotic aortic aneurysms. *J Vasc Surg*. 2009;50:269-274.

Pancreatic necrosectomy: North American mortality is much lower than expected

Parikh PY, Pitt HA, Kilbane M, et al (Indiana Univ, Indianapolis)
J Am Coll Surg 209:712-719, 2009

Background.—The aim of this analysis was to explore the American College of Surgeons National Surgical Quality Improvement Program (ACS-NSQIP) database to determine outcomes of patients undergoing debridement for pancreatic and peripancreatic necrosis. Single-institution series suggest that the mortality of patients undergoing pancreatic necrosectomy has improved but remains at 15% to 20%. But no national data have been available for patients with necrotizing pancreatitis. In 2007, a CPT code specific for debridement of pancreatic necrosis became available.

Study Design.—The ACS-NSQIP Participant Use File was queried for all patients who had debridement of pancreatic and peripancreatic necrosis (CPT code 48105) from January 1, 2007, through December 31, 2007. Patient demographics, observed (O) and expected (E) morbidity and mortality, and indices (O/E) were evaluated. A multivariate stepwise logistic regression was performed to determine predictors of mortality.

Results.—During this 12-month period, data were accumulated on 161 patients. The mean age was 54 years; 71% were male; and 75% were Caucasian. The mean body mass index was 30.3 kg/m^2; 29% had diabetes; and 11% abused alcohol. Forty-two percent were transferred to NSQIP hospitals from other facilities. Overall morbidity was 62%, and 30-day mortality was 6.8%, but morbidity and mortality indices were 0.86 and 0.33, respectively. Increased age and blood urea nitrogen were independent predictors of mortality.

Conclusions.—These data suggest that patients undergoing debridement for pancreatic and peripancreatic necrosis at ACS-NSQIP hospitals provide a new North American sample and have better than predicted outcomes. We concluded that ACS-NSQIP is a powerful tool to assess contemporary outcomes of uncommon, high-risk procedures.

▶ Necrotizing pancreatitis is also an infection that has been within the purview of the surgeon. Traditional mortality associated with this disease has been significant. This article reviews recent experience with surgical debridement of the pancreas and peripancreatic necrotic material. While the American College of Surgeons National Surgical Quality Improvement Program database does not discern the true rate of infection, the surgical approach (either retroperitoneal or transabdominal), or other intensive care unit-associated variables, the recent mortality associated with pancreatic necrosectomy has decreased to less than 7%. These numbers are very important as a comparator for the NOTES approach to the treatment of the disease. Open debridement of the necrotic tissue is very effective in reducing the risk of death. The endoscopic approach yields similar results, if such an approach is to be embraced.

T. Pruett, MD

Anaphylaxis Caused by Recurrent Hydatid Disease

Jamshidi R, Hill A, Harris H, et al (Univ of California–San Francisco)
Surg Infect (Larchmt) 10:155-157, 2009

Background.—Tapeworms of the genus *Echinococcus* cause hydatidosis, which is endemic in Asia and the Mediterranean region. Immigration and travel have contributed to an increase in cases found in North America.

The ingested larvae penetrate the small intestine and enter the portal circulation, producing liver cysts in 50% to 90% of cases, but also affecting the lungs, heart, central nervous system, and other areas. It may take over 20 years to produce signs and symptoms. Anaphylaxis caused by recurrent hydatid disease was reported.

Case Report.—Man, 54, from Iran drank nonpotable water 25 years ago, developed hepatic echinococcal infection, and was treated with laparotomy and cyst enucleation. Years later he was diagnosed with recurrent hydatid cysts and underwent 6 months of mebendazole therapy. Nearly 2 years later he suffered sudden-onset upper abdominal pain followed by urticaria and dyspnea. At the emergency department he was given epinephrine, diphenhydramine, and methylprednisolone. A few days later he suffered respiratory arrest while searching for an epinephrine pen and required tracheal intubation, defibrillation, and vasoactive drugs. Intra-abdominal cystic fluid collections that had enlarged since previous scans were found on computed tomography (CT). The liver and suprapancreatic retroperitoneum contained the most prominent lesions. Radiographs showed peripheral calcifications and septations consistent with daughter cysts, leading to a diagnosis of disseminated recurrent hydatid disease with sporadic anaphylaxis caused by partial cyst rupture.

Treatment involved continuing steroids and adding albendazole along with surgery to extirpate the cysts. For the liver lesion, a right posterolateral thoracostomy was performed; the operative field was surrounded by towels soaked in the scolicidal agent 23% sodium chloride. A phrenotomy was performed and the cysts and gelatinous debris removed to prevent dissemination. A pericystectomy left the cyst lining cored out, then the saline solution was instilled in the cavity and left for 10 minutes to promote lysis of the scolices.

Abdominal exploration was performed through an upper midline celiotomy to manage the two liver cysts and one between the pancreas and transverse mesocolon. Hypertonic saline-soaked towels were applied and interrogated needle aspiration used, then the site was drained and marsupialized. Throughout surgery the patient's serum sodium concentration was monitored, with furosemide encouraging natriuresis.

Praziquantel was given for 1 week and albendazole for 6 months postoperatively. The patient's recovery was gradual, with no evidence of recurrence 2 years later.

Conclusions.—Because of the risk of IgE-mediated anaphylaxis, it is important to treat all cases of hydatid disease. Antihelminthic drugs alone plus close follow up and interval imaging are sufficient for small cysts. Some patients may require percutaneous drainage. For complex hydatid disease, an operative approach is preferred to avoid cyst spillage and anaphylaxis or seeding. A scolicidal agent such as hypertonic saline solution, chlorhexidine gluconate, or cetrimide is used intraoperatively to minimize recurrence.

▶ As travel continues to allow regional diseases to present anywhere in the world, it is important that the practicing surgeon knows the fundamentals of management of common diseases. Hydatid disease is seen worldwide. Management of the disease will often include preoperative mebendazole, but that rarely cures the disease. Surgical management is planned with the goal of (1) evacuating the cyst contents without spillage; (2) sterilization of the cyst through instillation of the scolicidal agents; and (3) postsurgical anti-echinococcal therapy. The reviews that show up in the medical literature should not equate to the presumption that these are rare diseases.

T. Pruett, MD

Postexposure Prophylaxis for HIV Infection

Landovitz RJ, Currier JS (Univ of California at Los Angeles [UCLA] Ctr for Clinical AIDS Res and Education; David Geffen School of Medicine at UCLA, Los Angeles, CA)

N Engl J Med 361:1768-1775, 2009

A 24-year-old man presents to an outpatient clinic, reporting that 36 hours previously he had receptive anal intercourse without the use of a condom with an anonymous male partner who was known to have had sex with other men. The patient is known to the clinical practice and has had several negative tests for human immunodeficiency virus (HIV) infection, most recently 6 months previously. How should he be evaluated and treated?

▶ People in the operating room can get unintentional exposure to human immunodeficiency virus (HIV). The risk of contracting the disease is fairly proportional to the amount of virus to which one is exposed. While most surgical splashes and solid needle sticks carry a lower risk of acquisition than hollow needle sticks, the risk is not zero. Early treatment with antivirals can significantly reduce the risk of acquiring HIV infection. Some strains of HIV are now often resistant to many of the commonly used antiviral agents. This means that postexposure prophylaxis treatments should optimally be tailored to susceptibility of the virus. However, the most important theme after any exposure is to promptly seek care from an HIV specialist.

T. Pruett, MD

7 Endocrine

---

^{18}F-Fluorodeoxyglucose Positron Emission Tomography for the Diagnosis of Adrenocortical Tumors: A Prospective Study in 77 Operated Patients

Groussin L, Bonardel G, Silvéra S, et al (Centre Natl de la Recherche Scientifique Unité Mixte de Recherche, Paris, France; Hôpital d'Instruction des Armées du Val de Grâce, Paris, France; Université Paris Descartes, France; et al)

J Clin Endocrinol Metab 94:1713-1722, 2009

Context.—Most adrenal incidentalomas are nonfunctioning adrenocortical adenomas (ACAs). Adrenocortical carcinomas (ACCs) are rare but should be recognized at an early stage.

Objective.—The objective of the study was to evaluate the usefulness of ^{18}F-fluorodeoxyglucose positron emission tomography (^{18}F-FDG PET) to predict malignancy in patients without a previous history of cancer.

Design.—This was a prospective, multicenter study from 2001 to 2006.

Setting.—The study was conducted at a network of seven university hospitals in Paris.

Patients.—Seventy-seven patients were included. All underwent surgery because of hypersecretory and/or growing benign lesions ($n = 18$), obvious ACCs ($n = 21$), or radiologically indeterminate lesions ($n = 38$).

Main Outcome Measure.—The degree of ^{18}F-FDG PET uptake [maximum standardized uptake value (maxSUV)] was related to the pathological findings serving as a reference, and its diagnostic value was compared with that of computerized tomography (CT) scan.

Results.—Pathology eventually diagnosed 43 ACAs, 22 ACCs, and 12 nonadrenocortical lesions. Using a cutoff value above 1.45 for adrenal to liver maxSUV ratio, the sensitivity and specificity to distinguish ACAs from ACCs were, respectively, 1.00 (95% confidence interval 0.85–1.00) and 0.88 (95% confidence interval 0.75–0.96). Among the 38 indeterminate lesions at CT scan, we could analyze a subgroup of 16 adrenocortical tumors with high unenhanced density (>10 HU) and an inappropriate washout: ^{18}F-FDG PET correctly predicted the benignity in 13 of 15 ACAs.

Conclusions.—In a multidisciplinary team approach, ^{18}F-FDG PET helps to manage suspicious CT scan lesions. An adrenal to liver maxSUV ratio less than 1.45 is highly predictive of a benign lesion.

▶ The article by Groussin et al demonstrates the usefulness of positron emission tomography (PET) in helping to discriminate between benign and malignant adrenocortical tumors. PET was highly sensitive for malignancy (100%) with slightly lower specificity. However, by excluding the nonadrenocortical lesions—which comprised nearly one-third of the indeterminate lesions—the true value of PET in the diagnosis of these indeterminate lesions is unknown. While the authors suggest that surgery might be avoided in the PET-negative lesions, this conclusion cannot be accepted without the knowledge of what the 12 nonadrenocortical tumors were and how they would have affected the decision to ultimately manage the patient.

T. J. Fahey, MD

Bilateral Adrenalectomy for Refractory Cushing Disease: A Safe and Definitive Therapy

Smith PW, Turza KC, Carter CO, et al (Univ of Virginia, Charlottesville)

J Am Coll Surg 208:1059-1064, 2009

Background.—Refractory Cushing disease (CD) is associated with considerable morbidity and mortality. Bilateral adrenalectomy (BA) offers effective permanent treatment. Both open and laparoscopic approaches have been used, but longterm comparisons are few.

Study Design.—We reviewed 40 consecutive BA for refractory CD from 1995 through 2007. Surgical results were evaluated. A Short Form-36 Quality-of-Life (QOL) survey was performed.

Results.—Eighty-five percent (34 of 40) of patients were women, and median age was 41.9 years (range, 22.2 to 78.3 years). All had persistent CD after transsphenoidal operation (mean, 1.7; range, 1 to 3). Median followup was 5.0 years. Thirty-eight percent (15 of 40) of procedures were performed laparoscopically; 1 was converted to open. There were no operative or 30-day mortalities, and there was 1 90-day mortality. Morbidities occurred in 7 of 40 (18%) patients. Median length of stay was shorter in the laparoscopic group (4 versus 6 days; $p < 0.001$). All patients achieved clinical reversal of hypercortisolism, including the 5 (13%) with ectopic adrenal tissue. Elevated serum ACTH (>200 ng/mL) was present during followup in 33% (13 of 40). A QOL survey demonstrated 86% of patients felt good to excellent compared with 1 year pre-BA. Chronic fatigue was present most or all of the time in 46%, and patients were below population norms on 7 of 8 Short Form-36 scales. No difference was evident in QOL between laparoscopic and open adrenalectomy.

Conclusions.—Our experience demonstrates excellent survival and clinical results, despite the inherent risk in patients with CD. There are persistent fatigue and QOL deficits that are not ameliorated by laparoscopic compared with open resection.

▶ Management of patients with persistent Cushing disease is particularly challenging. This report demonstrates that bilateral adrenalectomy for patients with refractory Cushing improves the overall health status of the vast majority of patients at very low surgical risk, despite the fact that the majority of the patients in this series had open bilateral adrenalectomies. These patients continue to require intensive follow-up and medical management as attested to by the incidence of Nelson syndrome. Nevertheless, bilateral adrenalectomy can and should be considered as part of the long-term management of patients with refractory Cushing disease.

T. J. Fahey, MD

Bilateral Adrenalectomy for Refractory Cushing Disease: A Safe and Definitive Therapy

Smith PW, Turza KC, Carter CO, et al (Univ of Virginia, Charlottesville)
J Am Coll Surg 208:1059-1064, 2009

Background.—Refractory Cushing disease (CD) is associated with considerable morbidity and mortality. Bilateral adrenalectomy (BA) offers effective permanent treatment. Both open and laparoscopic approaches have been used, but longterm comparisons are few.

Study Design.—We reviewed 40 consecutive BA for refractory CD from 1995 through 2007. Surgical results were evaluated. A Short Form-36 Quality-of-Life (QOL) survey was performed.

Results.—Eighty-five percent (34 of 40) of patients were women, and median age was 41.9 years (range, 22.2 to 78.3 years). All had persistent CD after transsphenoidal operation (mean, 1.7; range, 1 to 3). Median followup was 5.0 years. Thirty-eight percent (15 of 40) of procedures were performed laparoscopically; 1 was converted to open. There were no operative or 30-day mortalities, and there was 1 90-day mortality. Morbidities occurred in 7 of 40 (18%) patients. Median length of stay was shorter in the laparoscopic group (4 versus 6 days; $p < 0.001$). All patients achieved clinical reversal of hypercortisolism, including the 5 (13%) with ectopic adrenal tissue. Elevated serum ACTH (>200 ng/mL) was present during followup in 33% (13 of 40). A QOL survey demonstrated 86% of patients felt good to excellent compared with 1 year pre-BA. Chronic fatigue was present most or all of the time in 46%, and patients were below population norms on 7 of 8 Short Form-36 scales. No difference was evident in QOL between laparoscopic and open adrenalectomy.

Conclusions.—Our experience demonstrates excellent survival and clinical results, despite the inherent risk in patients with CD. There are persistent fatigue and QOL deficits that are not ameliorated by laparoscopic compared with open resection.

▶ Patients with persistent Cushing's disease after failed transsphenoidal resection or other therapy represent one of the most challenging groups of surgical patients. The decision to operate on these patients, who are prone to multiple, potentially devastating complications is difficult, and operative therapy must be precise with little tissue trauma. Smith et al present a series of patients who were obviously well-selected and had excellent surgical care. Their results are outstanding, both in terms of a limited number of major complications and long-term outcome. However, their quality of life indicators suggest that Cushing's disease remains a systemic condition and that patients never achieve the quality of life of nonaffected controls. This does not appear to be related to the surgical outcome. Of note, in this series less than one-half of the patients were treated by a laparoscopic approach. Although the authors advocate laparoscopic resection, one wonders if the quality of life outcomes would have been better with the laparoscopic approach if more patients had been treated by this approach. Because the quality of life outcomes were determined at a single point in time (duration of follow-up at this point was not stated), the value of the laparoscopic approach on quality of life was not determined. Given the propensity of poor healing and wound complications in these patients, the laparoscopic approach should be strongly considered because these patients can develop significant wound infections that result in difficult-to-treat hernias.

K. E. Behrns, MD

Clinical Predictors and Algorithm for the Genetic Diagnosis of Pheochromocytoma Patients

Erlic Z, for the European-American Pheochromocytoma Study Group (Albert-Ludwigs-Univ, Freiburg, Germany; et al)

Clin Cancer Res 15:6378-6385, 2009

Purpose.—Six pheochromocytoma susceptibility genes causing distinct syndromes have been identified; approximately one of three of all pheochromocytoma patients carry a predisposing germline mutation. When four major genes (*VHL, RET, SDHB, SDHD*) are analyzed in a clinical laboratory, costs are ~$3,400 per patient. The aim of the study is to systematically obtain a robust algorithm to identify who should be genetically tested, and to determine the order in which genes should be tested.

Experimental Design.—DNA from 989 apparently nonsyndromic patients were scanned for germline mutations in the genes *VHL, RET, SDHB, SDHC*, and *SDHD*. Clinical parameters were analyzed as potential predictors for finding mutations by multiple logistic regression, validated by bootstrapping. Cost reduction was calculated between prioritized gene testing compared with that for all genes.

Results.—Of 989 apparently nonsyndromic pheochromocytoma cases, 187 (19%) harbored germline mutations. Predictors for presence of mutation are age <45 years, multiple pheochromocytoma, extra-adrenal location, and previous head and neck paraganglioma. If we used the presence of any one predictor as indicative of proceeding with gene testing, then 342 (34.6%) patients would be excluded, and only 8 carriers (4.3%) would be missed. We were also able to statistically model the priority of genes to be tested given certain clinical features. E.g., for patients with prior head and neck paraganglioma, the priority would be *SDHD>SDHB>RET>VHL*. Using the clinical predictor algorithm to prioritize gene testing and order, a 44.7% cost reduction in diagnostic process can be achieved.

Conclusions.—Clinical parameters can predict for mutation carriers and help prioritize gene testing to reduce costs in nonsyndromic pheochromocytoma presentations.

▶ The incidence of germline mutations in patients with apparently sporadic pheochromocytoma runs from 10% to 30% and is reported as 20% in this large series. Who to test and what genes to test for to rule out a germline predisposition to the development of pheochromocytoma is now an important issue. Given the cost involved with generic testing, an algorithm for deciding who to test and what genes to test for is highly desirable and supplied in this large collaborative study. Fig 1 in the original article outlines the order of gene testing to pursue. Importantly, it also identifies who should undergo testing. The guidelines did miss 8 carriers, but to alter the algorithm to catch all carriers would nearly eliminate any cost reduction associated with applying the algorithm.

T. J. Fahey, MD

Clinical Predictors for Germline Mutations in Head and Neck Paraganglioma Patients: Cost Reduction Strategy in Genetic Diagnostic Process as Fall-Out

Neumann HPH, Erlic Z, Boedeker CC, et al (Albert-Ludwigs Univ, Freiburg, Germany; et al)

Cancer Res 69:3650-3656, 2009

Multiple genes and their variants that lend susceptibility to many diseases will play a major role in clinical routine. Genetics-based cost reduction strategies in diagnostic processes are important in the setting of multiple susceptibility genes for a single disease. Head and neck paraganglioma (HNP) is caused by germline mutations of at least three succinate dehydrogenase subunit genes (*SDHx*). Mutation analysis for all 3 costs ~US$2,700 per patient. Genetic classification is essential for downstream management of the patient and preemptive management of family members. Utilizing HNP as a model, we wanted to determine predictors to prioritize the most heritable clinical presentations and which gene to begin testing in HNP presentations, to reduce costs of genetic screening. Patients were tested for *SDHB*, *SDHC*, and *SDHD* intragenic mutations and large deletions. Clinical parameters were analyzed as potential predictors for finding germline mutations. Cost reduction was calculated between prioritized gene testing compared with that for all genes. Of 598 patients, 30.6% had *SDHx* germline mutations: 34.4% in *SDHB*, 14.2% *SDHC*, and 51.4% *SDHD*. Predictors for an *SDHx* mutation are family history [odds ratio (OR), 37.9], previous pheochromocytoma (OR, 10.9), multiple HNP (OR, 10.6), age ≤40 years (OR, 4.0), and male gender (OR, 3.5). By screening only preselected cases and a stepwise approach, 60% cost reduction can be achieved, with 91.8% sensitivity and 94.5%

negative predictive value. Our data give evidence that clinical parameters can predict for mutation and help prioritize gene testing to reduce costs in HNP. Such strategy is cost-saving in the practice of genetics-based personalized health care.

▶ Head and neck paragangliomas are rare neuroendocrine tumors that are associated with germline mutations in the succinate dehydrogenase (SDH) genes B, C, and D. (A recent report in *Science* now also implicates *SDH5*.) Mutations are found in nearly one-third of patients (30.6% of 598 patients in this study). Mutation analysis is expensive. This study provides an excellent algorithm for which patients with head and neck paragangliomas should be tested and in what order the genes should be analyzed (Fig 2 in the original article). The proposed algorithm would be 92% sensitive for picking up a carrier and have a 94% negative predictive value. Although there will likely be changes in the recommendations over time, this is an excellent guide to advising patients with these tumors regarding genetic testing at this time.

T. J. Fahey, MD

Focused parathyroidectomy guided by intra-operative parathormone monitoring does not miss multiglandular disease in patients with sporadic primary hyperparathyroidism: A 10-year outcome

Lew JI, Irvin GL III (Univ of Miami Leonard M. Miller School of Medicine, FL)

Surgery 146:1021-1027, 2009

Background.—There remains concern that focused parathyroidectomy guided by intra-operative parathormone monitoring (IPM) will miss multiglandular disease (MGD) leading to a higher recurrence rate. This study reports the 10-year outcome of patients with sporadic primary hyperparathyroidism treated by focused parathyroidectomy guided by IPM.

Methods.—From 1993 to 1998, 173 consecutive patients with sporadic primary hyperparathyroidism underwent focused parathyroidectomy guided by IPM. When IPM showed >50% decrease 10 minutes after abnormal gland excision, the operation was completed. Recurrent hyperparathyroidism was defined as elevated serum calcium and parathormone (PTH) levels >6 months after successful parathyroidectomy.

Results.—There were 164 patients with a mean follow-up of 83 months. In this group, 96% patients had single gland disease (SGD) and 4% had MGD. Five (3%) patients developed recurrent hyperparathyroidism at 2, 4, 9, 10, and 12 years. In 43 eucalcemic patients followed for >10 years, PTH levels remained normal in 54%, were constantly above normal range in 2%, or varied between normal and above normal range in 44%.

Conclusion.—In patients 10 years after treatment, IPM-guided parathyroidectomy does not fail to identify MGD, allows for limited dissection in

SGD, and shows that various sized parathyroid glands left in situ do not cause higher recurrence rates.

▶ This long-term follow-up study of patients undergoing focused parathyroidectomy from the Miami group is in essence a response to the recent work by the Cleveland Clinic group published last year that suggested there was a substantial incidence of multigland disease even in patients who would have had a successful focused approach by IOPTH numbers. Lew and Irvin demonstrate that the recurrence rate with focused parathyroidectomy is low (3%), and argue that focused parathyroidectomy does not miss hyperfunctioning glands. Proponents of a 4-gland exploration might point to the relatively high percentage of patients with 10-yr follow-up who had persistent or intermittent elevation of parathyroid hormone as a possible reflection of large glands that were left behind. Finally, as noted by Dr Prinz in the comments, this cohort of patients is a highly selected group of patients to begin with, as attested to by the very low incidence of multigland disease at the outset.

T. J. Fahey, MD

Individualization of Lymph Node Dissection in RET (Rearranged During Transfection) Carriers at Risk for Medullary Thyroid Cancer: Value of Pretherapeutic Calcitonin Levels

Machens A, Lorenz K, Dralle H (Martin Luther Univ Halle-Wittenberg, Germany)

Ann Surg 250:305-310, 2009

Objective.—This study sought to define the need for lymph node dissection in Rearranged during Transfection (RET) carriers at risk for hereditary medullary thyroid cancer.

Summary Background Data.—Controversy surrounds the need for lymph node dissection to complement thyroidectomy in RET carriers.

Methods.—Integration of molecular, biochemical, histopathologic, and clinical information from 308 RET carriers referred for (re-)operation to a specialist surgical center.

Results.—The carriers differed significantly in age at thyroidectomy when stratified by histopathology (tumor-free thyroid, node-negative, and node-positive medullary thyroid cancer) and mutated codon (611, 618, 620, 634, 768, 790, 804, 891, and 918). The wide overlap among the 3 histopathologic groups compromised individual predictions based on age alone. There was a significant relationship between the presence of lymph node metastases and increased pretherapeutic basal calcitonin levels. All 46 carriers with node-positive medullary thyroid cancer, who harbored 1 to 68 positive nodes, exhibited increased pretherapeutic basal calcitonin levels (91.4 pg/mL or higher). Conversely, 74 (44%) of 168 carriers with normal thyroids, C-cell hyperplasia, or node-negative medullary thyroid cancer displayed normal pretherapeutic basal calcitonin levels (negative predictive value 100%). Prediction of lymph node metastasis was better in carriers of codon 918 mutations (positive predictive value, PPV, 80%–100%) and those older than 20 years of age (PPV, 50%).

Discussion.—In the absence of clinical evidence to the contrary, RET carriers with normal pretherapeutic basal calcitonin levels may forgo lymph node dissection. The usefulness of calcitonin thresholds to break down the block of carriers with increased calcitonin levels should be explored further.

► This article addresses the question regarding the extent of thyroidectomy ± neck dissection in patients with hereditary medullary thyroid cancer (MTC). The authors reviewed their large experience with familial MTC and demonstrated that patients with normal basal calcitonin levels can forego central neck dissection at the time of thyroidectomy as the incidence of lymph node (LN) metastases in this group was 0. In fact, they report that all carriers with LN metastases had basal calcitonin levels of >91 pg/mL. Although there is some additional risk (mainly of hypoparathyroidism) with performing central neck dissection over just thyroidectomy alone, it may be hard to not include a central neck dissection in the surgical approach to familial MTC, especially in older patients. Nevertheless, a normal preoperative calcitonin level would certainly enable a limited CND in patients with hereditary MTC.

T. J. Fahey, MD

Ipsilateral Versus Bilateral Central Neck Lymph Node Dissection in Papillary Thyroid Carcinoma

Moo T-AS, Umunna B, Kato M, et al (New York Presbyterian Hospital - Cornell, NY; et al)

Ann Surg 250:403-408, 2009

Objective.—Many patients undergoing thyroidectomy for papillary thyroid carcinoma (PTC) have subclinical nodal disease at the time of surgery. Prophylactic bilateral central neck dissection (CND) is gaining acceptance in the treatment of PTC as studies have shown nodal disease increases the rate of local recurrence and may alter postsurgical radioactive iodine dosing. Given the potential complications of bilateral CND, we undertook a prospective study to determine the adequacy of prophylactic ipsilateral CND for PTC.

Methods.—A total of 116 patients with PTC underwent total thyroidectomy and routine prophylactic CND at a tertiary referral center. Of these, 45 had right and left central neck lymph node basins submitted separately for pathologic examination. We examined the laterality of positive lymph nodes based on tumor location and size.

Results.—Overall, positive lymph nodes were found in 45% of patients. Of the patients having a lateralized CND, 33% had ipsilateral positive nodes only, while 20% had bilateral positive nodes. None of the patients with tumor size ≤1 cm had bilateral positive lymph nodes compared with 31% of patients with tumors >1 cm ($P = 0.02$). Multifocality did not affect lymph node metastasis in tumors ≤1 cm. Parathyroids were found in the pathology specimen of 34% of patients, 40% had parathyroids autotransplanted, 47% had temporary hypocalcemia, and 0% had permanent hypocalcemia. Rates of temporary and permanent recurrent laryngeal nerve injury were 5% and 0% respectively.

Conclusions.—Ipsilateral CND appears to be sufficient in patients with tumors ≤1 cm. In tumors >1 cm, bilateral CND should be considered as these patients are more likely to have bilateral positive nodes. If tumor size is used as criteria for prophylactic CND, approximately one-third of patients can be spared a bilateral CND.

▶ The debate over whether to perform a routine prophylactic central neck dissection (CND) for papillary thyroid carcinoma (PTC) has heated up over the past year. Those in favor argue that lymph node metastases are found in central neck lymph nodes approximately 40% of the time and 25% of the time, even in the presence of papillary microcarcinoma. It has been well documented that there are increased risks associated with CND, particularly with regard to the parathyroid glands. This prospective study was undertaken to determine whether ipsilateral CND might be adequate for patients with PTC, with an ultimate goal of trying to achieve what is achieved with bilateral CND with the lower morbidity of a unilateral CND. The results suggest that, at least for papillary microcarcinoma, an ipsilateral CND may be adequate, though certainly additional data need to be accrued. Due to the additional risks involved in CND and the absence of strong data documenting a therapeutic advantage of CND, the inclusion of routine CND as a part of the surgical treatment of PTC should probably be restricted to experienced thyroid surgeons.

T. J. Fahey, MD

Localization of Insulinomas to Regions of the Pancreas by Intraarterial Calcium Stimulation: The NIH Experience

Guettier J-M, Kam A, Chang R, et al (Natl Insts of Health, Bethesda, MD)

J Clin Endocrinol Metab 94:1074-1080, 2009

Context.—Selective intraarterial calcium injection of the major pancreatic arteries with hepatic venous sampling [calcium arterial stimulation (CaStim)] has been used as a localizing tool for insulinomas at the National Institutes of Health (NIH) since 1989. The accuracy of this technique for localizing insulinomas was reported for all cases until 1996.

Objectives.—The aim of the study was to assess the accuracy and track record of the CaStim over time and in the context of evolving technology and to review issues related to result interpretation and procedure complications. CaStim was the only invasive preoperative localization modality used at our center. Endoscopic ultrasound (US) was not studied.

Design and Setting.—We conducted a retrospective case review at a referral center.

Patients.—Twenty-nine women and 16 men (mean age, 47 yr; range, 13–78) were diagnosed with an insulinoma from 1996–2008.

Intervention.—A supervised fast was conducted to confirm the diagnosis of insulinoma. US, computed tomography (CT), magnetic resonance imaging (MRI), and CaStim were used as preoperative localization studies. Localization predicted by each preoperative test was compared to surgical localization for accuracy.

Main Outcome.—We measured the accuracy of US, CT, MRI, and CaStim for localization of insulinomas preoperatively.

Results.—All 45 patients had surgically proven insulinomas. Thirty-eight of 45 (84%) localized to the correct anatomical region by CaStim. In five of 45 (11%) patients, the CaStim was falsely negative. Two of 45 (4%) had false-positive localizations.

Conclusion.—The CaStim has remained vastly superior to abdominal US, CT, or MRI over time as a preoperative localizing tool for insulinomas. The utility of the CaStim for this purpose and in this setting is thus validated.

▶ This article provides a nice summary of the modern National Institutes of Health (NIH) experience in localizing insulinomas by intra-arterial calcium stimulation. The results reported are quite good, and, as demonstrated, selective arterial stimulation is far superior to US, CT, or MRI. However, the lack of comparison with endoscopic US (EUS) limits the scope of the study substantially. EUS is really the primary modality for localizing pancreatic neuroendocrine tumors, and in most studies EUS is equivalent or superior to arterial stimulation and considered less invasive. Nevertheless, the study provides a detailed review of how to plan selective arterial stimulation, in addition to reporting expected results.

T. J. Fahey, MD

Long-Term Outcome after Total Parathyroidectomy for the Management of Secondary Hyperparathyroidism

Stracke S, Keller F, Steinbach G, et al (Univ Hosp Greifswald, Germany; Univ Hosp Ulm, Germany)

Nephron Clin Pract 111:c102-c109, 2009

In patients with chronic renal failure, secondary hyperparathyroidism (sHPT) is a common problem requiring surgical parathyroidectomy (PTX) if medical treatment with active vitamin D and calcimimetics fails. To minimize the risk for recurrence, we perform total PTX (tPTX) without autotransplantation. From October 1997 to January 2004, 46 patients (31 men and 15 women) underwent tPTX without autotransplantation (median age 51 years; range 19–80 years; median dialysis time before PTX 5 years; range 0–25 years). Indications for PTX were hyperparathyroid bone disease in 41 cases and calciphylaxis in 5 cases. Postoperatively, all patients were supplemented with vitamin D analogues, both calcitriol and cholecalciferol. Patients were followed up for 4–107 months (median 63 months). Although tPTX was intended in all cases, we saw recurrent or persistent hyperparathyroidism in 26% and supernumerary glands in 15% of cases. In 7 patients (15%), five or more glands were documented and in another four suspected confirming the clinical relevance of intraoperative parathyroid hormone (PTH) measurement. In our study, the positive predictive value of a low intraoperative PTH (<20 pg/ml) for a successful tPTX was 92%. 15 patients received a renal transplant after tPTX without autotransplantation. Here, an uncomplicated hypocalcaemia was noted in 3 patients. Last available calcium levels were between 1.72 and 2.66 mmol/l (median 2.35 mmol/l). After follow-up, active vitamin D was given in a median daily dose of 0.5 µg calcitriol (range 0–2.5 µg/day). There was no evidence of clinical bone disease and no pathological fractures after tPTX after a median observation period of 63 months. tPTX still offers the highest percentage of cure for sHPT, it is safe and postoperatively easily manageable. It allows for adequate supplementation with active vitamin D, and it is the most cost-effective procedure. It should be reconsidered an option for the treatment of sHPT.

▶ The management of patients with renal hyperparathyroidism can be challenging. Patients with recurrent secondary hyperparathyroidism can be particularly difficult to manage, and the option of performing a total parathyroidectomy at times is an attractive one—especially in retrospect. This report suggests that total parathyroidectomy is an effective treatment strategy and is not associated with the development of severe bone disease over (relatively) long-term follow-up. Importantly, patients who subsequently underwent renal transplant did not develop significant post-transplant problems with hypocalcemia. Finally, intraoperative parathyroid hormone (IOPTH) was of some use in predicting a successful long-term outcome, with patients below the cutoff value of 60 pg/mL identifying successful long-term resolution of hyperparathyroidism.

T. J. Fahey, MD

Molecular Testing for Mutations in Improving the Fine-Needle Aspiration Diagnosis of Thyroid Nodules

Nikiforov YE, Steward DL, Robinson-Smith TM, et al (Univ of Cincinnati College of Medicine, OH; et al)

J Clin Endocrinol Metab 94:2092-2098, 2009

Context.—Thyroid nodules are common in adults, but only a small fraction of them are malignant. Fine-needle aspiration (FNA) with cytological evaluation is the most reliable tool for cancer diagnosis in thyroid nodules.

However, 10–40% of nodules are diagnosed as indeterminate by cytology, making it difficult to optimally manage these patients.

Objective.—The aim of this study was to establish the feasibility and role of testing for tumor-specific mutations in improving the FNA diagnosis of thyroid nodules.

Design.—The prospective study included 470 FNA samples of thyroid nodules from 328 patients. At the time of aspiration, a small portion of the material was collected and tested for *BRAF*, *RAS*, *RET/PTC*, and *PAX8/PPARγ* mutations. The mutational status was correlated with cytology and either surgical pathology diagnosis or follow-up (mean, 34 months).

Results.—A sufficient amount of nucleic acids were isolated in 98%of samples. Thirty-two mutations were found, including 18 *BRAF*, eight *RAS*, five *RET/PTC*, and one *PAX8/PPARγ*. The presence of any mutation was a strong indicator of cancer because 31 (97%) of mutation-positive nodules had a malignant diagnosis after surgery. A combination of cytology and molecular testing showed significant improvement in the diagnostic accuracy and allowed better prediction of malignancy in the nodules with indeterminate cytology.

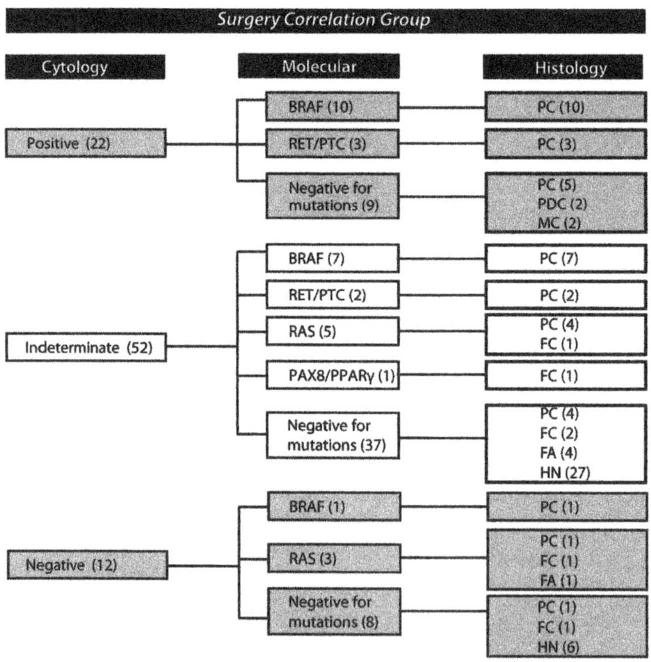

FIGURE 2.—Correlation between cytology, molecular findings, and histological diagnosis in the surgery correlation group. (Reprinted from Nikiforov YE, Steward DL, Robinson-Smith TM, et al. Molecular testing for mutations in improving the fine-needle aspiration diagnosis of thyroid nodules. *J Clin Endocrinol Metab*. 2009;94:2092-2098, Copyright © 2009, The Endocrine Society.)

TABLE 2.—Probability of Cancer in Thyroid Nodules Depending on the Results of Cytological and Molecular Analysis

Results of Cytology and Molecular Analysis	Cancer Probability (%)
Positive cytology and positive for mutation	100
Indeterminate cytology alone	40.4
Indeterminate cytology and positive for mutation	100
Indeterminate cytology and negative for mutation	16.2
Negative cytology alone	2.1
Negative cytology and negative for mutation	0.9

Conclusions.—These results indicate that molecular testing of thyroid nodules for a panel of mutations can be effectively performed in a clinical setting. It enhances the accuracy of FNA cytology and is of particular value for thyroid nodules with indeterminate cytology.

▶ As noted in the abstract, mutation detection has the potential to improve the accuracy of fine needle aspiration (FNA) diagnosis of thyroid nodules. This multicenter trial looking at mutation detection of the genes that are known to be commonly mutated in papillary and follicular thyroid cancers in FNA samples gives us a good idea of what we can expect to be the success of a broad approach to mutation identification as shown in Fig 2. What we can conclude is that the detection of a mutation is highly—though not 100%—correlated with the presence of cancer. So with the application of this strategy, initial surgery can be more appropriately directed. Table 2 indicates that when a mutation is found in a sample with an indeterminate cytology, the final diagnosis was cancer 100% of the time. The sensitivity for cancer in the indeterminate nodules was 75% (15/20), which is a substantial potential benefit.

T. J. Fahey, MD

Optimizing surgical treatment of papillary thyroid carcinoma associated with BRAF mutation

Yip L, Nikiforova MN, Carty SE, et al (Univ of Pittsburgh School of Medicine)
Surgery 146:1215-1223, 2009

Background.—To date, a mutation of the BRAF oncogene is the most common genetic alteration found in papillary thyroid carcinoma (PTC) and is associated with extrathyroidal extension, lymph node metastasis, and tumor recurrence. It is not known whether pre-operative identification of BRAF mutations in cytologic specimens should alter surgical management.

Methods.—From 2006 to 2008, the clinical, cytologic, and pathologic parameters of 106 consecutive surgically treated patients with BRAF-positive PTC were compared with a concurrent cohort of 100 patients with BRAF-negative PTC.

Results.—In all, 99 BRAF-positive PTC patients underwent initial treatment, and 7 BRAF-positive patients had surgical resection of recurrent/persistent PTC. BRAF mutations were identified on preoperative cytologic samples (31 patients) or after thyroidectomy (75 patients). All 31 patients with BRAF-positive fine-needle aspiration (FNA) had PTC at thyroidectomy (specificity 100%). At short-term follow-up, 11/106 BRAF-positive patients have required reoperation for recurrent/persistent disease compared with 3 BRAF-negative patients ($P = .04$). Preoperative knowledge of BRAF mutation positivity could have productively altered initial PTC surgical management in 24% of patients.

Conclusion.—In PTC, BRAF mutations are associated with cervical recurrence and with reoperation. Pre-operative cytologic identification of BRAF mutation has high specificity and may guide the initial extent of thyroidectomy and node dissection.

▶ The use of BRAF mutation analysis in thyroid fine-needle aspiration (FNA) is likely to become part of the standard evaluation for patients presenting with suspicious thyroid nodules. This report from a group that has been at the forefront of bringing this technology to the clinic indicates that there is potential value in knowing BRAF status preoperatively. However, the conclusion that knowledge of BRAF status could have altered the surgical management is overstated. The study documents that BRAF status is not accurately predicted by the determination of BRAF status of the FNA sample in 13/44 patients in their hands—these are the patients seen and evaluated by FNA at Pittsburgh. Yet they inappropriately exclude 8 of these 13 patients for technical reasons, and they report a false-negative rate of only 11%! It should be 30%! And they include these patients in those that could have benefited from knowledge of BRAF status preoperatively. So while BRAF testing promises to be useful, it may not have as significant an impact on surgical management as proposed, and will probably require a prospective analysis to determine the cost-benefit as we become increasingly cost conscious in our health care delivery.

T. J. Fahey, MD

Post-surgical hypocortisolism after removal of an adrenal incidentaloma: is it predictable by an accurate endocrinological work-up before surgery?

Eller-Vainicher C, Morelli V, Salcuni AS, et al (Univ of Milan, Italy; et al)
Eur J Endocrinol 162:91-99, 2010

Objective.—Few data are available regarding the need of steroid substitutive therapy after unilateral adrenalectomy for adrenal incidentaloma (AI). It is unknown whether, before surgery, the hypothalamic–pituitary–adrenal (HPA) axis secretion parameters can predict post-surgical hypocortisolism.

Aim.—This study aimed to evaluate whether, in AI patients undergoing unilateral adrenalectomy, post-surgical hypocortisolism could be predicted by the parameters of HPA axis function.

Design.—Prospective, multicenter.

Methods.—A total of 60 patients underwent surgical removal of AI (surgical indication: 29 subclinical hypercortisolism (SH); 31 AI dimension). Before surgery, SH was diagnosed in patients presenting at least three criteria out of urinary free cortisol (UFC) levels > 60 μg/24 h, cortisol after 1-mg dexamethasone suppression test (1 mg-DST) > 3.0 μg/dl, ACTH levels < 10 pg/ml, midnight serum cortisol (MSC) > 5.4 μg/dl.

Two months after surgery, HPA axis function was assessed by low dose ACTH stimulation test or insulin tolerance test when needed: 39 patients were affected (Group B) and 21 were not affected (Group A) with hypocortisolism. The accuracy in predicting hypocortisolism of pre-surgical HPA axis parameters or their combinations was evaluated.

Results.—The presence of > 2 alterations among 1 mg-DST > 5.0 μg/dl, ACTH < 10 pg/ml, elevated UFC and MSC has the highest odds ratio (OR) for predicting post-surgical hypocortisolism (OR 10.45, 95% confidence interval, CI 2.54–42.95, $P = 0.001$). Post-surgical hypocortisolism was predicted with 100% probability by elevated UFC plus MSC levels, but not ruled out even in the presence of the normality of all HPA axis parameters.

Conclusion.—Post-surgical hypocortisolism cannot be pre-surgically ruled out. A steroid substitutive therapy is indicated after unilateral adrenalectomy for SH or size of the adenoma.

▶ This is a well-done, thorough study examining whether postoperative adrenal insufficiency can be predicted from preoperative testing. The authors conclude that this cannot be done well with current tests to identify subclinical Cushing's syndrome. None of the 4 tests, either individually or combined, had an accuracy of greater than 72%, and while several combinations had a specificity of > 90%, the sensitivity reached over 90% only if any one of the 4 tests was abnormal (at the expense of specificity of < 10%). The point is that surgery for patients with adrenal incidentalomas has to be accompanied by a healthy suspicion for the development of adrenal insufficiency postoperatively. All patients should be instructed on the signs and symptoms of early adrenal insufficiency after the laparoscopic adrenal surgery for an incidentaloma.

T. J. Fahey, MD

Predicting Neuroendocrine Tumor (Carcinoid) Neoplasia Using Gene Expression Profiling and Supervised Machine Learning

Drozdov I, Kidd M, Nadler B, et al (Yale Univ School of Medicine, New Haven, CT; Weizmann Inst of Science, Rehovot, Israel)

Cancer 115:1638-1650, 2009

Background.—A more accurate taxonomy of small intestinal (SI) neuroendocrine tumors (NETs) is necessary to accurately predict tumor behavior and prognosis and to define therapeutic strategy. In this study, the authors identified a panel of such markers that have been implicated in tumorigenicity, metastasis, and hormone production and hypothesized that transcript levels of the genes melanoma antigen family D2 (*MAGE-D2*), metastasis-associated 1 (*MTA1*), nucleosome assembly protein 1-like (*NAP1L1*), *Ki-67* (a marker of proliferation), *survivin*, frizzled homolog 7 (*FZD7*), the Kiss1 metastasis suppressor (*Kiss1*), neuropilin 2 (*NRP2*), and chromogranin A (*CgA*) could be used to define primary SI NETs and to predict the development of metastases.

Methods.—Seventy-three clinically and World Health Organization pathologically classified NET samples (primary tumor, n = 44 samples; liver metastases, n = 29 samples) and 30 normal human enterochromaffin (EC) cell preparations were analyzed using real-time polymerase chain reaction. Transcript levels were normalized to 3 NET housekeeping genes (asparagine-linked glycosylation 9 or *ALG9*, transcription factor CP2 or *TFCP2*, and zinc finger protein 410 or *ZNF410*) using geNorm analysis. A predictive gene-based model was constructed using supervised learning algorithms from the transcript expression levels.

Results.—Primary SI NETs could be differentiated from normal human EC cell preparations with 100% specificity and 92% sensitivity. Well differentiated NETs (WDNETs), well differentiated neuroendocrine carcinomas, and poorly differentiated NETs (PDNETs) were classified with a specificity of 78%, 78%, and 71%, respectively; whereas poorly differentiated neuroendocrine carcinomas were misclassified as either WDNETs or PDNETs. Metastases were predicted in all cases with 100% sensitivity and specificity.

Conclusions.—The current results indicated that gene expression profiling and supervised machine learning can be used to classify SI NET subtypes and accurately predict metastasis. The authors believe that the application of this technique will facilitate accurate molecular pathologic delineation of NET disease, better define its extent, facilitate the assessment of prognosis, and provide a guide for the identification of appropriate strategies for individualized patient treatment.

▶ Prediction of behavior of GI neuroendocrine tumors purely on standard histopathologic criteria remains lacking. This study by Modlin's group attempts to refine the classification of carcinoids using a 9-gene model. The authors report enhanced ability to predict tumor behavior using this 9-gene model, though the accuracy does not reach 80% for most tumor types. Nevertheless, this is an important start to achieve more accurate staging of carcinoids using molecular classification. Future studies are required to refine (perhaps by broadening the number of genes being analyzed) the technique, but ultimately these data will be important for designing treatment protocols for individual patients.

T. J. Fahey, MD

Predictive Factors For Ipsilateral or Contralateral Central Lymph Node Metastasis in Unilateral Papillary Thyroid Carcinoma

Koo BS, Choi EC, Yoon Y-H, et al (Chungnam Natl Univ College of Medicine, Daejeon, Korea; Yonsei Univ College of Medicine, Seoul, Korea)

Ann Surg 249:840-844, 2009

Objectives.—To investigate the incidence and the risk factors for occult ipsilateral or contralateral central neck lymph node (LN) metastasis in patients with unilateral papillary thyroid carcinoma (PTC) and a clinically negative neck.

Summary Background Data.—Elective central lymph node dissection (CLND) in patients with PTC remains controversial. There have been few prospective studies assessing accurate histopathologic information and predictive factors for the presence of metastasis to the ipsilateral or contralateral central compartment of the neck in patients with PTC and clinically negative neck nodes.

Methods.—We reviewed a prospective protocol of 111 unilateral PTC patients with clinically node-negative necks who have received total thyroidectomy and elective bilateral CLND from 2005 to 2007. The relationships between LN metastasis to the ipsilateral or contralateral central neck compartment and clinico-pathologic factors such as age, sex, size of primary tumor, perithyroidal invasion, lymphovascular invasion, and capsular invasion were analyzed.

Results.—Occult central neck LN metastasis was present in 54.1% (60/111). Of these patients, bilateral central LN metastases were present in 50% (30/60), unilateral ipsilateral central LN metastasis in 43.3% (26/60), and unilateral contralateral central LN metastasis in 6.7% (4/60). In the univariate analysis, the rate of ipsilateral central LN metastasis was significantly higher in male patients, high risk MACIS score, carcinoma with a maximal diameter of greater than 1 cm, and carcinoma with lymphovascular invasion ($P < 0.05$). The rate of contralateral central LN metastasis was significantly higher in cases of carcinoma with a maximal diameter of greater than 1 cm, lymphovascular invasion or histologically proven metastasis to the ipsilateral central LN ($P < 0.05$). Multivariate analysis showed that the tumor size was an independent risk factor for the presence of ipsilateral central LN metastasis, and the presence of ipsilateral central LN metastasis was the only independent predictor for the presence of contralateral central LN metastasis.

Conclusions.—Unilateral PTC with a maximal diameter of greater than 1 cm is associated with a high rate of ipsilateral central neck LN metastasis. Moreover, ipsilateral central LN metastasis is a potential independent predictor of synchronous contralateral central LN metastasis. These findings suggest that contralateral as well as ipsilateral elective CLND, performed during the initial thyroid operation, may be effective in the management of patients with unilateral PTC having a maximal diameter of greater than 1 cm and ipsilateral central LN metastasis.

▶ This study documents findings that are very similar to the study by Moo et al.[1] The risk of occult central neck lymph node (LN) metastases in patients with papillary thyroid carcinoma (PTC) was 54% overall and 25% in patients with papillary microcarcinoma. Furthermore, the risk of contralateral central LN metastases was very low in patients with papillary microcarcinoma (3/28, 11%)—though clearly not zero. However, the technique for central neck dissection (CND) was different from that as performed in the Moo et al study. In this study, the authors did the central neck clearance and then divided the specimen. In the Moo et al study, the ipsilateral central neck contents were dissected en bloc from the ipislateral carotid to the contralateral anterolateral border of the trachea. It is uncertain if this affected the distribution of LNs. Overall, the findings support the conclusions of the study by Moo et al that contralateral CND may be unnecessary in patients with microcarcinomas. Certainly, when dealing with a papillary microcarcinoma and uncertain parathyroid viability of the ipsilateral parathyroids, a contralateral CND may be considered as very low yield and, therefore, not performed.

T. J. Fahey, MD

Reference

1. Moo TA, Umunna B, Kato M, et al. Ipsilateral versus bilateral central neck lymph node dissection in papillary thyroid carcinoma. *Ann Surg*. 2009;250:403-408.

Prophylactic Lymph Node Dissection for Papillary Thyroid Cancer Less Than 2 cm: Implications for Radioiodine Treatment

Bonnet S, Hartl D, Leboulleux S, et al (Institut Gustave Roussy, Villejuif Cedex, France)

J Clin Endocrinol Metab 94:1162-1167, 2009

Objective.—Prophylactic neck dissection for small papillary carcinoma remains controversial. Radioiodine ablation is not recommended for tumors less than 10 mm and depends on various factors for tumors between 10 and 20 mm.The aim was to determine the effect of lymph node (LN) staging on the indication for treatment with radioiodine.

Patients and Methods.—We conducted a retrospective study of 115 patients presenting with papillary thyroid carcinoma less than 2 cm without ultrasonographically detectable cervical LN treated by total thyroidectomy and complete selective dissection of the central and lateral compartment. Radioiodine treatment was based on definitive pathology (tumor and LN). Follow-up was based on neck ultrasound and thyroglobulin levels.

Results.—LN were found for 41.7% of cases. Radioiodine was not used for 42% of patients with tumors less than 20 mm and no metastatic LN. Fifty-eight percent of patients were treated with radioiodine due to LN metastasis, extracapsular thyroid invasion, or unfavorable histological subtype. LN status affected the indication for radioiodine in 30.5% of cases classified as T1, 12 cases with tumors less than 10 mm but with LN metastases (who received radioiodine), and 13 cases with tumors between 10 and 20 mm but without LN metastases (who did not receive radioiodine). Definitive vocal fold paralysis and hypoparathyroidism each occurred in 0.9% of cases. At 1 yr, ultrasound was normal in all patients, and recombinant human TSH-stimulated thyroglobulin was undetectable for 97% of the patients.

Conclusion.—Precise LN staging by prophylactic neck dissection for tumors initially staged T1N0 modified the indication for radioiodine ablation for 30% of patients.

▶ One of the arguments for doing prophylactic central neck dissection (CND) is that the information learned can help to guide subsequent treatment decisions. This study documents that this is, in fact, the case—especially for smaller papillary thyroid carcinomas. In the absence of lymph node (LN) metastases, the recurrence rate for micropapillary carcinomas is very low (<1%), while positive LNs are associated with a near 20% recurrence rate. Additionally, recent reports associating radioactive iodine (RAI) treatment with a higher risk of secondary malignancy—even if only very slightly increased—mean that if additional surgery can be done to reduce or eliminate the need for postoperative RAI without increasing the risk of recurrence, this is highly desirable. Thus, this is an important article to consider when weighing the merits of prophylactic CND.

T. J. Fahey, MD

Randomized clinical trial of visualization *versus* neuromonitoring of recurrent laryngeal nerves during thyroidectomy

Barczyński M, Konturek A, Cichoń S (Jagiellonian Univ College of Medicine, Kraków, Poland)

Br J Surg 96:240-246, 2009

Background.—The aim of this study was to test the hypothesis that identification of the recurrent laryngeal nerve (RLN) during thyroid surgery reduces injury, and that intraoperative nerve monitoring may be of additional benefit.

Methods.—One thousand consenting patients scheduled to have bilateral thyroid surgery were randomized to standard protection or additional nerve monitoring. The primary outcome measure was prevalence of RLN injury.

Results.—Of 1000 nerves at risk in each group, transient and permanent RLN injuries were found respectively in 38 and 12 nerves without RLN monitoring ($P = 0{\cdot}011$) and 19 and eight nerves with RLN monitoring ($P = 0{\cdot}368$). The prevalence of transient RLN paresis was lower in patients who had RLN monitoring by 2·9 per cent in high-risk patients ($P = 0{\cdot}011$) and 0·9 per cent in low-risk patients ($P = 0{\cdot}249$). The negative and positive predictive values of RLN monitoring in predicting postoperative vocal cord function were 98·9 and 37·8 per cent respectively.

Conclusion.—Nerve monitoring decreased the incidence of transient but not permanent RLN paresis compared with visualization alone, particularly in high-risk patients. Registration number: NCT00661024 (http://www.clinicaltrials.gov).

▶ The debate over the use of routine nerve monitoring in thyroid surgery continues. This study is a large, prospective trial of nerve monitoring. The authors demonstrate that there is a deduction in the incidence of temporary recurrent laryngeal nerve (RLN) injuries, though not permanent injuries. While this is encouraging for nerve monitoring proponents, in reality the intraoperative application is somewhat troubled. The sensitivity for a RLN injury when one occurred was only 63% at best (44% if directly stimulating the RLN as opposed to the vagus), and the positive predictive value (PPV) was only 33%. So one cannot be sure that you do not have a nerve injury before proceeding to the other side, and if you rely on the nerve stimulator, you will stop the exploration prematurely without a RLN injury two-thirds of the time. Finally, in the days of progressively smaller incisions for thyroid surgery, one wonders what the average length of the incision was for patients in this series who had nerve monitoring because every one of them had the vagus nerve identified before starting the thyroid dissection. The bottom line is that the RLN still has to be visualized, and one must suspect that the nerve branches at an early point in every case.

T. J. Fahey, MD

Relation of Final Intraoperative Parathyroid Hormone Level and Outcome Following Parathyroidectomy

Heller KS, Blumberg SN (NYU Langone Med Ctr, New York)
Arch Otolaryngol Head Neck Surg 135:1103-1107, 2009

Objective.—To determine if final intraoperative parathyroid hormone (IOPTH) level predicts those at risk for recurrence after parathyroidectomy. Minimally invasive parathyroid exploration guided by preoperative imaging and IOPTH level is an accepted alternative to bilateral exploration for the treatment of primary hyperparathyroidism (HPT). However, additional enlarged, hypercellular parathyroid glands are present in some patients in whom IOPTH levels fall to normal after excision of a single adenoma. At least 15% of patients are normocalcemic with elevated PTH levels (PPTH) after parathyroidectomy. In these patients, a higher risk of recurrent HPT has been found.

Design.—Retrospective review of medical records.

Setting.—University teaching hospital.

Patients.—The records of all 194 patients who underwent successful initial parathyroidectomy for nonfamilial HPT in 2007 and 2008 by 1 surgeon were reviewed.

Main Outcome Measures.—Intraoperative PTH level was measured prior to incision (baseline); at excision of the abnormal gland; at 5, 10, 15, and 20 minutes after excision; and at various additional times as needed. Of the patients, 71% underwent minimally invasive parathyroid exploration. Calcium, PTH, and 25-hydroxyvitamin D levels were measured during the first month after surgery in all patients and after 3 months or more in 80%. Patients were divided into 5 groups depending on the following final IOPTH levels: lower than 10 pg/mL (group 1) (to convert PTH to nanograms per liter, multiply by 1.0); 10 to 19 pg/mL (group 2); 20 to 29 pg/mL (group 3); 30 to 39 pg/mL (group 4); and 40 pg/mL or higher (group 5).

Results.—Of the patients, 82% had a single adenoma, 9% had double adenomas, and 9% had 3 or more abnormal glands. The final IOPTH/baseline IOPTH value in groups 1 to 5 was 7%, 11%, 16%, 23%, and 26%, respectively. There was no significant difference in the preoperative calcium among the groups. All 3 patients with persistent HPT and 5 patients with PPTH were in group 5. One of the 96 patients in groups 1 and 2 and 5 of the 72 patients in groups 3 and 4 had PPTH at the last evaluation.

Conclusion.—Patients with a final IOPTH level of 40 pg/mL or higher are at higher risk of having persistent HPT and should be followed up closely and indefinitely following parathyroidectomy.

▶ This study reports a relatively short-term follow-up following parathyroidectomy. Similar to the study by Chen,[1] the authors are trying to identify the factors associated with the development of persistent elevation in parathyroid hormone or the development of recurrent hyperparathyroidism. Here, Heller reports that a final intraoperative parathyroid hormone (IOPTH) level of > 40 pg/ml is associated with a higher risk of persistence. The study is a bit confusing in that the data are reported as a percentage of the baseline IOPTH level, but the final recommendation is noted as an absolute level. In any case, the data suggest that IOPTH levels that do not drop below 40 pg/ml warrant additional exploration. This is a study that is both feasible and begs to be done.

T. J. Fahey, MD

Reference

1. Ning L, Sippel R, Schaefer S, Chen H. What is the clinical significance of an elevated parathyroid hormone level after curative surgery for primary hyperparathyroidism? *Ann Surg*. 2009;249:469-472.

Role of Unilateral Adrenalectomy in Bilateral Primary Aldosteronism: A 22-Year Single Center Experience

Sukor N, Gordon RD, Ku YK, et al (Univ of Queensland School of Medicine, Australia)
J Clin Endocrinol Metab 94:2437-2445, 2009

Objective.—The aim of the study was to examine blood pressure and biochemical responses to unilateral adrenalectomy in patients with bilateral primary aldosteronism (PA) and identify predictive parameters.

Context.—PA considered due to bilateral autonomous production of aldosterone is usually treated medically. Unilateral adrenalectomy has been considered ineffective. Because quality outcome data are lacking and medical treatment may cause adverse effects or fail to control hypertension, defining the role for unilateral adrenalectomy in bilateral PA is an important clinical issue.

Design and Setting.—Between 1984 and 2004, 51 of 684 patients diagnosed with bilateral PA underwent unilateral adrenalectomy. This report is based on the records of the 40 considered suitable for inclusion, who were followed for at least 12 (median, 56.4) months.

Results.—Hypertension was cured in 15% of patients and improved in 20%, usually within 1 yr of unilateral adrenalectomy. The proportion with controlled hypertension was significantly ($P < 0.001$) higher after adrenalectomy (65%) than before (25%). Mean systolic ($P < 0.001$) and diastolic ($P < 0.001$) blood pressure, left ventricular mass index ($P < 0.05$), plasma upright aldosterone ($P < 0.05$), and aldosterone/renin ratio ($P < 0.001$) fell. Serum creatinine independently predicted hypertension cure.

Conclusion.—Although this retrospective analysis of patients from a single center does not permit prediction of response rates among patients diagnosed elsewhere, it suggests that unilateral adrenalectomy can be beneficial in some patients with apparent bilateral PA and should not be dismissed as a treatment option.

▶ This study from the Endocrine Hypertension Group in Queensland is a nice analysis of patients with bilateral primary aldosteronism who underwent unilateral adrenalectomy. The data are perhaps surprising to the authors themselves in that there was a clear benefit in 35% of the patients. The authors' criteria for lateralization happens to be particularly strict, raising the question as to whether the response is seen in just patients who would be considered candidates for surgery by other adrenal vein sampling criteria. Fortunately, the authors address this and show that the response rate would be virtually identical even if some patients were eliminated as having unilateral disease. Although the expectation was that the effect might be seen most in patients with out-of-control blood pressure, in fact, patients with earlier stages of hypertension appeared to have the best response. While these data will not change current treatment algorithms regarding management of patients with bilateral primary hyperaldosteronism, they demonstrate that further study of the role of surgery is necessary in these patients.

T. J. Fahey, MD

Surgical Versus Conservative Management for Subclinical Cushing Syndrome in Adrenal Incidentalomas: A Prospective Randomized Study

Toniato A, Merante-Boschin I, Opocher G, et al (Univ of Padua School of Medicine, Padova, Italy; Familial Cancer Clinic, Padua, Italy)

Ann Surg 249:388-391, 2009

Objective.—To compare the clinical outcome of patients with subclinical Cushing syndrome (SCS) due to an adrenal incidentaloma (the autonomous hypersecretion of a small amount of cortisol, which is not enough to cause clinically-evident disease) who underwent surgery or were managed conservatively.

Summary Background Data.—The most appropriate management of SCS patients is controversial, either adrenalectomy or close follow-up being recommended for their treatment.

Methods.—Over a 15-year period, 45 SCS patients were randomly selected to undergo surgery (n = 23) or conservative management (n = 22). All surgical procedures were laparoscopic adrenalectomies performed by the same surgeon. All patients were followed up (mean, 7.7 years; range, 2–17 years) clinically by 2 experienced endocrinologists 6 and 12 months after surgery and then yearly, or yearly after joining the trial, particularly monitoring diabetes mellitus (DM), arterial hypertension, hyperlipidemia, obesity, and osteoporosis. The study end point was the clinical outcome of SCS patients who underwent adrenalectomy versus those managed conservatively.

Results.—All 23 patients in the surgical arm had elective surgery. Another 3 patients randomly assigned to conservative management crossed over to the surgical group due to an increasing adrenal mass >3.5 cm. In the surgical group, DM normalized or improved in 62.5% of patients (5 of 8), hypertension in 67% (12 of 18), hyperlipidemia in 37.5% (3 of 8), and obesity in 50% (3 of 6). No changes in bone parameters were seen after surgery in SCS patients with osteoporosis. On the other hand, some worsening of DM, hypertension, and hyperlipidemia was noted in conservatively-managed patients.

Conclusions.—Based on the results of this study, laparoscopic adrenalectomy performed by skilled surgeons appears more beneficial than conservative management for SCS patients complying with our selection

TABLE 3.—Long-Term Outcome in the Surgical Group

	Before Surgery	After Surgery Normalization	Improvement	No Changes	*P* Value
Low plasma ACTH, n (%)	7/23 (30.4)	7/7 (100)	—	—	—
Elevated UFC, n (%)	9/23 (39.1)	9/9 (100)	—	—	—
Post-DMX text, n (%)	23/23 (100)	23/23 (100)	—	—	—
DM, n (%)	8/23 (34.8)	2/8 (25)	3/8 (37.5)	3/8 (37.5)	.619
Hypertension, n (%)	18/23 (78.3)	5/18 (27.8)	7/18 (38.9)	6/18 (33.3)	.046
Hypercholesterolemia, n (%)	8/23 (34.8)	3/8 (37.5)	—	5/8 (62.5)	.619
BMI >30, n (%)	6/23 (26.1)	3/6 (50)	—	3/6 (50)	—
Osteoporosis, n (%)	5/23 (21.7)	—	—	5/5 (100)	—

ACTH = adrenocorticotropic hormone; UFC = urine-free cortisol; DXM = dexamethasone, DM = diabetes mellitus; BMI = body mass index.

criteria. This trial is registered with Australian Clinical Trials Registry number, ANZCTR12608000567325 (Table 3).

▶ This important study documents that laparoscopic adrenalectomy is both safe and effective at reducing morbidity associated with subclinical Cushing syndrome. Subclinical Cushing syndrome was diagnosed if patients had no overt clinical signs of excess hormone and had at least 2 biochemical hypothalamic-pituitary-adrenal (HPA) axis alterations. The strengths of the study are the prospective randomized format and long-term follow-up. The main weakness is the small size of each arm. The results for the surgically treated patients are shown in Table 3. The same parameters in patients in the observation arm remained the same or worsened over the same time period. Those who favor a conservative approach might be bolstered by the fact that none of the patients in the observation arm went on to obvious clinical Cushing syndrome. However, the data here convincingly support a surgical approach to reduce or stabilize complications of Cushing, including diabetes, hypertension, and excess weight.

T. J. Fahey, MD

The Effectiveness of Radioguided Parathyroidectomy in Patients With Negative Technetium Tc 99m–Sestamibi Scans

Chen H, Sippel RS, Schaefer S (Univ of Wisconsin, Madison)
Arch Surg 144:643-648, 2009

Background.—Many surgeons have shown that radioguided resection of parathyroid glands can facilitate intraoperative localization in selected patients with primary hyperparathyroidism, especially in the reoperative setting. However, in patients with negative technetium Tc 99m–sestamibi (hereafter referred to as "sestamibi") scans, the usefulness of the gamma probe is unclear. Thus, we were interested in determining the role of radioguided techniques in patients with primary hyperparathyroidism and negative or nonlocalizing sestamibi scans.

Design.—Retrospective analysis of a prospective parathyroid database.

Setting.—Academic medical center.

Patients.—Seven hundred sixty-nine patients with primary hyperparathyroidism who had a sestamibi scan and underwent surgical invention by a single surgeon. All patients had radioguided parathyroidectomy using a handheld gamma probe.

Main Outcome Measures.—Radioactive counts, eucalcemia rate, and complications were compared between patients with positive and patients with negative sestamibi scans.

Results.—All enlarged parathyroid glands were localized with the gamma probe in patients with a negative or with a positive sestamibi scan with similar sensitivities. This occurred despite the fact that smaller parathryoid glands were present, on average, in patients with negative sestamibi scans (428 mg vs 828 mg, $P = .001$). Equivalent high postoperative eucalcemia rates (>98%) and low complication rates (0.5%) were achieved with radioguided techniques in both patient populations.

Conclusions.—Radioguided techniques are equally effective in patients with negative (nonlocalizing) sestamibi scans undergoing parathyroidectomy for primary hyperparathyroidism. Moreover, use of the gamma probe led to the detection of all parathyroid glands, including ectopically located ones. These data suggest that the gamma probe has an important role for localization of parathyroid glands in patients with negative preoperative sestamibi scans.

► Many endocrine surgeons have shunned the use of MIP based on MIBI + gamma probe due to the fact that MIBI scans localize disease in only 50% to 60% of patients with primary hyperparathyroidism (despite reports of successful localization in 70%-80%). This report by Chen suggests that a positive scan is not necessary for successful use of the probe intraoperatively. While the numbers reported seem quite convincing, it is not clear that the gamma probe is not simply being used to confirm an enlarged gland once it has been found surgically in these MIBI-negative cases, which is a substantially different use than using it to identify the offending gland. In other words, a 4-gland exploration by an expert parathyroid surgeon leads to a high rate of success in MIBI-negative cases independent of the MIBI or the gamma probe, not because of the gamma probe.

T. J. Fahey, MD

The limited role of midnight salivary cortisol levels in the diagnosis of subclinical hypercortisolism in patients with adrenal incidentaloma

Masserini B, Morelli V, Bergamaschi S, et al (Univ of Milan, Italy; et al)
Eur J Endocrinol 160:87-92, 2009

Objective.—The criteria for defining subclinical hypercortisolism (SH) are debated and a real gold standard test or combination of tests is lacking. Recently, late-night salivary cortisol (MSC) has been described as a sensitive and easy-to-perform marker for diagnosing overt hypercortisolism. No data are available on the role of MSC in the diagnosis of SH. The aim of this study was to evaluate the sensitivity and specificity of MSC levels in the diagnosis of SH in patients with adrenal incidentalomas (AI).

Methods.—In 103 (females/males, 69/34) patients with AI, MSC levels were studied. One milligram overnight dexamethasone suppression test (DST), urinary-free cortisol (UFC), and ACTH plasma levels were also evaluated. Patients were defined as affected by SH if they showed two of the following criteria: DST > 83 nmol/l, ACTH < 2.2 pmol/l, and UFC > 193 nmol/24 h.

Results.—No difference in MSC levels in patients with SH (3.1 ± 3.1 nmol/l) compared with patients without SH (2.2 ± 2.8 nmol/l) was observed. In patients with SH, MSC levels were significantly correlated with DST ($r = 0.4$, $P < 0.05$). Using the cut-off of 5.1 nmol/l, the sensitivity and specificity of MSC levels for diagnosis of SH is 22.7 and 87.7% respectively.

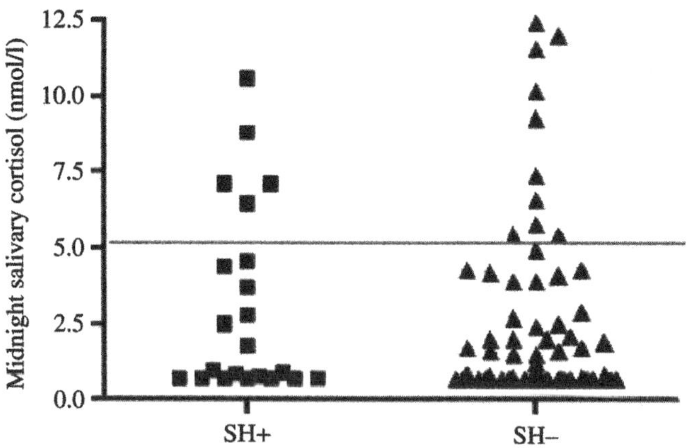

FIGURE 1.—Midnight salivary cortisol levels distribution in patients affected with adrenal incidentalomas with (SH+) and without subclinical hypercortisolism (SH−). Subclinical hypercortisolism was diagnosed if two of the following criteria were present: DST > 83 nmol/l, 24-hour urinary-free cortisol > 193 nmol/24 h, and ACTH < 2.2 pmol/l. The cut-off of 5.1 nmol/l corresponds to the 95th percentile of our reference population. (Courtesy of Masserini B, Morelli V, Bergamaschi S, et al. The limited role of midnight salivary cortisol levels in the diagnosis of subclinical hypercortisolism in patients with adrenal incidentaloma. *Eur J Endocrinol*. 2009;160:87-92.)

Conclusion.—In patients with AI, normal levels of MSC do not exclude SH, whereas high levels may suggest the presence of SH identified by conventional tests. Thus, MSC is not suitable as a screening test, although it may be used in conjunction with other tests as the confirming test in selected patients.

▶ The use of midnight or bedtime salivary cortisol levels to help in the diagnosis of overt Cushing's syndrome is now well established and has a sensitivity and specificity of > 90%. This study analyzes whether bedtime salivary cortisol can be useful in the diagnosis of subclinical hypercortisolism. As shown in Fig 1, there is virtually no difference in the distribution of salivary cortisol levels in patients with and without subclinical hypercortisolism. The authors acknowledge that the study only analyzed a single salivary cortisol level and that it is possible that the test could be more sensitive with analysis of additional samples.

T. J. Fahey, MD

Unrecognized adrenal insufficiency in patients undergoing laparoscopic adrenalectomy

Mitchell J, Barbosa G, Tsinberg M, et al (The Cleveland Clinic, OH)
Surg Endosc 23:248-254, 2009

Background.—Subclinical Cushing's syndrome (SCS) is a well-described phenomenon where abnormalities of the hypothalamic–pituitary–adrenal axis exist in the absence of overt signs and symptoms of classic Cushing's syndrome. While this has been shown to exist in 5–20% of patients with adrenal lesions, no standardized biochemical regimen exists to screen for SCS. Consequently, many of these patients may not be diagnosed prior to adrenalectomy with the risk of postoperative adrenal insufficiency. We began checking morning (a.m.) serum cortisol levels on postoperative day 1 (POD1) following unilateral adrenalectomy for nonfunctioning adrenal lesions to determine the incidence of unrecognized adrenal insufficiency (AI) in these patients.

Methods.—One hundred and five patients undergoing adrenalectomy at a tertiary care center from 1999 to 2007 were retrospectively evaluated. Patients with Cushing's syndrome, conditions associate with bilateral disease, and those receiving perioperative steroids were excluded, leaving 41 patients for analysis. A.m. serum cortisol levels were obtained in all patients POD1. Multiple factors were analyzed as possible predictors of AI. Analysis of variance (ANOVA), *t*-test, and chi-square test were used to determine statistical significance.

Results.—The 41 patients' diagnoses included 13 pheochromocytomas, 15 nonsecreting adenomas, 5 aldosteronomas, 5 metastatic lesions, 1 adrenocortical carcinoma, and 2 other benign lesions. Three groups were identified based on POD1, a.m. cortisol levels: sufficient (>10 μg/dl; $n = 25$,

61%), low-normal (3.4–10 μg/dl; $n=7$, 17%), and insufficient (<3.4 μg/dl; $n=9$, 22%). Tumor size and presence of diabetes, hypertension, and obesity were predictive of postoperative AI ($p < 0.05$).

Conclusions.—AI after unilateral adrenalectomy without evidence of cortisol hypersecretion on preoperative screening was present in a significant number of patients in our series. Patients with diabetes, hypertension, obesity, and larger tumors may be at higher risk for postoperative AI. More thorough screening for cortisol hypersecretion may be warranted in patients with these characteristics, and obtaining routine postoperative cortisol levels may avoid potentially dangerous unrecognized adrenal insufficiency following adrenalectomy.

▶ The results reported here are interesting, though somewhat perplexing. The study appropriately focuses attention on unrecognized adrenal insufficiency after unilateral adrenalectomy. In most cases, however, this occurs in patients who are undergoing resection of a presumed nonfunctioning adenoma with subclinical hypercortisolism. Although there are plausible explanations presented for why adrenal insufficiency may appear in the setting of pheos and other tumors where it would not be expected, in practical terms, symptomatic adrenal insufficiency would seem unlikely and has not been seen by this reviewer (after pheo resection), raising the question as to the accuracy of a single postoperative morning serum cortisol level measurement for the diagnosis of adrenal insufficiency. Additionally, though not addressed in the article, the group that perhaps warrants the most scrutiny is the patients who receive perioperative steroids, which can mask adrenal insufficiency prior to discharge.

T. J. Fahey, MD

What is the Clinical Significance of an Elevated Parathyroid Hormone Level After Curative Surgery for Primary Hyperparathyroidism?

Ning L, Sippel R, Schaefer S, et al (Univ of Wisconsin, Madison; Univ of Wisconsin Paul P. Carbone Comprehensive Cancer Ctr, Madison)

Ann Surg 249:469-472, 2009

Objectives.—Recent reports have demonstrated that between 8%–40% of patients after curative surgery for primary hyperparathyroidism (HPT) have an elevated parathyroid hormone level (ePTH). To determine the clinical significance of ePTH and if it is a potential risk factor for recurrent HPT, we reviewed our experience.

Methods.—611 consecutive patients underwent curative parathyroidectomy for primary HPT by one surgeon. Patients with ePTH [defined as postoperative parathyroid hormone (PTH) levels ≥65 pg/mL at least 1 week after surgery with normal calcium levels] were compared with those with normal PTH.

Results.—ePTH occurred in 111/611 (18.2%) patients. When compared with those with normal PTH, ePTH patients were older and had higher preoperative PTH and alkaline phosphatase levels ($P < 0.05$). Importantly, recurrent HPT was significantly higher in patients with ePTH (5.4% versus 1.2%, $P < 0.05$). Further analysis of the ePTH patients revealed that serum calcium 1-week after surgery was predictive of recurrent HPT. In ePTH patients with postoperative calcium ≥9.7 mg/dL, the recurrence rate was 16% compared with 0% in those whose calcium was <9.7 mg/dL.

Conclusions.—Most of patients (95%) with ePTH after curative parathyroidectomy for primary HPT will not develop recurrent HPT. However, recurrent disease is significantly more common among patients with ePTH and was always associated with postoperative calcium ≥9.7 mg/dL. Thus, these data suggest that streamlining postoperative surveillance to this subset of patients may optimize resource utilization.

▶ Persistent elevation of parathyroid hormone after parathyroidectomy has been recognized for some time. Whether this is associated with a higher incidence of recurrence has been debated for almost as long. This single surgeon series documents that there is a higher risk of recurrence in patients who have postoperative hyperparathormonemia, and furthermore documents that this occurs in the subset of patients who have postoperative calcium levels in the higher range of normal. It is an important study, and raises the question as to whether this group of patients that is more prone to recurrence is the same group that the Cleveland Clinic group has identified as having additional enlarged glands, despite an appropriate intraoperative parathyroid hormone (IOPTH) response to the excision of a single enlarged gland. This will be a difficult prospective study to ever perform, and I am not sure we will ever have an answer to this question.

T. J. Fahey, MD

Identification of Borderline Thyroid Tumors by Gene Expression Array Analysis

Arora N, Scognamiglio T, Lubitz CC (New York Presbyterian Hosp-Weill Cornell Med Ctr)

Cancer 115:5421-5431, 2009

Background.—A subset of follicular lesions of the thyroid is encapsulated similar to follicular adenomas but with partial nuclear features suggestive of papillary thyroid carcinoma (PTC), raising the possibility of biologically borderline tumors.

Methods.—Gene expression profiling and advanced significance analyses were performed on 50 histologically unequivocal benign and malignant tumors, and a list of 61 differentially expressed genes was generated. By using this 61-gene list, unsupervised hierarchical and K-means cluster analyses were performed on 40 additional tumors, including 15 histologically borderline tumors, 11 benign tumors, and 14 PTCs.

Results.—Analysis revealed 3 distinct tumor groups—benign, malignant, and intermediate. Tumors in the intermediate group (n = 15) were mostly histologic borderline tumors and had an expression profile overlapping with the benign and malignant groups. Twenty-seven genes were expressed differentially between the benign and intermediate groups, including the cyclic AMP response element-binding protein/p300-interactivator with glutamic acid/aspartic acid-rich carboxy-terminal domain 1 or *CITED1* gene and the fibroblast growth factor receptor 2 or *FGFR2* gene. Fourteen genes were expressed differentially between the intermediate group and malignant tumors, notably overexpression of the *met* proto-oncogene and of the high-mobility group adenine/thymine-hook 2 or *HMGA2* gene in malignancies. Mutations of the v-raf murine sarcoma viral oncogene homolog B1 or *BRAF* gene were identified in 4 of 14 malignant tumors but not in benign or intermediate tumors. Patients who had either histologically or molecularly borderline tumors did not have metastasis or recurrences.

Conclusions.—Gene expression profiling supported the finding that encapsulated thyroid follicular lesions with partial nuclear features of PTC are biologically borderline tumors that are distinct molecularly from benign and malignant tumors.

▶ Classification of borderline thyroid tumors is a perplexing problem with substantial implications for patient treatment. These tumors may have been the minimally invasive follicular carcinomas according to previous classification, but are now designated as encapsulated follicular lesions with some of the nuclear features of papillary thyroid carcinoma. They are frequently designated as carcinomas and treated as such—including complete thyroidectomy and postoperative radioactive iodine (RAI) therapy. The authors propose that molecular classification be added to traditional histopathologic criteria for determining malignancy, and that consideration be given to classifying these tumors as premalignant lesions. Long-term studies need to be completed to confirm the benign behavior of this class of tumors, but I suspect that this will confirm what the gene expression data are telling us.

T. J. Fahey, MD

8 Nutrition

Determining small intestinal transit time and pathomorphology in critically ill patients using video capsule technology

Rauch S, Krueger K, Turan A, et al (Univ of Louisville, KY)

Intensive Care Med 35:1054-1059, 2009

Purpose.—Gastrointestinal motility can be impaired by serious illness or medications, compromising enteral feeding in critical care patients. We compared small bowel transit time and morphology in neurosurgical critical care (ICU) patients with those in healthy subjects.

Methods.—We evaluated small intestinal transit time, quality of visualization and intestinal morphology in 16 ICU patients (Glasgow Coma Scale score from 6 to 14) and 16 healthy ambulatory patients. Video data were obtained with PillCam SB capsules (Given Imaging Ltd., Yoqneam, Israel).

Results.—Transit time was 5.1 h (3.9–7.7) (median [IQR]) in ICU and 4.3 (4.1–5.3 h) in ambulatory patients ($P = 0.481$). Six ICU patients (37%) and two ambulatory patients (12%) had pathological findings (ulcers, petechia, erosions) ($P = 0.10$).

Conclusions.—Median small bowel transit times in critically ill neurosurgical patients were similar to those in ambulatory subjects, although transit times were more variable in the critically ill patients.

▶ Patients in critical care settings may have difficulty tolerating enteral feeding. A variety of causes such as infection, medications, and underlying critical condition are often cited. Yet, it is well known that after major abdominal surgery with manipulation of the small intestine, peristalsis seems normal and jejunal feedings can be accomplished. Thus, this randomized controlled study is very important. Median small bowel transit time was not significantly different between patients and controls, although there was a greater variation in transit times in patients compared with controls. At times, while the small bowel motility is normal, there can be gastric and colonic dysmotility in critically ill patients. Interestingly, there was no correlation between small bowel transit and the degree of critical illness as determined by APACHE scores, and so forth.

This study lends importance to our understanding of the small bowel's response to major injury, particularly brain injury.

J. M. Daly, MD

Enteral Nutrition Enriched With Eicosapentaenoic Acid (EPA) Preserves Lean Body Mass Following Esophageal Cancer Surgery: Results of a Double-Blinded Randomized Controlled Trial

Ryan AM, Reynolds JV, Healy L, et al (St James's Hosp, Ireland)
Ann Surg 249:355-363, 2009

Background.—Esophagectomy represents an exemplar of controlled major trauma, with marked metabolic, immunologic, and physiologic changes as well as an associated high incidence of complications. Eicosapentaenoic acid (EPA) enriched enteral nutrition (EN) modulates immune function and limits catabolism in patients with advanced cancer, but its impact in the peri-operative period is unclear.

Objectives.—To examine the effects of perioperative EPA enriched EN on the metabolic, nutritional, and immuno-inflammatory response to esophagectomy, and on postoperative complications.

Methods.—In a double-blind design, patients were randomized to a standard EN formula or a formula enriched with 2.2 g EPA/d for 5 days preoperatively (orally) and 21 days postoperatively (jejunostomy). Segmental bioelectrical impedance analysis was performed preoperatively and on POD 21. Postoperative complications were monitored, as well as the acute phase response, coagulation markers, and serum cytokines.

Results.—Fifty-three patients (28 EPA, 25 standard) completed the study, and both groups were well matched. Serum and peripheral blood mononuclear cell (PBMC) membrane EPA levels were significantly increased in the EPA group. There was no difference in the incidence of major complications. The EPA group maintained all aspects of body composition postoperatively, whereas patients in the standard EN group lost significant amounts of fat-free mass (1.9 kg, $P \leq 0.030$) compared with the EPA group [leg (0.3 kg, $P \leq 0.05$), arm (0.17 kg, $P \leq 0.01$), and trunk (1.44 kg, $P \leq 0.03$)]. The EPA group had a significantly ($P < 0.05$) attenuated stress response for TNFα, IL-10, and IL-8 compared with the standard group.

Conclusions.—EPA supplemented early EN is associated with preservation of lean body mass post esophagectomy compared with a standard EN. These properties may merit longer-term study to address its impact on recovery of function and quality of life in models of complex surgery or multimodal cancer treatment regimens.

▶ Multiple animal, in vitro, and some human studies have evaluated the effects of eicosapentaenoic acid (EPA) supplementation on host cellular inflammatory responses. Cellular studies show early incorporation of EPA into monocyte membranes, which are related to changes in stimulated cytokine production. In human studies, often other nutrients have been provided along with supplemented omega-3-fatty acids perhaps confounding the results. In addition, the patients undergoing operation have often been heterogeneous.

Thus, Dr Reynolds' study is quite important, as one type of major operation was used for evaluation. In addition, the EPA-enriched enteral nutrition (EN) formula was begun 5 days before the operation, allowing some time for the formula to potentially alter the host's response to surgery. In these 53 patients studied, there was no mortality and there were few differences in morbidity between the 2 groups. There were differences noted in the plasma levels of cytokine responses to operation. Interestingly, there was significantly less lean body mass lost in the EPA supplemented group than in the standard fed group.

J. M. Daly, MD

High Rates of Mortality and Morbidity Occur in Infants With Parenteral Nutrition–Associated Cholestasis

Willis TC, Carter BA, Rogers SP, et al (Baylor College of Medicine, Houston, TX; Baylor College of Medicine and Texas Children's Hosp, Houston)

JPEN J Parenter Enteral Nutr 34:32-37, 2010

Background.—Extremely few data are available about the natural history of parenteral nutrition (PN)–associated cholestasis. The authors evaluated a cohort of infants at a large center to determine the outcome of PN-associated cholestasis in infants with some gastrointestinal function.

Methods.—The authors reviewed the records of all infants admitted to a level 3 neonatal intensive care unit over a 16-month period who had the diagnosis of PN-associated cholestasis. Records were reviewed in these infants for course of cholestasis, laboratory values, outcome, and infection rate.

Results.—Sixty-six patients were admitted who met the study criteria. There were 10 deaths and 1 referral for liver transplant (Death/TPlant) (17%) in the first year of life. All Death/TPlant infants had at least 1 positive blood culture after the onset of cholestasis. Maximum conjugated bilirubin (MaxCB) in Death/TPlant infants was 15.7 ± 2.2 (SEM) compared to 8.4 ± 1.0 mg/dL in babies who recovered. Of 21 infants with a MaxCB ≥10.0, Death/TPlant occurred in 8/21 (38%). Of 40 babies with positive blood cultures, 11 were in the Death/TPlant group vs no deaths among the 25 without positive blood cultures. Average time to resolution from the MaxCB to a CB <2.0 mg/dL was 66 ± 7 days (n = 49).

Conclusions.—Infants with PN-associated cholestasis have high rates of mortality despite the presence of some gastrointestinal function. These data support further evaluation and the development of novel forms of therapy for babies with parenteral-associated CB ≥2 mg/dL with emphasis on interventions for infants with a CB >10 mg/dL.

▶ The authors performed a retrospective review of infants who developed parenteral nutrition-associated cholestasis in an attempt to define the risk factors for mortality and morbidity. They noted that when conjugated bilirubin (CB) levels exceeded 10 mg/dL, the mortality and requirement for transplant risk was 38% compared with 7% in the group with CB < 10 mg/dL. The rate of necrotizing enterocolitis was also quite high (52%) in the group with CB

>10 mg/dL compared with 18% in the group with lower CB. This study is useful in that it provides some quantitative parameters to define very ill infants at high risk for mortality in association with the administration of parenteral nutrition. It may be that the use of other lipid formulations may reduce the incidence and degree of cholestasis along with the aggressive treatment of underlying conditions. As further data accumulate on alternative nutritional constituents, infants with CB >10 mg/dL or slightly less would be eligible to receive such therapy.

J. M. Daly, MD

Impact of Fish Oil-Based Lipid Emulsion on Serum Triglyceride, Bilirubin, and Albumin Levels in Children With Parenteral Nutrition-Associated Liver Disease

Lee SI, Valim C, Johnston P, et al (Harvard Med School, Boston, MA; Children's Hosp Boston, MA)

Pediatr Res 66:698-703, 2009

Parenteral nutrition is known to cause liver injury in babies. The aim of this study is to investigate the effects of different lipid emulsions on parenteral nutrition-associated cholestasis in infants. In addition, there may be a relationship between the lipid emulsion and triglyceride levels. Furthermore, triglyceride levels may correlate with direct bilirubin and albumin, as markers of liver impairment and nutritional status. Patients with parenteral nutrition-associated cholestasis who were treated with a fish oil-based lipid emulsion ($n = 18$) were prospectively followed for triglyceride, direct bilirubin, and albumin levels and compared with patients who were maintained on a soy-based lipid emulsion ($n = 59$). Triglyceride levels decreased in the fish oil cohort from a mean of 140 mg/dL at wk 0 to 40 mg/dL at wk 20 but remained unchanged at ~140 mg/dL in the soybean cohort. Triglyceride levels of patients treated with fish oil declined over time, while those receiving soybean oil did not. Also, changes in triglyceride levels over time were directly correlated with direct bilirubin and inversely related to albumin levels. These findings may indicate an added benefit of reduced triglyceride levels for patients treated with fish oil and this effect coincides with markers for improved liver function and nutritional status.

▶ As has been noted, parenteral nutrition-associated cholestasis is a major problem in low-birth-weight infants and is associated with increased mortality and morbidity, especially when bilirubin levels exceed 10 mg/dL. This study prospectively evaluated 18 infants receiving a fish oil-based (FO) lipid emulsion compared with 59 infants who continued with soybean-based (SB) lipid emulsion as part of their total parenteral nutrition (TPN). The authors noted that bilirubin and triglyceride levels decreased significantly in the FO group compared with the SB group, which maintained their triglyceride levels at approximately 140 mg/dL. In addition, serum albumin levels climbed as the triglyceride levels decreased in the FO group.

While not a randomized trial, this prospective evaluation provides ample evidence to initiate a randomized trial in infants with parenteral nutrition-associated cholestasis in an effort to improve their outcomes.

J. M. Daly, MD

Inhibition of Gastroesophageal Reflux by Semi-solid Nutrients in Patients With Percutaneous Endoscopic Gastrostomy

Nishiwaki S, Araki H, Shirakami Y, et al (Nishimino Kosei Hosp, Gifu, Japan; Gifu Univ, Japan)

JPEN J Parenter Enteral Nutr 33:513-519, 2009

Background.—Aspiration is one of the major complications after percutaneous endoscopic gastrostomy (PEG). The administration of semi-solid nutrients by means of gastrostomy tube has recently been reported to be effective in preventing aspiration pneumonia. The effects of semi-solid nutrients on gastroesophageal reflux, intragastric distribution, and gastric emptying were evaluated.

Methods.—Semi-solid nutrients were prepared by liquid nutrients mixed with agar at the concentration of 0.5%. The distribution of the administered radiolabeled liquid and semi-solid nutrients was monitored by a scintillation camera for 15 post-PEG patients. The percentage of esophageal reflux, the distribution of the proximal and distal stomach, and the gastric emptying time were evaluated.

Results.—The percentage of gastroesophageal reflux was significantly decreased in semi-solid nutrients (0.82 ± 1.27%) compared with liquid nutrients (3.75 ± 4.25%), whereas the gastric emptying time was not different. The distribution of semi-solid nutrients was not different from liquid nutrients in the early phase, whereas higher retention of liquid nutrients in the proximal stomach was observed in the late phase.

Conclusions.—Gastroesophageal reflux was significantly inhibited by semi-solid nutrients. One of the mechanisms of the inhibition is considered to be an improvement in the transition from the proximal to distal stomach in semi-solid nutrients.

▶ Percutaneous endoscopic gastrostomy is a very common procedure to maintain enteral nutrition in those unable to swallow properly because of a variety of underlying conditions. Unfortunately, gastric dysmotility and reduced lower esophageal sphincter pressures result in a high incidence of gastric content pulmonary aspiration. This interesting study evaluated the use of semisolid nutrients instead of liquid nutrients on GI reflux and gastric emptying. Importantly, use of semisolid nutrients resulted in a greater passage of nutrients from the proximal to the distal stomach. Gastric emptying was not different between groups, but GI reflux was less with semisolid nutrients.

Results of this study should be taken to more routine use in patients who cannot inherently protect their airways from aspiration. It is possible that use of gastric motility pro-kinetic agents may be synergistic with the use of semisolid nutrients to improve outcomes in these patients.

J. M. Daly, MD

Nutrition Support With Glutamine Dipeptide in Patients Undergoing Liver Transplantation

Qiu Y, Zhu X, Wang W, et al (Med School of Nanjing Univ, China)

Transplant Proc 41:4232-4237, 2009

Aim.—The effect of total parenteral nutrition (TPN) support supplemented with alanyl-glutamine (Ala-Gln) dipeptide was investigated in a randomized, controlled clinical trial.

Methods.—Sixty-five patients with the diagnosis of end-stage liver disease or hepatic cellular carcinoma admitted for orthotopic liver transplantation were randomly divided into 3 groups: diet group ($n = 21$), TPN group ($n = 22$), and Gln group ($n = 22$). Patients in the TPN and Gln groups received isocaloric and isonitrogenous TPN for 7 days. Venous heparin blood samples were obtained for assay on days 2 and 9 after surgery; we performed routine pathologic tests.

Results.—Compared with the results on day 9 in the TPN group, there was a significant increase in the prognostic nutrition index and in prealbumin among the Gln group. Aspartate aminotransferase improved significantly by Gln treatment compared with traditional TPN support ($P < .05$). The pathologic results also showed Gln supplementation to reduce hepatic cell injury. A significant decrease in postoperative hospital stay was observed in the Gln group.

Conclusions.—Posttransplant TPN support greatly improved protein metabolism and nutritional state of patients. TPN with Ala-Gln helped to improve synthetic function and to reduce the injury to a transplanted liver.

▶ Glutamine supplementation in cellular and animal studies has shown clear benefits. Human studies have been less clear. Thus, this prospective, randomized trial of total parenteral nutrition (TPN) versus glutamine dipeptide-supplemented TPN versus control patients undergoing hepatic transplantation is very important. It is powered with 65 patients entered into a 3-arm trial only to evaluate the metabolic parameters. The trial did demonstrate an improvement in the Prognostic Nutritional Index and prealbumin levels. Interestingly, despite no difference in the postoperative morbidity or mortality, hospital length of stay was shorter in the Gln group. There was a suggestion of less hepatic cellular injury in the Gln group as well. It would have been interesting if the authors had studied immune function in the 3 groups before and at intervals after surgery. It would also be important to understand the benefits of enteral supplementation after transplantation perhaps compared with TPN. Previous studies have not shown a clear-cut benefit to nutritional supplementation surrounding hepatic transplantation.

J. M. Daly, MD

Parenteral and enteral nutrition in the management of neurosurgical patients in the intensive care unit

Oertel MF, Hauenschild A, Gruenschlaeger J, et al (Univ Hosp Giessen and Marburg, Klinikstrasse, Germany)

J Clin Neurosci 16:1161-1167, 2009

The iatrogenic malnutrition of neurosurgical patients in intensive care units (ICU) is an underestimated problem. It may cause a decrease in plasma albumin and oncotic pressure, leading to an increase in the amount of water entering the brain and increased intracranial pressure (ICP). This study was conducted to test the hypothesis that combined high-protein parenteral and enteral nutrition is beneficial for neurosurgical patients in ICU. A total of 202 neurosurgical patients in ICU (mean age ± standard deviation, 56 years ± 16 years; male:female = 1.2:1) were studied. Two consecutive 1-year time periods were compared, during which two different nutritional regimens were followed. In the first time period (Y1) patients were given a low-protein/high-fat formulation parenterally, followed by a standard enteral regimen. In the second time period (Y2) a protein-rich, combined parenteral and enteral diet was prospectively administered. The Glasgow Outcome Score was measured at 3–6 months after discharge. The following clinical parameters were recorded during the first 2 weeks after admission: ICP; albumin; cholinesterase (CHE); daily hours of ICP > 20 mmHg and cerebral perfusion pressure < 70 mmHg; and Acute Physiology and Chronic Health Evaluation II (APACHE II) score. It was found that overall albumin (32.4 g/L ± 4.1 g/L *vs.* 27.5 g/L ± 3.6 g/L) and CHE was higher during Y2, although the total energy supply, glucose and fat intake was lower. Higher GOS scores were seen when patients had lower APACHE II scores and received the Y2 nutritional regimen. During Y2, the total hours of ICP > 20 mmHg were fewer. With the Y2 nutrition, maintenance of adequate cerebral perfusion required less catecholamine medication and colloidal fluid replacement. Therefore, adequate nutrition is an important parameter in the management of neurosurgical patients in ICU.

► The use of nutritional support of some sort is widespread in neurosurgical units. However, the true value is unclear, as there may be little effect on ultimate outcome, which is determined more from the type, extent, and duration of brain injury. This interesting clinical study used a methodology of 2 consecutive time periods in which a standard low-calorie, low-nitrogen diet was given in period 1, while combined parenteral and enteral nutrition was given in period 2. It appeared that cerebral recovery was better in period 2 when a nutritional support team monitored the nutritional intake. The quantity of calories was less in period 2 than in period 1. Nevertheless, albumin levels appeared to increase and were higher in period 2 than in period 1. Improvement in brain function was positively associated with serum albumin levels and Acute Physiology and Chronic Health Evaluation II (APACHE II) scores.

There are a number of possibilities for improvement in one period versus another period, despite what appears to be a very similar population in both periods. For example, blood glucose monitoring may have improved with the nutritional consultant team in period 2. Thus, to truly determine whether one form or degree of nutrition is equivalent, better, or worse than another, a prospective, randomized, blinded trial must be carried out.

J. M. Daly, MD

Parenteral Feeding Depletes Pulmonary Lymphocyte Populations

Hermsen JL, Gomez FE, Sano Y, et al (Univ of Wisconsin School of Medicine and Public Health, Madison)

JPEN J Parenter Enteral Nutr 33:535-540, 2009

Background.—The effect of parenteral nutrition (PN) on lymphocyte mass in the lung is unknown, but reduced mucosal lymphocytes are hypothesized to play a role in the reduced immunoglobulin A–mediated immunity in both gut and lung. The ability to transfer and track cells between mice may allow study of diet-induced mucosal immune function. The objectives of this study are to characterize lung T-cell populations following parenteral feeding and to study distribution patterns of transferred donor lung T cells in recipient mice.

Methods.—In experiment 1, cannulated male Balb/c mice are randomized to receive chow or PN for 5 days. Lung lymphocytes are obtained via collagenase digestion, and flow cytometric analysis is used to identify total T (CD3+) and B (CD45/B220+) cells. In experiment 2, isolated lung T cells from chow-fed male Balb/c mice are pooled and labeled in vitro with a fluorescent dye (carboxyfluorescein diacetate succinimidyl ester [CFSE]), and 1.1×10^8 CFSE+ cells (3.1×10^6 T cells) are transferred to chow-fed Balb/c recipients. Cells recovered from recipient lungs and intestinal lamina propria (LP) are analyzed by flow cytometry to determine CFSE/ CD3+ T cells at 1, 2, and 7 days. In experiment 3, cells are transferred to PN-fed recipients.

Results.—In experiment 1, PN significantly decreases lung T- and B-cell populations compared with chow feeding. In experiment 2, CFSE+ T-cell retention is highest on day 1 in lung and LP, and decreases on day 2. Cells are gone by day 7; 98.1% of retained donor lung T cells migrate to recipient lungs and 1.9% to the intestine on day 1. Similar results are seen in experiment 3 after transfer of cells to PN-fed recipients.

Conclusions.—PN reduces pulmonary lymphocyte populations consistent with impaired respiratory immunity. Transferred lung T cells preferentially localize to recipient lungs rather than intestine with maximal accumulation at 24 hours. Limited cross-talk of transferred lung T cells to the intestine indicates that mucosal lymphocyte traffic might be programmed to localize to specific effector sites.

▶ This article is one of a series of terrific articles from the laboratory of the senior author, Dr Kudsk. Previously he has shown that animals receiving total parenteral nutrition (TPN) show increased mortality to infection and have diminished immunity in the lungs as well as inability to handle endotoxin. He has also demonstrated decreased secreted IgA and decreased lymphocyte mass in the small intestine of TPN-fed animals. This study seeks to answer the questions as to the lung lymphocyte response to TPN. It also seeks to answer whether or not transferred pulmonary lymphocytes localize to the lung or the intestine. Clearly, administration of TPN results in a decrease in the number of lung lymphocytes rapidly. In addition, transference of pulmonary lymphocytes from chow-fed animals into either chow-fed or TPN-fed animals results in the tracking of these lymphocytes into the lung and not into the intestine. Thus, tissue specificity is critically important. Studies such as these may help explain the previously noted increased infection rates, particularly pneumonia, in the TPN-fed patients.

J. M. Daly, MD

Parenteral Fish Oil as Monotherapy Prevents Essential Fatty Acid Deficiency in Parenteral Nutrition–Dependent Patients

de Meijer VE, Le HD, Meisel JA, et al (Children's Hosp Boston and Harvard Med School, MA)

J Pediatr Gastroenterol Nutr 50:212-218, 2010

Objective.—The use of fish oil–based emulsions as the sole source of fat for patients receiving parenteral nutrition (PN) has raised concerns for the development of essential fatty acid deficiency (EFAD), hindering its adoption into clinical practice. The purpose of the present study was to examine fatty acid profiles of patients receiving no enteral energy, while completely dependent on PN and an intravenous fish oil–based lipid emulsion, for onset of EFAD and maintenance of growth.

Patients and Methods.—Prospectively collected data from 10 patients were reviewed for evidence of EFAD, defined as a triene:tetraene ratio >0.2. Gestational age–adjusted z scores for length, growth, and head circumference at baseline were compared with the corresponding z scores at time of censoring. All of the patients received PN with a fish oil–based lipid emulsion at $1\ g \cdot kg^{-1} \cdot day^{-1}$ as the sole source of fat energy for at least 1 month. The fish oil monotherapy was used under a compassionate use protocol.

Results.—Median gestational age at the time of birth was 35 weeks, and median age at the start of treatment was 3.5 months. After a median time of 3.8 months on exclusive PN and fish oil–based lipid emulsion, none of the patients developed biochemical or clinical evidence of EFAD. *z* scores were not statistically different, indicating no growth impairment. Median direct bilirubin levels improved in 9 patients from 6.8 to 0.9 mg/dL ($P = 0.009$).

Conclusions.—When dosed appropriately, fish oil–based lipid emulsions contain sufficient amounts of essential fatty acids to prevent EFAD and sustain growth in patients who are completely dependent on PN.

▶ As previous studies have indicated, parenteral nutrition-associated liver disease is a major problem in low-birth-weight infants and can be addressed by combinations of treatment, including TPN cycling and changing the fat source used in lipid emulsions. This compassionate use study prospectively evaluated 10 infants who required TPN starting at a median age of 3.5 months. After a median time of 3.8 months on exclusive TPN, there was no evidence of essential fatty acid deficiencies. In addition, after a median time of 3.8 months on TPN and Omegaven therapy, total bilirubin levels decreased significantly in 9 of 10 patients from approximately 6 mg/dL to 0.9 mg/dL.

Thus, use of fish oil-based lipid therapy did not result in clinical signs of or biochemical ratios predictive of essential fatty acid deficiencies. These studies should be expanded to larger numbers, as safety of these fish oil lipid infusions has been assured in infants of this number, with the studies done in a prospective and randomized fashion.

J. M. Daly, MD

Parenteral Fish Oil Improves Outcomes in Patients With Parenteral Nutrition-Associated Liver Injury

Puder M, Valim C, Meisel JA, et al (Children's Hosp Boston and Harvard Med School, MA)

Ann Surg 250:395-402, 2009

Objective.—The objective was to determine the safety and efficacy of a fish oil-based intravenous lipid emulsion (ILE) in the treatment of parenteral nutrition-associated liver disease (PNALD).

Summary and Background Data.—PNALD can be a lethal complication in children with short bowel syndrome (SBS). ILE based on soybean oil administered with parenteral nutrition (PN) may contribute to its etiology.

Methods.—We performed an open-labeled trial of a fish oil-based ILE in 42 infants with SBS who developed cholestasis (serum direct bilirubin >2 mg/dL) while receiving soybean oil-based ILE. Safety and efficacy outcomes were compared with those from a contemporary cohort of 49 infants with SBS and cholestasis whose PN course included soybean ILE only. The primary efficacy end-point was time to reversal of cholestasis (direct bilirubin ≤2 mg/dL).

Results.—Three deaths and 1 liver transplantation occurred in the fish oil cohort, compared with 12 deaths and 6 transplants in the soybean oil cohort ($P = 0.005$). Among survivors not transplanted during PN, cholestasis reversed while receiving PN in 19 of 38 patients in the fish oil cohort versus 2 of 36 patients in the soybean oil cohort. Based on Cox models, subjects receiving fish oil-based ILE experienced reversal of cholestasis 6 times faster (95% CI: 2.0–37.3) than those receiving soybean oil-based ILE. The provision of fish oil-based ILE was not associated with hypertriglyceridemia, coagulopathy, or essential fatty acid deficiency. Moreover, hypertriglyceridemic events and abnormal international normalized ratio levels were more common among controls.

Conclusions.—Fish oil-based ILE is safe, may be effective in treating PNALD, and may reduce mortality and organ transplantation rates in children with SBS.

▶ Development of liver disease in infants receiving parenteral nutrition can be devastating. Thus, methods to reduce its occurrence are critically important. Use of fish oil-based lipid emulsions is 1 method believed to positively impact this development. In this study, 42 infants with short bowel syndrome who developed cholestasis while receiving soybean-based lipid emulsions as part of total parenteral nutrition (TPN) were followed up after switching to a fish oil-based lipid solution. Serum bilirubin and alanine aminotransferase (ALT) levels decreased significantly in the fish oil group compared with a historical cohort of patients. Cholestasis was reversed in 50% of infants receiving the fish oil-based lipid compared with 5.6% of infants in the soybean oil-based group. Administration of fish oil-based lipid also decreased triglyceride levels while there were no safety concerns related in tests of international normalized ratio (INR) or platelet counts. The results of this study, if confirmed in a prospective trial, would appear to have a major impact on the outcomes of these infants with short bowel syndrome.

J. M. Daly, MD

Plasma citrulline is a biomarker of enterocyte mass and an indicator of parenteral nutrition in HIV-infected patients

Crenn P, De Truchis P, Neveux N, et al (Université de Versailles-Saint Quentin en Yvelines, Garches, France; Université Paris Descartes, France)

Am J Clin Nutr 90:587-594, 2009

Background.—Plasma citrulline is a biomarker of enterocyte mass and function in humans.

Objective.—We evaluated citrulline in the reemerging context of diarrhea in HIV-infected patients receiving highly active antiretroviral therapy.

Design.—This study prospectively measured citrulline in 6 groups of HIV-1 patients ($n = 115$): *1*) undetectable viral load without chronic diarrhea (a; $n = 40$) and with protease inhibitor–associated toxic chronic diarrhea (b; $n = 26$), *2*) detectable viral load and CD4 >200/mm^3 (a; $n = 6$) and with (b; $n = 11$) chronic diarrhea, and *3*) detectable viral load and

CD4 <200/mm^3 without chronic diarrhea (a; $n = 7$) and with opportunistic intestinal infections or HIV enteropathy (b; $n = 25$). The influence of diarrhea on citrulline was assessed by comparing the a and b subgroups with healthy control subjects ($n = 100$).

Results.—Citrulline was slightly decreased (22–30 μmol/L) in groups 1b and 2b and was <22 μmol/L in 19 of 25 patients in group 3b. In group 3b, a citrulline concentration <10 μmol/L was associated with a clinical indication for parenteral nutrition ($n = 6$ of 8 compared with 2 of 17 if the citrulline concentration was >10 μmol/L; $P < 0.05$). Citrulline correlated positively with albumin ($P < 0.01$) and BMI ($P < 0.05$) and negatively with C-reactive protein ($P < 0.01$). When antiinfectious and nutritional therapies were successful ($n = 18$ of 25), citrulline normalized in 2–12 wk. Neither chronic hepatic or pancreatic disease nor lipodystrophy and the metabolic syndrome affected citrulline. Compared with control subjects (38 ± 8 μmol/L), patients without chronic diarrhea (groups 1a, 2a, and 3a) had normal citrulline concentrations (36 ± 6 μmol/L).

Conclusions.—Plasma citrulline is a reliable biomarker of enterocyte functional mass in HIV patients. Citrulline does not allow the etiologic diagnosis of enteropathy, but it can discriminate between protease inhibitor toxic diarrhea and infectious enteropathy and quantify the functional consequences, which makes it an objective tool for indicating the need for parenteral nutrition.

▶ This very interesting study evaluated prospectively the plasma citrulline levels in HIV-infected patients with and without diarrhea. In patients, low citrulline levels were associated with decreased enterocyte mass and with a need for parenteral nutrition. Low plasma citrulline levels were also associated with chronic diarrhea. Importantly, as patients improved either with parenteral nutrition or with antimicrobial therapy, plasma citrulline levels normalized. Thus, measurement of these levels provided prognostic information as to the results of therapy.

Studies such as these are critical to our ability to develop good biomarkers of the extent of disease, avoiding more invasive methods to ascertain the physiologic and anatomic status of the small intestine. It would also be important to determine whether measurement of plasma citrulline levels could be used to evaluate other diseases of the small intestine.

J. M. Daly, MD

Reversal of intestinal failure–associated liver disease in infants and children on parenteral nutrition: experience with 93 patients at a referral center for intestinal rehabilitation

Cowles RA, Ventura KA, Martinez M, et al (Morgan Stanley Children's Hosp of New York-Presbyterian and Columbia Univ Med Ctr)

J Pediatr Surg 45:84-88, 2010

Purpose.—Intestinal failure (IF)–associated liver disease (IFALD) complicates the treatment of children with IF receiving parenteral nutrition (PN). We hypothesized that prevention or resolution of IFALD was possible in most children and that this would result in improved outcomes.

Methods.—We reviewed prospectively gathered data on all children referred to the intestinal rehabilitation and transplantation center at our institution. Total bilirubin level (TB) was used as the marker for IFALD. Patients were grouped based on TB at referral and at subsequent inpatient stays and outpatient visits. Standard treatment consisted of cycling of PN, limiting lipid infusion, enteral stimulation, use of ursodeoxycholic acid, and surgical intervention when necessary. Outcomes such as mortality, dependence on PN, and need for transplantation were assessed. Statistical analyses were performed using Fisher's exact, Mann-Whitney *U*, and Wilcoxon signed rank tests.

Results.—Ninety-three patients with intestinal failure and on PN were treated at our center from 2003 to 2009. Median age at referral was 5 months (0.5-264 months). Prematurity was a complicating factor in 63 patients and necrotizing enterocolitis was the most common diagnosis. Eighty-two children had short bowel syndrome, whereas the remaining 11 had extensive motility disorders. 97% of children required significant alteration of their PN administration. At referral, 76 of 93 children had TB 2.0 mg/dL or higher, and 17 had TB below 2.0 mg/dL. TB normalized in 57 of 76 children with elevated TB at referral, and TB remained elevated in 19. Normalization of TB was associated with a mortality of 5.2%, and transplantation was needed in 5.2%. Conversely, when TB remained elevated, mortality was 58% ($P = .0002$ vs TB normalized), and transplantation occurred in 58% owing to failure of surgical and medical rehabilitation.

Conclusions.—Most children referred for treatment of IF have IFALD. A dedicated IF rehabilitation program can reverse IFALD in many children, and this is associated with improved outcome.

▶ As stated by the authors, liver disease associated with intestinal failure is also associated with administration of parenteral nutrition in these children. The authors used a multipronged approach by cycling total parenteral nutrition (TPN), limiting lipid infusions, using enteral feedings to stimulate the intestinal tract, use of ursodeoxycholic acid, and sometimes surgery. This concerted effort resulted in significant reduction in serum bilirubin levels in 57 of 76 children and was associated with a major reduction in mortality. Other authors have not found consistent results using single-handed approaches to this problem and have sought other means such as changing the composition of the lipid emulsion. Nevertheless, Cowles et al have shown in their retrospective review that multiple interventions may cumulatively have a beneficial outcome in these severely ill infants.

J. M. Daly, MD

Slow versus rapid enteral feeding advancement in preterm newborn infants 1000–1499 g: a randomized controlled trial

Krishnamurthy S, Gupta P, Debnath S, et al (Univ College of Med Sciences and Guru Tegh Bahadur Hosp, Delhi, India)

Acta Paediatr 99:42-46, 2010

Aim.—To evaluate whether preterm neonates weighing 1000–1499 g at birth receiving rapid enteral feeding advancement at 30 mL/kg/day attain full feedings (180 mL/kg/day) earlier than those receiving slow enteral feeding advancement at 20 mL/kg/day without increase in the incidence of feeding intolerance or necrotizing enterocolitis.

Methods.—A total of 100 stable intramural neonates weighing between 1000 and 1499 g and gestational age less than 34 weeks were randomly allocated to enteral feeding (expressed human milk or formula) advancement of 20 mL/kg/day ($n = 50$) or 30 mL/kg/day ($n = 50$).

Results.—Neonates in the rapid feeding advancement group achieved full volume feedings before the slow advancement group (median 7 days vs. 9 days) ($p < 0.001$), had significantly fewer days of intravenous fluids (median 2 days vs. 3.4 days) ($p < 0.001$), shorter length of stay in hospital (median 9.5 days vs. 11 days) ($p = 0.003$) and regained birth weight earlier (median 16 days vs. 22 days) ($p < 0.001$). There were no statistical differences in the proportion of infants with apnea, feed interruption or feed intolerance.

Conclusion.—Rapid enteral feeding advancements of 30 mL/kg/day are well tolerated by stable preterm neonates weighing 1000–1499 g.

▶ There is always the desire to accelerate the feeding of preterm infants weighing less than 1500 g at birth. "If a little helps, then more is better." However, there is great trepidation that necrotizing enterocolitis, aspiration and distention with bloating, and poor respiratory function may develop if feedings are increased too rapidly. This prospective randomized trial compared more rapid advancement of feeding starting at 30 mL/kg/day with a lower amount (20 mL/kg/day). Better weight gain and shorter hospital length of stay occurred in the 30-mL group compared with the 20-mL group without increasing complications, such as apnea or feeding intolerance. In addition, infants started at 30 mL regained their birth weight faster than the 20-mL group. Thus, it appears to be just as safe to start at a higher rate, and there are many metabolic advantages. One has to remember that very close attention to detail is necessary to be certain that complications do not ensue with the use of a higher rate of enteral feeding.

J. M. Daly, MD

Whole-blood–free Choline and Choline Metabolites in Infants Who Require Chronic Parenteral Nutrition Therapy

Sentongo TA, Kumar P, Karza K, et al (Univ of Chicago, IL; Children's Memorial Hosp, Chicago, IL; et al)

J Pediatr Gastroenterol Nutr 50:194-199, 2010

Background and Aim.—Choline deficiency is associated with hepatic dysfunction. Parenteral nutrition (PN) and lipid emulsions contain phosphatidylcholine (PtdCho) but insignificant free choline (FCho). PtdCho is sequentially degraded to glycerolphosphocholine (GPCho), phosphocholine (PCho), and finally to FCho. Biosynthesis of FCho may be insufficient during PN therapy. The aim of the study was to examine the status of FCho and related metabolites in infants on prolonged (≥4 weeks) PN.

Methods.—Whole blood concentrations of FCho, PtdCho, GPCho, and PCho were measured and compared in infants on PN and infants on enteral feeds (controls).

Results.—Infants on PN (n = 14) had higher birth weight but same postnatal age as controls (n = 14) (mean ± standard deviation) 8.3 ± 3.9 versus 7.4 ± 3.6 weeks. Parenteral nutrition was associated with increased PtdCho 1761 ± 452 versus 1471 ± 221 nmol/mL, $P = 0.04$. Mean whole blood FCho, GPCho, and PCho concentrations did not differ significantly in PN versus controls: 40.0 ± 15.4 versus 50.8 ± 49.7, 16.4 ± 14.5 versus 25.2 ± 29.3, and 15.3 ± 13.5 versus 22.0 ± 14.8 nmol/mL, respectively. However, PCho was positively correlated with GPCho in controls ($r = 0.91$, $P < 0.01$) but not PN ($r = 0.24$, $P =$ NS), and infants receiving >90% of daily energy intake from PN (n = 6) had decreased PCho, 5.7 ± 4.1 nmol/mL, compared with those receiving <90% of daily energy intake (n = 8) 22.5 ± 13.7 nmol/mL, $P < 0.05$, and controls, 22.0 ± 14.8 nmol/mL, $P < 0.01$.

Conclusions.—Decreased whole-blood concentrations of choline suggest possible evidence of choline deficiency as illustrated by decreased whole-blood PCho. Choline supplementation should be investigated in infants who require prolonged PN, and whole-blood PCho can be used to monitor response.

▶ Monitoring low-birth-weight infants for metabolic deficiencies, particularly those receiving parenteral nutrition is critical. The authors noted that whole blood choline levels as depicted by phosphocholine levels were lower in infants receiving parenteral nutrition compared with control infants receiving enteral feedings. This may indicate choline deficiencies in total parenteral nutrition (TPN) infants. The importance of this finding is that infants receiving TPN may develop severe TPN-associated liver disease. Studies reviewed herein suggest that the type of lipid infusion may be the culprit. This study suggests a biochemical metabolic mechanism whereby liver dysfunction may occur.

J. M. Daly, MD

A 6-year review of total parenteral nutrition use and association with late-onset acute respiratory distress syndrome among ventilated trauma victims

Plurad D, Green D, Inaba K, et al (Univ of Southern California and Los Angeles County Hosp Division of Trauma/Surgical Critical Care)

Injury 40:511-515, 2009

Aim.—To establish whether total parenteral nutrition (TPN) for ventilated trauma victims is associated with late-onset acute respiratory distress syndrome (ARDS) independent of ventilation and transfusion parameters.

Method.—Intensive care unit data over 6 years from a level I centre regarding all trauma victims ≥16 years old who underwent mechanical ventilation within the first 48 h of admission were examined. Patients were prospectively followed for late ARDS. Variables were examined for significant changes over time and independent associations with late ARDS were determined.

Results.—Of 2346 eligible patients among whom 404 (17.2%) were exposed to TPN, 192 (8.2%) met criteria for late ARDS. The incidence of late ARDS among those exposed to TPN was 28.7% (116/404) compared with 3.9% (76/1942) among those not so exposed. Adjustments for potential confounding associated risk factors were made.

Conclusions.—TPN administration is independently associated with late ARDS, and its use among critically ill trauma victims should be carefully scrutinised.

▶ The authors performed a retrospective review of patients admitted to their ICU who were exposed to total parenteral nutrition (TPN) during their therapy. They noted that those who received TPN were older, sicker (higher Injury Severity Score [ISS]), more often received transfusions, were more commonly hypotensive in the emergency room, and were more commonly obese. These same variables were associated with late-onset acute respiratory distress syndrome (ARDS). However, the authors concluded that a logistic regression analysis showing that TPN was an independent factor meant that TPN should be severely restricted or not be used at all in ICU patients.

Retrospective analyses such as these provide suggestions, but rarely definitive conclusions because of the multiplicity of variables not controlled for in the study. Statistical analytic techniques cannot do this well enough to lead to definitive conclusions. All would agree that sicker patients are at risk for late-onset ARDS. The authors note in their article that the incidence of late-onset ARDS fell dramatically before there was any substantial decline in the use of TPN (Figs 1 and 2 in the original article). Why? How is this explained?

Were other ICU treatment protocols put in place during these years such as different ventilator management, better control of hyperglycemia, etc?

The authors should be lauded for the dramatic decline in late-onset ARDS from 14% to 4% as shown in Fig 1 in the original article, in their patients during the study period. I certainly agree that early and more aggressive use of enteral nutrition in this population is warranted. In fact, the authors note that their protocol calls for 10 days without adequate enteral intake before TPN is used in ICU patients. What happens then?

J. M. Daly, MD

Randomized clinical trial to compare the effects of preoperative oral carbohydrate *versus* placebo on insulin resistance after colorectal surgery

Wang ZG, Wang Q, Wang WJ, et al (Second Military Med Univ, Shanghai, China; et al)

Br J Surg 97:317-327, 2010

Background.—Preoperative oral carbohydrate (OCH) reduces postoperative insulin resistance (PIR). This randomized trial investigated whether this effect is related to insulin-induced activation of the phosphatidylinositol 3-kinase (PI3K)/protein kinase B (PKB) signalling pathway.

Methods.—Patients with colorectal cancer scheduled for elective open resection were randomly assigned to preoperative OCH, fasting or placebo. Preoperative general well-being, insulin resistance before and immediately after surgery, and postoperative expression of PI3K, PKB, protein tyrosine kinase (PTK) and glucose transporter 4 (GLUT4) in rectus abdominis muscle were evaluated.

Results.—Patient and operative characteristics did not differ between groups. Subjective well-being was significantly better in OCH and placebo groups than in the fasting group, primarily because of reduced thirst ($P = 0{\cdot}005$) and hunger ($P = 0{\cdot}041$). PIR was significantly greater in fasting and placebo groups ($P < 0{\cdot}010$). By the end of surgery, muscle PTK activity as well as PI3K and PKB levels were significantly increased in the OCH group compared with values in fasting and placebo groups ($P < 0{\cdot}050$), but GLUT4 expression was unaffected.

Conclusion.—PIR involves the PI3K/PKB signalling pathway. Preoperative OCH intake improves preoperative subjective feelings of hunger and thirst compared with fasting, while attenuating PIR by stimulation of the PI3K/PKB pathway. Registration number: NCT00755729 (http://www.clinicaltrials.gov)

▶ This prospective, randomized trial enlisted 52 patients who received preoperatively either oral carbohydrate solution or noncarbohydrate fluids, or were kept without drinking before general abdominal colorectal surgery. Postoperative insulin resistance was significantly diminished in the carbohydrate group compared with the others. The study is important, as there is a greater trend to reduce hyperglycemia in postoperative patients. Clinical trials have shown normalization of blood glucose levels to be associated with less morbidity in surgical intensive care patients and others. Other studies have noted the importance of immediate postoperative control of blood glucose levels along with oxygenation and warming to maximize each patient's response to surgery. Improving postoperative insulin resistance through a simple method of offering a glucose drink seems intuitively the correct thing to do. In addition, patients like it.

J. M. Daly, MD

9 Wound Healing

A multicenter clinical trial of recombinant human GM-CSF hydrogel for the treatment of deep second-degree burns

Zhang L, Chen J, Han C (Zhejiang Univ College of Medicine, Hangzhou, China; The Third Affiliated Hosp, Wenzhou, China)

Wound Repair Regen 17:685-689, 2009

Wound healing is a complex and dynamic biological process. The efficacy and safety of a recombinant human granulocyte-macrophage colony-stimulating factor (rhGM-CSF) hydrogel to promote deep-second-degree burn wound healing is evaluated in this study. In this multicenter, randomized, double-blind, and placebo-controlled clinical trial, 90 patients with deep second-degree burns were randomly assigned into two groups. Complete healing time and percentage of wound healing at different time points were observed and side effects were recorded. A statistically significant difference was noted at each time point ($p < 0.01$). No side effects were observed. These results suggest that rhGM-CSF hydrogel can significantly accelerate deep second-degree burn wound healing and is considered to be safe.

▶ The authors performed a multicenter, randomized, blinded, and controlled study of recombinant human granulocyte-macrophage colony-stimulating factor (rhGM-CSF) in a gel applied to patients ($n = 60$) who had superficial and deep second-degree burns, and compared healing results with a control group ($n = 30$) who simply had a gel applied. As shown in Table 1 in the original article, results demonstrated significantly improved wound healing in the treated burn patients compared with controls. Previous authors have demonstrated an altered hormonal milieu in burn patients, which does not recover until the burn wound is healed. Systemic administration of rhGM-CSF maintains neutrophil levels, which normally decrease following major burn injury. Local application to wounds of a number of agents in animal studies have demonstrated improved healing by increasing concentrations at the local site. This well-conducted study in humans reaffirms that principle. It would be important to understand whether scarring was better, worse, or the same in the treated patients versus controls if systemic infections were increased, decreased, or the same, and if metabolic improvements were noted in the treated patients. Although not yet the standard of care, this study provides good evidence that rhGM-CSF is helpful in these very ill patients.

J. M. Daly, MD

A Novel Polypeptide Derived From Human Lactoferrin in Sodium Hyaluronate Prevents Postsurgical Adhesion Formation in the Rat

Nilsson E, Björn C, Sjöstrand V, et al (PharmaSurgics AB, Gothenburg, Sweden; et al)

Ann Surg 250:1021-1028, 2009

Objective.—The objective of the study was to evaluate whether a peptide derived from human lactoferrin, PXL01 could act safely to reduce the formation of peritoneal adhesions in the rat model and to map the molecular mechanisms of its action.

Summary Background Data.—Adhesion formation is a significant problem within every surgical discipline causing suffering for the patients and major cost for the society. For many decades, attempts have been made to reduce postsurgical adhesions by reducing surgical trauma. It is now believed that major improvements in adhesion prevention will only be reached by developing dedicated antiscarring products, which are administrated in connection to the surgical intervention.

Methods.—Anti-inflammatory as well as fibrinolytic activities of PXL01 were studied in relevant human cell lines. Using the sidewall defect-cecum abrasion model in the rat, the adhesion prevention properties of PXL01 formulated in sodium hyaluronate were evaluated. Large bowel anastomosis healing model in the rat was applied to study if PXL01 would have any negative effects on intestine healing.

Results.—PXL01 exhibits an inhibitory effect on the most important hallmarks of scar formation by reducing infections, prohibiting inflammation, and promoting fibrinolysis. PXL01 formulated in sodium hyaluronate markedly reduced formation of peritoneal adhesions in rat without any adverse effects on wound healing.

Conclusions.—A new class of synthetically derived water soluble low molecular weight peptide compound, PXL01 showed marked reduction of peritoneal adhesion formation in an animal model without any negative effects on healing. On the basis of these data, a comprehensive adhesion prevention regimen in clinical situation is expected.

▶ This interesting in vitro and in vivo study evaluated a novel peptide derived from human lactoferrin for its effects on intermediate biomarkers of inflammation and adhesion formation after injury. An animal intraperitoneal adhesion model was also used to assess its effects. Using human cell lines, the compound appeared very effective. Its use also reduced intraperitoneal adhesions while maintaining bursting pressures in a rat intestinal anastomosis model.

The authors argue for human testing as the next step; however, I would be more circumspect. The model should be further tested in controlled animal models not only of adhesion formation and wound healing (there are numerous models available), but also models of intraperitoneal infection to determine if abscess localization occurs normally and that mortality is unaffected. Other models of wound healing (fascia and skin) should also be used to be certain that there are no unwarranted side effects.

There are clear advantages in that the peptide is derived from human lactoferrin, so clearly further studies of this interesting molecule are indicated.

J. M. Daly, MD

Accelerated Wound Healing in Healing-Impaired *db/db* Mice by Autologous Adipose Tissue-Derived Stromal Cells Combined With Atelocollagen Matrix

Nambu M, Kishimoto S, Nakamura S, et al (Natl Defense Med College, Saitama, Japan; et al)

Ann Plast Surg 62:317-321, 2009

Adipose tissue-derived stromal cells (ATSCs) have recently gained widespread attention as a potential alternate source to bone marrow-derived mesenchymal stem cells with a proliferative capacity and a similar ability to undergo multilineage differentiation. In this study, we evaluated the effectiveness of freshly isolated autologous ATSCs-containing atelocollagen matrix with silicon membrane (ACMS) on wound healing of diabetic (*db/db*) mice.

Cultured ATSCs from (*db/db*) mice secreted significant amounts of growth factors and cytokines, which are suitable for wound repair. Two full thickness round skin defects were made on the backs of healing-impaired db/db mice. Freshly isolated autologous ATSCs-containing ACMS or ACMS alone were applied to the wounds. Twelve mice were treated and then killed at 1 or 2 weeks ($n = 6$ each). Histologic sections of the wounds were prepared at each time period after treatment.

Histologic examination demonstrated significantly advanced granulation tissue formation, capillary formation, and epithelialization in diabetic healing-impaired wounds treated with autologous ATSCs-containing ACMS, compared with mice treated with ACMS alone. These results suggested that transplantation of autologous ATSCs-containing ACMS significantly accelerated wound healing in diabetic healing-impaired *db/db* mice.

▶ Impairment of wound healing occurs in many conditions, such as impaired vascularity due to diabetes, smoking, radiation, etc. Thus, methods to improve wound healing due to administration of growth factors and other biologic factors have important potential benefits for many patients. Use of adipose tissue-derived stromal cells (ATSCs) seems to have the potential to improve healing when it would otherwise be impaired.

The authors used a well-known *db/db* animal model of impaired wound healing. They used freshly isolated ATSCs containing atelocollagen matrix with silicon membrane implanted in these wounds and showed significant benefit in terms of granulation tissue formation, capillary formation, and epithelialization.

This study provides important information, in that autologous cells were used from these diabetic mice, obviating any need for immunosuppression. As obesity often occurs concomitantly with diabetes, ATSCs should be abundantly available. It is a very promising approach.

J. M. Daly, MD

Acute Effects of Nicotine and Smoking on Blood Flow, Tissue Oxygen, and Aerobe Metabolism of the Skin and Subcutis

Sørensen LT, Jørgensen S, Petersen LJ, et al (Bispebjerg Hosp, Copenhagen, Denmark; et al)

J Surg Res 152:224-230, 2009

Background.—Nicotine released from tobacco smoke causing reduction in blood flow has been suggested as causative for postoperative wound complications in smokers, but the mechanism remains unknown.

Materials and Methods.—In eight healthy male smokers and eight ex-smokers, the cutaneous and subcutaneous blood flow (QBF, SqBF) was assessed by Laser Doppler and 133Xe clearance. Tissue oxygen tension (TO_2) was measured by a LICOX O_2-electrode. Tissue glucose and lactate (Tgluc, Tlact) were assessed by microdialysis. The parameters were studied after intravenous infusion of 1.0 mg nicotine, smoking of one cigarette, arterial occlusion, and reperfusion.

Results.—Nicotine infusion decreased SqBF from 4.2 ± 2.0 to 3.1 ± 1.2 mL/100 g tissue/min ($P < 0.01$), whereas QBF was 21.7 ± 8.6 and 22.7 ± 9.6 Arbitrary Units (AU), respectively ($P = 0.21$). TO_2 increased from 49.3 ± 12.0 to 53.9 ± 12.0 mm Hg ($P = 0.01$). Tgluc and Tlact remained unaffected. Smoking decreased SqBF from 4.2 ± 2.0 to 2.7 ± 1.2 mL/100 g tissue/min ($P < 0.01$). QBF decreased from 23.4 ± 9.2 to 20.3 ± 7.4 AU ($P < 0.01$), and TO_2 decreased from 53.9 ± 12.0 to 48.4 ± 11.1 mm Hg ($P < 0.01$). Following smoking, Tgluc decreased from 0.7 ± 0.1 to 0.6 ± 0.1 ng/mL ($P < 0.01$), and Tlact increased from 0.2 ± 0.1 to 0.3 ± 0.2 ng/mL ($P < 0.01$). The observed alterations were similar in smokers and ex-smokers.

Conclusions.—Nicotine has a limited vasoactive effect in the skin and subcutis unlikely to be explained by smoking, which distinctly decreases tissue blood flow, oxygen tension, and aerobe metabolism independent of smoking status.

▶ It is well known that smoking inhibits wound healing and substantially increases the morbidity of surgical patients. Greater numbers of patients are using nicotine substitutes in an effort to curb or eliminate smoking. Thus, it is important to try and define the mechanisms whereby smoking adversely affects tissue oxygenation.

This study conducted in humans evaluated the role of nicotine, smoking 1 cigarette, as well as arterial occlusion and reperfusion in current and ex-smokers on cutaneous and subcutaneous blood flow, oxygenation, glucose, and lactate. Importantly, the authors found that nicotine only transiently impaired blood flow in both smokers and nonsmokers. However, in keeping with other studies, smoking 1 cigarette demonstrated significantly decreased blood flow, oxygen tension, and aerobe metabolism in both smokers and nonsmokers.

Results of this study suggest that use of nicotine as a substitute to inhibit craving, thereby reducing or eliminating smoking, should have a positive outcome on wound healing by eliminating the adverse consequences of smoking in those undergoing surgery.

J. M. Daly, MD

Adipose Stromal Cells and Platelet-Rich Plasma Therapies Synergistically Increase Revascularization during Wound Healing

Blanton MW, Hadad I, Johnstone BH, et al (Indiana Univ School of Medicine, Indianapolis)

Plast Reconstr Surg 123:56S-64S, 2009

Background.—The authors examined the efficacy of adipose stem cells, when supplied either alone or in platelet-rich fibrin gels, to improve wound healing.

Methods.—A porcine full-thickness wound model was used to compare six topical treatments: platelet-poor plasma; platelet-rich plasma; autologous adipose stem cells plus platelet-poor plasma; autologous adipose stem cells plus platelet-rich plasma; allogeneic adipose stem cells containing green fluorescent protein plus platelet-poor plasma; and saline (control). One week after isolation, adipose stem cells were applied to full-thickness wounds on the paraspinal and thoracic regions of three pigs (44 wounds per pig; each treatment was applied to eight separate wounds). Each wound was monitored over 21 days for closure, cosmesis, and histopathology.

Results.—There was no significant difference in the reepithelialization rate, but treatments containing adipose stem cells demonstrated increased microvessel densities (31.75 ± 5.73 vessels/cm^2 versus 7.93 ± 3.61 vessels/cm^2) compared with groups without adipose stem cells. Wound cosmesis was improved in the adipose stem cell plus platelet-rich plasma group compared with other treatment groups ($p < 0.05$). Vascular endothelial growth factor levels detected in matrices containing adipose stem cells were approximately 7-fold higher compared with platelet-rich plasma or platelet-poor plasma ($p < 0.05$). Localization of transgenic green fluorescent protein plus adipose stem cells indicated incorporation near neovasculature.

Conclusions.—In normal healing wounds, adipose stem cells appear to enhance the healing process only when provided in a fibrin gel vehicle containing a number of complementary wound-healing trophic factors. Perivascular adipose stem cell localization suggests a function in enhancing blood supply through providing physical and paracrine support to newly forming vessels.

▶ The authors studied adipose stem cells plus platelet-rich plasma as a topical application to full-thickness wounds versus other combinations. Re-epithelialization wound healing in these 3 pigs was not affected by any combination, but cosmesis and wound vascular endothelial growth factor (VEGF) levels were improved in the treated group. The authors also noted that there appeared to be greater structural support for the microvessels in the wounded areas. Certainly, there is an abundance of adipose cells from which stem cells can be harvested. In this animal model, it required 7 days for the harvest. It is also interesting that for full benefit the stem cells had to be present with platelet-rich plasma, suggesting the synergy of growth factors with the adipose stem cells. It would be important to test this hypothesis regarding the efficacy of stem cells and platelet-rich plasma in wound models of impaired healing, such as in diabetic animals, those having undergone radiation or chemotherapy, and so forth.

J. M. Daly, MD

Blinded randomized clinical trial of botulinum toxin *versus* isosorbide dinitrate ointment for treatment of anal fissure

Festen S, Gisbertz SS, van Schaagen F, et al (Dept of Surgery, Onze Lieve Vrouwe Gasthuis, Oosterpark, Amsterdam, The Netherlands)

Br J Surg 96:1393-1399, 2009

Background.—Nitric oxide donors such as isosorbide dinitrate (ISDN) are considered the first choice of treatment for anal fissure. After reports of the successful treatment of such fissures with botulinum toxin, this randomized blinded trial compared botulinum toxin with ISDN in the treatment of chronic anal fissure.

Methods.—Patients were randomized to receive an injection of botulinum in the internal anal sphincter and a placebo ointment, or a placebo injection and ISDN ointment. The primary endpoint was macroscopic fissure healing after 4 months.

Results.—After 4 months macroscopic healing of the fissures was noted in 14 of 37 patients in the botulinum group and 21 of 36 in the ISDN group. Pain scores were lower among patients who received ISDN, although the difference was not significant. Side-effects were similar in the two groups.

Conclusion.—In contrast with previous reports on botulinum toxin as a therapeutic agent for anal fissure, this study found no advantage over treatment with a nitric oxide donor as regards fissure healing and fissure-related pain.

▶ Chronic anal fissure is a major problem causing pain and loss of productivity. The first step in medical therapy is to paralyze the internal anal sphincter; this is often done with botulinum toxin. This interesting prospective, randomized, and blinded human trial compared botulinum toxin injection with local application of a nitrous oxide donor (ISDN), which also affects muscle contraction and may improve local wound healing. Use of ISDN appeared to provide better results in terms of macro healing, although many patients were lost to follow-up, which was a major disadvantage of this study. Clearly, daily local application of cream to the affected area is less desirable than a single injection; however, there are side effects to the use of botulinum toxin. The results of this pilot study argue for a much larger multicenter trial to evaluate these treatments to provide the power to truly understand the efficacy of these therapies.

J. M. Daly, MD

Chronic Morphine Administration Delays Wound Healing by Inhibiting Immune Cell Recruitment to the Wound Site

Martin JL, Koodie L, Krishnan AG, et al (Univ of Minnesota, Minneapolis; Division of Basic and Translational Res, Minneapolis, MN; et al)
Am J Pathol 176:786-799, 2010

Patients prescribed morphine for the management of chronic pain, and chronic heroin abusers, often present with complications such as increased susceptibility to opportunistic infections and inadequate healing of wounds. We investigated the effect of morphine on wound-healing events in the presence of an infection in an *in vivo* murine model that mimics the clinical manifestations seen in opioid user and abuser populations. We show for the first time that in the presence of an inflammatory inducer, lipopolysaccharide, chronic morphine treatment results in a marked decrease in wound closure, compromised wound integrity, and increased bacterial sepsis. Morphine treatment resulted in a significant delay and reduction in both neutrophil and macrophage recruitment to the wound site. The delay and reduction in neutrophil reduction was attributed to altered early expression of keratinocyte derived cytokine and was independent of macrophage inflammatory protein 2 expression, whereas suppression of macrophage infiltration was attributed to suppressed levels of the potent macrophage chemoattractant monocyte chemotactic protein-1. When the effects of chronic morphine on later wound healing events were investigated, a significant suppression in angiogenesis and myofibroblast recruitment were observed in animals that received chronic morphine administration. Taken together, our findings indicate that morphine treatment results in a delay in the recruitment of cellular events following wounding, resulting in a lack of bacterial clearance and delayed wound closure.

▶ Chronic substance abuse has a multitude of untoward effects. This article demonstrates in an animal model that chronic morphine administration results in marked delay in the healing of an open wound, which appears to be caused by a substantial decrease in the infiltration of the wound with neutrophils and later by macrophages. This also results in lower chemoattractant production and dissemination of bacteria from the open wound systemically as demonstrated by positive organ cultures in the morphine-treated animals compared with controls. Taken together, these experimental results provide a basis for the clinical observation that chronic heroin, opium, and morphine users have difficulty healing after trauma and surgery.

It would have been valuable if the authors had measured food intake among the animals within the 3 groups: controls, chronic morphine administration, and the group given morphine and naloxone. It is known that morphine acts on satiety centers to decrease food intake. It is also known that malnutrition affects wound healing and the cellular events in the early processes of healing. Thus, controlled pair feeding may have been useful in the experimental design. In addition, it would be useful to extend this animal model to one where the chronic morphine administration is discontinued and at varying points in time the animals are wounded. This would give an idea as to how long the decrease in wound neutrophil and macrophage infiltration is inhibited.

Overall, this interesting article provides important cellular mechanisms whereby healing is inhibited by chronic morphine administration.

J. M. Daly, MD

Corticosterone exerts immunostimulatory effects on macrophages via endoplasmic reticulum stress

Zhou J-Y, Zhong H-J, Yang C, et al (Third Military Med Univ, Chongqing, China)

Br J Surg 97:281-293, 2010

Background.—Glucocorticoids are the central effector hormones for the hypothalamic–pituitary–adrenal axis. However, the effects of endogenous glucocorticoids on the immune system are not understood completely.

Methods.—Macrophage function (adherence, chemotaxis and cytokine production) was assessed in the presence of increasing concentrations of corticosterone. The role of endoplasmic reticulum (ER) stress in corticosterone immunoregulation was determined with thapsigargin and plasmid pGCL-GFP-siXBP1. Mifepristone was used to determine the role of glucocorticoid receptor in the corticosterone-induced ER stress response.

Results.—Corticosterone exerted immunostimulatory effects on macrophage function at low concentrations. No effects were observed at high concentrations in the absence of immunological stimulation. Low-dose corticosterone induced ER stress, which was correlated to the corticosterone immunostimulatory activities. Expression of X box-binding protein (XBP) 1, but not activating transcription factor 6, was significantly increased at both mRNA and protein levels only in the presence of low-dose corticosterone. Inhibition of XBP1 expression with small interfering RNA significantly inhibited the corticosterone immunostimulatory effects. In addition, pretreatment of macrophages with mifepristone significantly inhibited the expression of glucose response protein 78 and XBP1 in macrophages by low-dose corticosterone.

Conclusion.—At low concentrations, endogenous glucocorticoids exert immunostimulatory actions on macrophages. The underlying mechanisms may be correlated to ER stress via the glucocorticoid receptor, in which XBP1 plays an important role.

▶ This interesting in vitro macrophage study demonstrates that corticosterone can actually have immunostimulatory effects on these cells. Traditionally, we believe that all corticoids are immunosuppressive; however, our laboratory has also shown that under certain conditions they have stimulatory effects. For example, if human or mouse macrophages are exposed to low doses of corticosterone, washed, and then later stimulated, they show an increased production of superoxide anion and increased production of a variety of cytokines.

The authors here describe a mechanism related to endoplasmic reticulum stress in which X box-binding protein 1 (XBP1) plays a major role. Cellular studies such as these provide understanding as to the dual roles that corticoids may play in the response to stress.

J. M. Daly, MD

Decontamination of the Digestive Tract and Oropharynx in ICU Patients

de Smet AMGA, Kluytmans JAJW, Cooper BS, et al (Univ Med Ctr, Utrecht, the Netherlands; Amphia Hosp, Breda; Centre for Infections Health Protection Agency Statistics, London; et al)

N Engl J Med 360:20-31, 2009

Background.—Selective digestive tract decontamination (SDD) and selective oropharyngeal decontamination (SOD) are infection-prevention measures used in the treatment of some patients in intensive care, but reported effects on patient outcome are conflicting.

Methods.—We evaluated the effectiveness of SDD and SOD in a crossover study using cluster randomization in 13 intensive care units (ICUs), all in the Netherlands. Patients with an expected duration of intubation of more than 48 hours or an expected ICU stay of more than 72 hours were eligible. In each ICU, three regimens (SDD, SOD, and standard care) were applied in random order over the course of 6 months. Mortality at day 28 was the primary end point. SDD consisted of 4 days of intravenous cefotaxime and topical application of tobramycin, colistin, and amphotericin B in the oropharynx and stomach. SOD consisted of oropharyngeal application only of the same antibiotics. Monthly point-prevalence studies were performed to analyze antibiotic resistance.

Results.—A total of 5939 patients were enrolled in the study, with 1990 assigned to standard care, 1904 to SOD, and 2045 to SDD; crude mortality in the groups at day 28 was 27.5%, 26.6%, and 26.9%, respectively. In a random-effects logistic-regression model with age, sex, Acute Physiology and Chronic Health Evaluation (APACHE II) score, intubation status, and medical specialty used as covariates, odds ratios for death at day 28 in the SOD and SDD groups, as compared with the standard-care group, were 0.86 (95% confidence interval [CI], 0.74 to 0.99) and 0.83 (95% CI, 0.72 to 0.97), respectively.

Conclusions.—In an ICU population in which the mortality rate associated with standard care was 27.5% at day 28, the rate was reduced by an estimated 3.5 percentage points with SDD and by 2.9 percentage points with SOD. (Controlled Clinical Trials number, ISRCTN35176830.)

▶ This is an excellent multidisciplinary study evaluating nearly 6000 ICU patients regarding selective digestive tract decontamination (SDD) and selective oropharyngeal decontamination (SOD). The eligibility criteria were well defined in the 13 institutions that took part. The end result was a 2.9% to 3.5% reduction in day 28 mortality compared with the control group.

As the authors have noted, multiple studies have evaluated SDD and SOD as methods to decrease morbidity from infectious complications, especially ventilator-associated pneumonia. Many studies have shown benefit while others have not demonstrated improved outcome. This is the largest multi-institutional randomized controlled study to date where these 2 treatment methods have evaluated mortality as the specific outcome and compared the 2 modalities with each other and a control group. In the study, the estimated cost of SOD was $1 per day compared with $12 per day for SDD. These costs pale in comparison with other costs in the ICU. Nevertheless, SOD does not require a 4-day infusion of cephalosporin and has less risk of the host developing antibiotic-resistant bacteria. Thus, with a similar reduction in mortality, there appears to be a benefit to the use of SOD in ICU patients at risk for ventilator-associated pneumonia.

As the authors have noted, multiple studies have evaluated SDD and SOD.

J. M. Daly, MD

Does smoking influence outcome after autologous chondrocyte implantation? A case-controlled study

Jaiswal PK, Macmull S, Bentley G, et al (Royal Natl Orthopaedic Hosp, Stanmore, England)

J Bone Joint Surg Br 91:1575-1578, 2009

Smoking is known to have an adverse effect on wound healing and musculoskeletal conditions. This case-controlled study looked at whether smoking has a deleterious effect in the outcome of autologous chondrocyte implantation for the treatment of full thickness chondral defects of the knee.

The mean Modified Cincinatti Knee score was statistically significantly lower in smokers ($n = 48$) than in non-smokers ($n = 66$) both before and after surgery ($p < 0.05$). Smokers experienced significantly less improvement in the knee score two years after surgery ($p < 0.05$). Graft failures were only seen in smokers ($p = 0.016$). There was a strong negative correlation between the number of cigarettes smoked and the outcome following surgery (Pearson's correlation coefficient −0.65, $p = 0.004$).

These results suggest that patients who smoke have worse pre-operative function and obtain less benefit from this procedure than non-smokers. The counselling of patients undergoing autologous chondrocyte implantation should include smoking, not only as a general cardiopulmonary risk but also because poorer results can be expected in smokers following this procedure.

▶ The authors retrospectively reviewed a prospective database evaluating the results of autologous chrondocyte implantation (ACI) in smokers, ex-smokers, and nonsmokers. Nonsmokers had better implantation and healing as well as greater improvement and less pain at 2 years after the procedure than either of the other 2 groups. Importantly, the graft failures were seen only in smokers.

Many studies have shown the impairment of smoking on wound healing of many sites and types. Cellular implantation is different inherently than development of skin flaps and other wounds. Nevertheless, successful implantation was severely inhibited. It would have been valuable for the authors to describe the ex-smokers in greater detail. Other studies have shown that quitting smoking for varying periods of time can return healing function back toward normal. In this study, that was not true. These results may be due to ACI versus other types of wound healing, or it may be due to the duration of nonsmoking in the ex-smokers.

J. M. Daly, MD

Effect of Stitch Length on Wound Complications After Closure of Midline Incisions: A Randomized Controlled Trial

Millbourn D, Cengiz Y, Israelsson LA (Sundsvall Hosp, Sweden; Umeå Univ, Sweden)

Arch Surg 144:1056-1059, 2009

Hypothesis.—In midline incisions closed with a single-layer running suture, the rate of wound complications is lower when a suture length to wound length ratio of at least 4 is accomplished with a short stitch length rather than with a long one.

Design.—Prospective randomized controlled trial.

Setting.—Surgical department.

Patients.—Patients operated on through a midline incision.

Intervention.—Wound closure with a short stitch length (ie, placing stitches <10 mm from the wound edge) or a long stitch length.

Main Outcome Measures.—Wound dehiscence, surgical site infection, and incisional hernia.

Results.—In all, 737 patients were randomized: 381 were allocated to a long stitch length and 356, to a short stitch length. Wound dehiscence occurred in 1 patient whose wound was closed with a long stitch length. Surgical site infection occurred in 35 of 343 patients (10.2%) in the long stitch group and in 17 of 326 (5.2%) in the short stitch group ($P = .02$). Incisional hernia was present in 49 of 272 patients (18.0%) in the long stitch group and in 14 of 250 (5.6%) in the short stitch group ($P < .001$). In multivariate analysis, a long stitch length was an independent risk factor for both surgical site infection and incisional hernia.

Conclusion.—In midline incisions closed with a running suture and having a suture length to wound length ratio of at least 4, current recommendations of placing stitches at least 10 mm from the wound edge should be changed to avoid patient suffering and costly wound complications.

Trial Registration.—clinicaltrials.gov Identifier: NCT00508053.

▶ For large intra-abdominal procedures, the midline incision continues to be the most widely used. The era of closure using interrupted nonabsorbable sutures has been largely replaced by using continuous, synthetic, and slowly absorbable sutures. There are many proponents of using large "deep" bites of fascia and muscle in closures, theorizing that this method provides better suture and tissue purchase. Thus, the authors performed a large, well-controlled study to determine whether a short suture technique or long suture technique was best for healing. Surgical site infection occurred twice as commonly using the long suture technique, and incisional hernia developed over 3 times as often using the long suture compared with the short suture technique. Sutures were pulled firmly but not tightly.

Presumably, the long suture technique led to greater tissue ischemia as well as sites between sutures where hernias could occur. A suture length ratio of at least 4 mm is recommended along with suturing only 5 to 8 mm from the wound edges. This important study should be reviewed by all general surgeons, as it may change one's approach to midline wound closures.

J. M. Daly, MD

Effects of medicinal mushroom (*Sparassis crispa*) on wound healing in streptozotocin-induced diabetic rats

Kwon A-H, Qiu Z, Hashimoto M, et al (Kansai Med Univ, Osaka, Japan; Res and Development Ctr, Kyoto, Japan)

Am J Surg 197:503-509, 2009

Background.—The impaired wound healing in diabetes mellitus is a major clinical problem. *Sparassis crispa* (SC) is a medicinal mushroom and its *β*-glucan content is more than 40%. This study investigated whether oral administration of SC could improve the impaired wound healing in diabetic rats.

Methods.—Full-thickness skin wounds were created on the backs of streptozotocin (STZ)-induced diabetic rats. Diabetic rats were then divided into 2 groups: SC-treated group that was orally administered doses of 1,000 mg/kg body weight per day of SC for 4 weeks and a control group without SC administration. Moreover, collagen synthesis of purified *β*-glucan from SC was estimated in vitro.

Results.—Wound closure was significantly accelerated by oral administration of SC. Furthermore, in SC-treated wounds there were significant increases in macrophage and fibroblast migration, collagen regeneration, and epithelialization compared with the control group. The levels of type I collagen synthesized by cultured human dermal fibroblasts for the SC group were significantly higher than those for the control group.

Conclusions.—SC can improve the impaired healing of diabetic wounds. This effect might involve an increase in the migration of macrophages and fibroblasts, and *β*-glucan from SC directly increases the synthesis of type I collagen. Therefore, the use of SC may be extended to the clinical setting and prove an effective promoter of wound healing in patients with diabetes.

► Improvement in wound healing is an important goal in diabetics. Many avenues are undergoing active investigation. These authors used the medicinal mushroom *Sparassis crispa* (SC) with a β-glucan content of more than 40%. In this study, rats were made diabetic using a well-known technique, and did demonstrate impaired wound contracture compared with normal controls. Administration of 1000 mg/kg of SC (a large dose) daily for 4 weeks after wounding did improve wound contracture, but only later in the contracture process on days 16 and 20. Early in the healing phase (before day 12) there appeared little difference in wound contracture due to SC administration. Differences in type I collagen content were observed on day 7.

There are a number of issues with this animal study that reflect on translating animal studies to humans. First, a large dose of SC was administered; the equivalent in man would be 70 000 mg per day. Second, there was no control group for the SC group, whereby β-glucan content was administered to eliminate any other factors in SC which might be responsible. Third, many methods have been described to investigate wound healing with contracture, type I collagen content, and histology being just a few of them. Clearly other methods such as wound tensile strength should be used in this model. Finally, the mechanisms of action of SC should be more clearly defined.

Much more work is needed before this approach should be tried in humans.

J. M. Daly, MD

Mechanism of Sustained Release of Vascular Endothelial Growth Factor in Accelerating Experimental Diabetic Healing

Brem H, Kodra A, Golinko MS, et al (New York Univ; et al)

J Invest Dermatol 129:2275-2287, 2009

In this study, we hypothesize that local sustained release of vascular endothelial growth factor (VEGF), using adenovirus vector (ADV)-mediated gene transfer, accelerates experimental wound healing. This hypothesis was tested by determining the specific effects of $VEGF_{165}$ application on multiple aspects of the wound healing process, that is, time to complete wound closure and skin biomechanical properties. After showing accelerated wound healing *in vivo*, we studied the mechanism to explain the findings on multiple aspects of the wound healing cascade, including epithelialization, collagen deposition, and cell migration. Intradermal treatment of wounds in non-obese diabetic and db/db mice with ADV/$VEGF_{165}$ improves healing by enhancing tensile stiffness and/or increasing epithelialization and collagen deposition, as well as by decreasing time to wound closure. $VEGF_{165}$, *in vitro*, stimulates the migration of cultured human keratinocytes and fibroblasts, thus revealing a non-angiogenic effect of VEGF on wound closure. In conclusion, ADV/VEGF is effective in accelerating wound closure by stimulating angiogenesis, epithelialization, and collagen deposition. In the future, local administration and sustained, controlled release of $VEGF_{165}$ may decrease amputations in patients with diabetic foot ulcers and possibly accelerate closure of venous ulcers and pressure ulcers.

▶ Multiple studies (see Table 1 in the original article) have suggested that local administration of vascular endothelial growth factor (VEGF) leads to improved wound healing in a variety of animal models. In this study, the authors used a model of adenovirus (ADV)-mediated gene transfer to enhance the local production of VEGF. They noted a marked shortening of healing in db/db diabetic animals in the treated animals versus controls. There was enhanced migration of keratinocytes but no increase in the stiffness of the healing wound.

This study has major relevance, as wound healing in diabetic patients is abnormal. However, other models should be tested, including those wound healing models with low blood flow, radiation, host immunosuppresion, etc.

It would be interesting to use sutured models of fascial or intestinal healing to learn the potential benefits on tensile and bursting strengths using ADV-mediated VEGF local injection.

J. M. Daly, MD

Midline Versus Transverse Incision in Major Abdominal Surgery: A Randomized, Double-Blind Equivalence Trial (POVATI: ISRCTN60734227)

Seiler CM, Deckert A, Diener MK, et al (Univ of Heidelberg, Germany)

Ann Surg 249:913-920, 2009

Objective.—There are 2 main types of access for patients requiring major open, elective abdominal surgery: the midline or the transverse approach. The aim of this study is to compare both approaches by focusing on postoperative pain, complications, and frequency of incisional hernias.

Summary Background Data.—A recent Cochrane review suggested that transverse incisions may be less painful but incisional hernia rates do not differ.

Methods.—Randomized, patient- and observer-blinded, monocentric, equivalence clinical trial. Patients were scheduled for elective primary abdominal incisions. Composite primary end point measured 48 hours after surgery was the total amount of analgesics (piritramide) required in the last 24 hours and pain (Visual Analogue Scale). Secondary end points were early-onset and late complications. This study is registered in the ISRCTN registry and has the ID number ISRCTN60734227.

Results.—Two hundred patients (101 midline and 99 transverse) were randomized. Both incision types resulted in similar amounts of required analgesics (95% confidence interval [−0.38; −0.33] was included in the equivalence level). For the Visual Analogue Scale, both the 95% and 90% CI (0–10) were neither within the equivalence levels nor were their differences significant at the 5% level. No relevant differences between midline and transverse incisions were observed for 30-day mortality (2 vs. 2, $P = 0.99$), mortality after one year (15 vs. 23, $P = 0.15$), pulmonary complications (13 vs. 17, $P = 0.43$), median length of hospital stay (11 vs. 12 days, $P = 0.08$), median time to tolerance of solid food (12 vs. 14 days, $P = 0.30$), and incisional hernias after one year (13 vs. 8, $P = 0.48$). More wound infections occurred in the transverse group (15 vs. 5, $P = 0.02$).

Conclusion.—The decision about the incision should be driven by surgeon preference with respect to the patient's disease and anatomy.

▶ Surgical lore suggests that transverse incisions are less subject to postoperative hernia development and the occurrence of infection. Some have suggested that fewer pulmonary complications occur. This randomized, prospective, equivalence trial in 200 patients evaluated midline vs transverse incisions for abdominal procedures. There was no significant difference noted, except for a higher wound infection rate in patients who underwent the transverse incisions. No differences were noted in the development of wound hernias or pulmonary complications.

Studies such as these are very important, as they subject lore to the scientific rigor of a clinical trial. It is also not common to see equivalence trials published because often reviewers are looking for the next breakthrough. Appropriately, the authors suggest that the choice of incision should be dictated by the intra-abdominal pathology and the operation to be performed.

J. M. Daly, MD

Poly-N-Acetyl Glucosamine Nanofibers: A New Bioactive Material to Enhance Diabetic Wound Healing by Cell Migration and Angiogenesis

Scherer SS, Pietramaggiori G, Matthews J, et al (Brigham and Women's Hosp, Boston, MA; et al)

Ann Surg 250:322-330, 2009

Introduction.—In several fields of surgery, the treatment of complicated tissue defects is an unsolved clinical problem. In particular, the use of tissue scaffolds has been limited by poor revascularization and integration. In this study, we developed a polymer, poly-N-acetyl-glucosamine (sNAG), with bioactive properties that may be useful to overcome these limitations.

Objective.—To develop a scaffold-like membrane with bioactive properties and test the biologic effects in vitro and in vivo in diabetic wound healing.

Methods.—In vitro, cells–nanofibers interactions were tested by cell metabolism and migration assays. In vivo, full thickness wounds in diabetic mice (n = 15 per group) were treated either with sNAG scaffolds, with a cellulosic control material, or were left untreated. Wound healing kinetics, including wound reepithelialization and wound contraction as well as microscopic metrics such as tissue growth, cell proliferation (Ki67), angiogenesis (PECAM-1), cell migration (MAP-Kinase), and keratinocyte migration (p 63) were monitored over a period of 28 days. Messenger RNA levels related to migration (uPAR), angiogenesis (VEGF), inflammatory response (IL-1β), and extracellular matrix remodeling (MMP3 and 9) were measured in wound tissues.

Results.—sNAG fibers stimulated cell metabolism and the in vitro migratory activity of endothelial cells and fibroblasts. sNAG membranes profoundly accelerated wound closure mainly by reepithelialization and increased keratinocyte migration (7.5-fold), granulation tissue formation (2.8-fold), cell proliferation (4-fold), and vascularization (2.7-fold) compared with control wounds. Expression of markers of angiogenesis (VEGF), cell migration (uPAR) and ECM remodeling (MMP3, MMP9) were up-regulated in sNAG treated wounds compared with controls.

Conclusions.—The key mechanism of the bioactive membranes is the cell-nanofiber stimulatory interaction. Engineering of bioactive materials may represent the clinical solution for a number of complex tissue defects.

▶ It is well known that wound healing is impaired in type II diabetes. Often, these patients suffer complex wounds that require methods for establishing artificial scaffolding to obtain wound closure in a timely fashion. The problem is that cell migration and angiogenesis is markedly decreased in these patients resulting in a chronically infected nonhealing wound. The authors have discovered a polymer that can be crafted into nanofibers and which in vitro stimulates cell migration and metabolism. In vivo, in diabetic mice, open surface wounds closed more quickly in the case of nanofiber-treated wounds compared with the 2 control groups.

This study is important for its use of a new polymer that stimulates cellular activity and for the use of nanotechnology increasing the polymer's surface area and providing the cellular stimulation and scaffolding for improved cell migration to occur.

J. M. Daly, MD

Prevention of postoperative adhesion formation by individual and combined administration of 4 per cent icodextrin and dimetindene maleate

Tepetes K, Asprodini EK, Christodoulidis G, et al (Larissa Univ Hosp, Greece; et al)

Br J Surg 96:1476-1483, 2009

Background.—To date, no single method has been successful in eliminating peritoneal adhesion formation after major abdominal surgery. This study evaluated the individual and possible synergistic effect of a local intraperitoneal barrier, 4 per cent icodextrin, and an intravenously administered antihistamine drug, dimetindene maleate, in the prevention of adhesion development following surgical trauma.

Methods.—*De novo* experimental adhesions were induced by standardized trauma of the peritoneum and large bowel in 120 New Zealand White rabbits. The animals were randomized into four groups receiving intraperitoneal saline, intraperitoneal 4 per cent icodextrin (60 ml), intravenous dimetindene maleate (0·1 mg/kg) and 4 per cent icodextrin–dimetindene in combination ($n = 30$ per group). Ten days later, adhesion scores and incidence were assessed by two independent surgeons and surface area by computer-aided planimetry.

Results.—Treatment with either icodextrin or dimetindene maleate significantly reduced adhesion scores and increased the incidence of adhesion-free animals in an equipotent manner. The effect of combined treatment on severity, incidence and surface area of adhesions was more pronounced than that of each drug administered separately.

Conclusion.—Combined administration of 4 per cent icodextrin and dimetindene maleate may be used safely and efficaciously to prevent surgically induced adhesions.

▶ The development of postoperative adhesions is very common after major abdominal surgery. In fact, adhesions often lead to secondary operations. Thus, there is a continual search for the correct products that can ameliorate adhesion formation while maintaining wound healing in the intestine and fascia and allow for the proper intra-abdominal localization of bacteria. It is quite a challenge. These authors have attempted to decrease adhesion through systemic and local approaches. Intraperitoneal administration of icodextrin alone is beneficial in reducing adhesion formation in experimental animals. The systemic administration of an antihistamine, dimetindene maleate, also reduces adhesion formation, while the combination is synergistic in effects.

It will be important for the authors to test their methods in wound healing models as well as several intraperitoneal models of intraperitoneal infection and sepsis to be certain that harm does not occur with the use of these agents.

J. M. Daly, MD

Randomized controlled trial and cost-effectiveness analysis of silver-donating antimicrobial dressings for venous leg ulcers (VULCAN trial)

Michaels JA, Campbell B, King B, et al (Univ of Sheffield, UK; Royal Devon and Exeter NHS Foundation Trust, UK; Sheffield Primary Care Trust, UK)

Br J Surg 96:1147-1156, 2009

Background.—Antimicrobial silver dressings are used beneath graduated compression in the treatment of venous ulceration. There is little information on whether their use is effective. This was a prospective randomized trial and cost-effectiveness analysis of silver-donating *versus* non-silver low-adherence dressings in the treatment of venous leg ulcers.

Methods.—Patients were randomized between the two types of dressing. The primary outcome measure was complete ulcer healing at 12 weeks. Secondary outcomes included time to healing, quality of life and cost-effectiveness.

Results.—A total of 213 patients were recruited. There was no difference between the dressings in the proportion of ulcers healed at 12 weeks (59·6 per cent for silver and 56·7 per cent for control dressings). Mean utility scores for the EuroQol 5D and Short Form 6D were similar in both groups at 1, 3, 6 and 12 months. Compared with the control group the antimicrobial group had an incremental cost of £97·85 and an incremental quality-adjusted life year gain of 0·0002, giving an incremental cost-effectiveness ratio of £489 250 for the antimicrobial dressings.

Conclusion.—No significant differences were found in either primary or secondary endpoints. There was no evidence to support the routine use of silver-donating dressings beneath compression for venous ulceration.

Registration number: ISRCTN 72485131 (http://www.controlled-trials.com).

▶ Patients with chronic venous ulcers are often vexing to the general surgeon. Individuals use a variety of methods—both surgical and nonsurgical—in an attempt to heal the ulcers more quickly. The type of dressing has been claimed by many to make substantial difference in the rates of healing; yet, few prospective randomized trials offer proof. These authors compared silver-donating dressings with nonsilver, low adherence dressings in over 200 patients following them for rates of healing. No differences were noted in the rates of healing, but the silver-donating dressing was much more expensive. Thus, the nonsilver, low-adherence dressing remains the standard of care. The *British Journal of Surgery* is to be commended for publishing an important trial that will save health care costs in the management of these patients. As newer modalities come along, they must be subjected to a randomized trial to determine their effectiveness.

J. M. Daly, MD

Selective and Specific Macrophage Ablation Is Detrimental to Wound Healing in Mice

Mirza R, DiPietro LA, Koh TJ (Univ of Illinois at Chicago)

Am J Pathol 175:2454-2462, 2009

Macrophages are thought to play important roles during wound healing, but definition of these roles has been hampered by our technical inability to specifically eliminate macrophages during wound repair. The purpose of this study was to test the hypothesis that specific depletion of macrophages after excisional skin wounding would detrimentally affect healing by reducing the production of growth factors important in the repair process. We used transgenic mice that express the human diphtheria toxin (DT) receptor under the control of the CD11b promoter (DTR mice) to specifically ablate macrophages during wound healing. Mice without the transgene are relatively insensitive to DT, and administration of DT to wild-type mice does not alter macrophage or other inflammatory cell accumulation after injury and does not influence wound healing. In contrast, treatment of DTR mice with DT prevented macrophage accumulation in healing wounds but did not affect the accumulation of neutrophils or monocytes. Such macrophage depletion resulted in delayed re-epithelialization, reduced collagen deposition, impaired angiogenesis, and decreased cell proliferation in the healing wounds. These adverse changes were associated with increased levels of tumor necrosis factor-α and reduced levels of transforming growth factor-$\beta 1$ and vascular endothelial growth factor in the wound. In summary, macrophages seem to promote both wound closure and dermal healing, in part by regulating the cytokine environment of the healing wound.

▶ The cellular cascade after wounding is critically important to maximize the healing potential and the timing of complete epithelialization. This is a very interesting experimental study in mice using a novel approach to local depletion of macrophages in healing tissue without disrupting neutrophil and monocyte infiltration. The authors noted that macrophage depletion severely decreased epithelialization, collagen deposition, and cell proliferation and impaired angiogenesis in the wound and markedly delayed wound healing. Thus, the macrophage and its infiltration into the healing wound is critical to its early healing. Administration of growth factors and chemoattractants may be very effective locally in accelerating the infiltration of wounds with macrophages. This knowledge and potential therapy may be particularly important in wounds created in radiated areas, in those individuals with diabetes or those patients receiving immunosuppressant drugs.

J. M. Daly, MD

A tissue-scale gradient of hydrogen peroxide mediates rapid wound detection in zebrafish

Niethammer P, Grabher C, Look AT, et al (Harvard Med School, Boston, MA)
Nature 459:996-999, 2009

Barrier structures (for example, epithelia around tissues and plasma membranes around cells) are required for internal homeostasis and protection from pathogens. Wound detection and healing represent a dormant morphogenetic program that can be rapidly executed to restore barrier integrity and tissue homeostasis. In animals, initial steps include recruitment of leukocytes to the site of injury across distances of hundreds of micrometres within minutes of wounding. The spatial signals that direct this immediate tissue response are unknown. Owing to their fast diffusion and versatile biological activities, reactive oxygen species, including hydrogen peroxide (H_2O_2), are interesting candidates for wound-to-leukocyte signalling. Here we probe the role of H_2O_2 during the early events of wound responses in zebrafish larvae expressing a genetically encoded H_2O_2 sensor. This reporter revealed a sustained rise in H_2O_2 concentration at the wound margin, starting ~3 min after wounding and peaking at ~20 min, which extended 100–200 μm into the tail-fin epithelium as a decreasing concentration gradient. Using pharmacological and genetic inhibition, we show that this gradient is created by dual oxidase (Duox), and that it is required for rapid recruitment of leukocytes to the wound. This is the first observation, to our knowledge, of a tissue-scale

H_2O_2 pattern, and the first evidence that H_2O_2 signals to leukocytes in tissues, in addition to its known antiseptic role.

▶ This is a very interesting biologic study in zebrafish looking at signaling mechanisms whereby phagocytic neutrophils rapidly enter tissue at the edges of the wound site. The authors used the zebrafish model because they could use novel techniques to follow H_2O_2 gradients after wounding. They demonstrated that such gradients do exist at the wound margins quickly (within 20 minutes) after wounding and then persist for at least 99 minutes. They also showed that a novel dual oxidase (dual oxidase [DUOX]) creates the gradient and is required for the recruitment of leukocytes.

While H_2O_2 is known to have antibacterial properties itself, this is the first time it has been shown to be at least partially responsible for the influx into wounded areas of phagocytic cells coming from other sites.

J. M. Daly, MD

10 Gastrointestinal

Introduction

This was an exciting year to review the gastrointestinal surgery literature because of several high-quality manuscripts that addressed issues in diagnostic approaches to gastrointestinal disease, evolving minimally invasive treatments, the assessment of surgical outcomes, and the examination of traditional challenging surgical problems. The most difficult task was to limit the number of papers that could be included. Many worthy contributions to the literature are excluded because the breadth and depth of the publications in gastrointestinal surgery continue to expand in number and quality. Nonetheless, I will share broad highlights of some noteworthy topics.

Diagnostic testing for gastrointestinal diseases continues to evolve at a rapid pace. Advances in the diagnostic techniques of benign and malignant esophageal disease have led to improvements in not only detecting disease but also refined management of esophageal motor disorders and esophageal cancer. For example, image-based high resolution manometry for diagnosis of esophageal motor disease and positron emission tomography for esophageal cancer are newer diagnostic modalities that are impacting the management of these diseases.

Not only are our diagnostic capabilities improving, but advances in minimally invasive treatment of nearly all gastrointestinal surgical diseases are changing quickly. Endoscopic approaches, minimally invasive surgical approaches, natural orifice transluminal endoscopic surgery, and transanal endoscopic microsurgery for anorectal diseases are increasingly used to treat diseases from the esophagus to the anus. Furthermore, even the minimally invasive surgical procedures have evolved from multi-incision approaches to single-incision laparoscopic surgery for a number of functional and extirpative procedures. The techniques and outcomes of these procedures are reported with increasing frequency—stay tuned to this evolving field.

Importantly, the gastrointestinal surgical literature, like that of other medical disciplines, has been increasingly populated with outcome studies that review the results from select practices or large administrative databases that are examined systematically. This burgeoning area of investigation should lead to improved patient care and outcomes. These publications, in comparing single-surgeon results (practice-based learning) to large data sets and examining system-based approaches to improving patient care, will advance the field of gastrointestinal surgery, and most importantly, improve care.

Finally, many studies have revisited some of our old foes like the multiply-repaired ventral hernia, persistent bowel obstruction from adhesions, and lower gastrointestinal bleeding. Though we do not have the cure to many of these vexing conditions, the continued review of outcomes and advancements in new ideas for alternative therapies continue to gradually move forward the surgical approaches to these diseases.

I hope you enjoy reviewing these publications as much as I did. Bountiful material exists to advance our knowledge and thought processes in the field of gastrointestinal surgery. I encourage you to read, review, and make your own contributions to the gastrointestinal surgical literature.

Kevin E. Behrns, MD

---

^{18}F-Fluorodeoxyglucose-Positron Emission Tomography for the Assessment of Histopathologic Response and Prognosis After Completion of Neoadjuvant Chemoradiation in Esophageal Cancer

Vallböhmer D, Hölscher AH, Dietlein M, et al (Univ of Cologne, Germany; Univ of Dusseldorf, Germany)

Ann Surg 250:888-894, 2009

Objective.—To evaluate the potential of [^{18}F]-fluorodeoxyglucose-positron emission tomography (FDG-PET) after the completion of neoadjuvant chemoradiation for the assessment of histopathologic response and prognosis in the multimodality treatment of patients with esophageal cancer.

Background.—Combined chemoradiation with and without surgery are widely accepted treatment options for patients with locally advanced esophageal cancer. Evidence suggests that patients with response to chemoradiation have no additional benefit from surgery compared with definitive chemoradiation. However, there is still a great lack in noninvasive markers for response assessment in patients with esophageal cancer undergoing multimodality treatment. Interestingly, recent studies imply that FDG-PET significantly correlates with histopathologic response and survival in patients with esophageal cancer undergoing neoadjuvant chemotherapy followed by surgical resection.

Methods.—Study patients were recruited from a prospective clinical observation trial on neoadjuvant chemoradiation for esophageal cancer between 1997 and 2006. The study included 119 (98 men, 21 women; median age, 59.4 years; squamous cell cancer: 66; adenocarcinoma: 53) patients with locally advanced esophageal cancer (cT2–4, N_x, M_0). All patients received neoadjuvant chemoradiation (cisplatin, 5-FU, 36 Gy) and subsequently underwent transthoracic en bloc esophagectomy. Histomorphologic regression was defined as major histopathologic response when resected specimens contained less than 10% vital residual tumor cells (major response: 47 patients [39.5%]; minor response: 72 patients [60.5%]). FDG-PET was performed before and 2 to 3 weeks after the end of chemoradiation with assessment of the intratumoral FDG-uptake (pretreatment standardized uptake value; post-treatment standardized uptake value; percentage change). These variables were correlated with histopathologic response and survival.

Results.—Major histomorphologic response was confirmed as an important prognostic factor ($P = 0.005$; log-rank test). Neoadjuvant chemoradiation led to a significant reduction of intratumoral FDG-uptake ($P < 0.0001$). A nonsignificant association was seen between major responders and FDG-PET results ($P = 0.056$). However, the receiver operating characteristic analysis could not identify a standardized uptake value threshold with a relevant predictive value for histomorphologic response. No significant association between metabolic imaging and prognosis was found.

Conclusion.—FDG-PET seems not to be an imaging system that effectively characterizes the groups of major and minor response as well as survival in patients with esophageal cancer after multimodality treatment.

▶ Over the last decade or more, neoadjuvant therapy for esophageal cancer has been favored in an attempt to downstage the tumor and improve the R0 resection rate. However, determining the response to neoadjuvant therapy has remained somewhat elusive. The use of positron emission tomography (PET) would appear to be a valuable modality to determine preoperative and postoperative metabolic function of the tumor, and thus, the response to neoadjuvant therapy. Several studies have suggested that PET is helpful in determining the response; however, many studies including this well-designed study by Vallböhmer et al refute the discriminating value of PET in the assessment of the response to neoadjuvant chemoradiotherapy. This article shows that PET was helpful only in those patients who had a complete response, and, in fact, there remained significant overlap between these patients and patients who had only a minor histopathologic response. Although PET, in theory, would seem to be an ideal modality to determine the response to neoadjuvant therapy, the reasons for the lack of discrimination are not clear, but may point to the marked heterogeneity of the esophageal tumors. PET is dependent on the uptake and metabolism of 18F-fluorodeoxyglucose (FDG), but even this seemingly simple cellular mechanism may be altered significantly and not easily captured by imaging. Furthermore, many recent studies of the tumor microenvironment suggest that the interplay between the cancer cell and the surrounding stroma may play an important role in tumor viability, yet PET does not address the stromal compartment. This study is further evidence of our need to acquire more knowledge of the cancer cell and its environment so that we can more clearly assess and kill cancer cells.

K. E. Behrns, MD

A New Era in Esophageal Diagnostics: The Image-Based Paradigm of High-Resolution Manometry

Salvador R, Dubecz A, Polomsky M, et al (Univ of Rochester, NY)

J Am Coll Surg 208:1035-1044, 2009

Background.—The development of high-resolution (HRM) catheters and software displays of manometric recordings in color-coded pressure plots has changed the diagnostic assessment of esophageal disease. HRM may offer advantages over conventional methods, including improved identification of motility disorders, hiatal hernia, and outflow obstruction, and ease interpretation.

Study Design.—HRM studies were obtained in 50 healthy volunteers and 106 patients. HRM was performed using a 36-channel catheter, with sensors spaced at 1-cm intervals. Manometric findings were classified into abnormalities of the gastroesophageal barrier and those of the esophageal body and validated by comparison with endoscopic and radiographic diagnostic methods.

Results.—The mean time for HRM was significantly lower than that for a conventional method (8.1versus 24.4 minutes; $p < 0.0001$). A structurally defective lower esophageal sphincter (LES) was present in 53 (57.3%) patients, a hypertensive LES in 6 (7.8%), and impaired LES relaxation in 17 patients (16.7%). Validating the LES findings, 86.3% (44 of 51) of patients with a defective sphincter by HRM had radiographic or endoscopic evidence of a hiatal hernia, and 80% (41 of 51) had a positive pH study, endoscopic erosive esophagitis, or Barrett's esophagus. Evidence of a hiatal hernia by HRM was seen in 33 (56%) patients; a hiatal hernia was seen in 91% (30 of 33) of these on endoscopy and 81% (17 of 21) on barium swallow. Fifty-eight patients (54.7%) had an abnormal body motility.

Conclusions.—HRM studies are shorter than those using conventional methods. Interpretation is image based, and correlation with objective endoscopic and physiologic findings confirms the accuracy of interpretation. The introduction of HRM is a significant advance in the outpatient evaluation of esophageal function.

▶ Salvador et al report an innovative, advanced functional assessment of the esophagus through the use of high-resolution manometry (HRM) that incorporates image generation. The HRM catheter is 4.2 mm in diameter and has 36 solid-state circumferential sensors spaced at 1-cm intervals. Ten swallows are administered following transnasal catheter placement. The data generated represent a marked advance over conventional manometry in that in addition to standard pressure data, image data are available through a usable software tool. This technology compares favorably with conventional manometry and permits the visual image identification of high- or low-pressure zones. Furthermore, the data are obtained in much less time than conventional manometry. The information generated appears to be particularly beneficial in patients with achalasia. How will this new technology change the evaluation of patients with esophageal disease? We hope this is a forerunner of even more advanced technologies that will combine functional manometric data with imaging data. Current evaluation of many patients with esophageal disease includes esophagogastroduodenoscopy, manometry, barium swallow, and a pH probe. Although often necessary, this complete evaluation causes considerable discomfort and inconvenience to the patient. Diagnostic procedures that integrate functional manometric assessment with imaging represent a major advance not only in providing useful information but also in providing patient comfort and convenience. Further evaluation of this diagnostic procedure in common diseases, such as gastroesophageal reflux disease, may shed light on its use and allow it to be a prototype diagnostic tool.

K. E. Behrns, MD

A Population-Based Study of Perforated Diverticular Disease Incidence and Associated Mortality

Humes DJ, Solaymani-Dodaran M, Fleming KM, et al (Nottingham Univ Hosp NHS Trust, UK; Univ of Nottingham, UK)

Gastroenterology 136:1198-1205, 2009

Background & Aims.—Perforated diverticular disease represents the most serious complication of diverticular disease, but little is known regarding its occurrence and mortality. We aimed to determine the incidence and mortality associated with diverticular perforation and the influence of comorbidity.

Methods.—We used a population based cohort study using patients with perforated diverticular disease and population controls identified from 1990 to 2005 in the General Practice Research Database (GPRD). Incidence and mortality rates were modelled using Poisson and Cox regression. Comorbidity was quantified using the Charlson index.

Results.—We identified 953 incident patients. The overall incidence was 2.66 (95% confidence interval [CI]: 2.49–2.83) per 100,000 person-years. The incidence rates increased 2.28-fold (95% CI: 1.79–2.95) when corrected for age and sex between 1990 and 2005. The risk of death was highest in the first year with a 6-fold increase (hazard ratio [HR], 5.63; 95% CI: 4.68–6.77). Adjusted for age and sex, the risk of death in the first year was highest in those with lowest comorbidity (HR, 11.11; 95% CI: 8.06–15.31), but the absolute mortality rates were greatest in those with the highest comorbidity (263.1 per 1000 person-years).

Conclusions.—The incidence of perforated diverticular disease has doubled over the period of the study. Patients presenting with a perforated diverticulum are 6 times more likely to die than the general population during the first year following perforation. Those who have the greatest comorbidity are the most likely to die; however, those with least comorbidity have an 11-fold increase in mortality in the first year.

▶ The population-based study of Humes et al examines the rate of perforation of diverticular disease of the colon and the risk of death in the United Kingdom. In this study, 963 index patients retrieved from the General Practice Research Database from 1990-2005 were examined, and the presence of a perforated diverticulum was validated. The results were compared with those persons in the general population. The results showed that the incidence of a perforated diverticulum was 2.66 per 100 000 person-years. Somewhat surprisingly, the incidence of perforated diverticula has doubled over the study period. More troubling, however, was the fact that patients with a perforated diverticulum are 6 times more likely to die than the general population in the first year. Although patients with comorbidities had an expected increased risk of death, even those patients with no comorbidities had an 11-fold increased risk of death compared with the general population. These data raise the question of whether our purported improvements in intensive care medicine have translated to true increased survivorship across multiple disciplines and diseases. Furthermore, are the results in the United Kingdom transferable to the United States and elsewhere? As the authors reference, some data suggest that the United Kingdom has higher initial rates of postoperative death compared with the United States, but no study has compared the rate of death from perforated diverticular disease in these 2 countries. Finally, what can or should we do to prevent perforation—should we hold to the time-honored, but data-poor dictum that patients should experience 2 bouts of diverticulitis before resection or are we exposing our patients to increased risks? A question worthy of further study.

K. E. Behrns, MD

A Prospective Evaluation of the Long-Term Outcome of Ileal Pouch-Anal Anastomosis in Patients with Inflammatory Bowel Disease-Unclassified and Indeterminate Colitis

Murrell ZA, Melmed GY, Ippoliti A, et al (Cedars-Sinai Med Ctr, Los Angeles, CA)

Dis Colon Rectum 52:872-878, 2009

Purpose.—The long-term outcome of ileal pouch-anal anastomosis in patients with indeterminate colitis is controversial. The aim of this study was to prospectively evaluate the long-term outcome of ileal pouch-anal anastomosis in a closely monitored cohort of patients with ulcerative colitis or indeterminate colitis.

Methods.—Prospectively generated clinical profiles on consecutive patients with ulcerative colitis or indeterminate colitis undergoing ileal pouch-anal anastomosis with close postoperative follow-up by one surgeon were reviewed. All patients were classified before surgery as either ulcerative colitis or inflammatory bowel disease-unclassified, and after surgery as either ulcerative colitis or indeterminate colitis. Long-term outcomes included acute pouchitis (antibiotic responsive), chronic pouchitis (antibiotic dependent or refractory), or *de novo* Crohn's disease (small inflammation above the pouch inlet or pouch fistula).

Results.—The study cohort of 334 patients were classified before surgery as ulcerative colitis in 237 (71 percent) and inflammatory bowel disease-unclassified in 97 (29 percent). After surgery, patients were classified as ulcerative colitis in 236 (71 percent) and indeterminate colitis in 98 (29 percent). After a median follow-up after stoma closure of 26 months, 53 patients (16 percent) developed acute pouchitis, 37 patients (11 percent) developed chronic pouchitis, and 40 patients (12 percent) developed *de novo* Crohn's disease. There was no significant difference in the incidence of acute pouchitis, chronic pouchitis, or *de novo* Crohn's disease between the ulcerative colitis, inflammatory bowel disease-unclassified, and indeterminate colitis patient groups.

Conclusion.—The incidence of acute pouchitis, chronic pouchitis, and *de novo* Crohn's disease after ileal pouch-anal anastomosis do not differ significantly between patients with ulcerative colitis, inflammatory bowel disease-unclassified, or indeterminate colitis. Patients with inflammatory bowel disease-unclassified and indeterminate colitis can undergo ileal pouch-anal anastomosis and expect a long-term outcome equivalent to patients with ulcerative colitis.

▶ Ileal pouch-anal anastomosis (IPAA) has been a major advance in the treatment of ulcerative colitis, and over the last several decades has provided thousands of patients with a stoma-free life. However, the indications for IPAA are not clear in up to nearly 1 in 3 patients. This substantial subgroup of patients does not carry a clear-cut diagnosis of ulcerative colitis; rather, they have indeterminate colitis (IC) or what is more recently called inflammatory bowel disease-unclassified (IBD-U). As expected, surgeons are somewhat reluctant to perform an IPAA on patients with IC or IBD-U for fear that patients will develop Crohn's disease. It has been well documented that patients with Crohn's fare poorly after an IPAA is performed. The article by Murrell et al provides some reassurance that patients with IC or IBD-U have no higher risk of acute or chronic pouchitis. Furthermore, patients that developed de novo Crohn's disease after IPAA were just as likely to have a preoperative or postoperative diagnosis of ulcerative colitis as a diagnosis of IC or IBD-U. It is, however, important to note that 10% to 15% of patients developed de novo Crohn's disease, and that even histologic sections may not be reliable in substantiating the correct preoperative diagnosis. This article highlights both the incredible advances that have been made in patients with inflammatory bowel disease and the profound disappointments resulting from our inability to correctly diagnose patients with inflammatory bowel disease. Even though genetic linkages between Crohn's and the NOD2 were established in 2001, we have not yet capitalized on this association to arrive at appropriate diagnoses. This article is a testament to both how far we have come surgically and how far we must travel to improve patient care.

K. E. Behrns, MD

Abdominal Wall Reconstruction: Lessons Learned From 200 "Components Separation" Procedures

Ko JH, Wang EC, Salvay DM, et al (Northwestern Univ, Chicago, IL; Feinberg School of Medicine, Chicago, IL)

Arch Surg 144:1047-1055, 2009

Objectives.—To determine the efficacy and describe the evolution of the "components separation" technique for abdominal wall repair in 200 consecutive patients.

Design.—Retrospective medical record review.

Setting.—Northwestern Memorial Hospital, Chicago, Illinois.

Patients.—Two hundred consecutive patients who underwent ventral hernia repair using the components separation technique.

Interventions.—Biological and permanent meshes were used in select patients to augment the repair of the midline fascial closure but were not used as "bridging" materials.

Main Outcome Measures.—Hernia recurrence rates and major and minor complication rates for the overall series and for the different techniques.

Results.—Primary components separation (n = 158) yielded a 22.8% recurrence rate. Closure of the midline tissues with augmentation of the repair using an acellular cadaveric dermis underlay (n = 18) had a 33.3% recurrence rate requiring a second operation, whereas intra-abdominal soft polypropylene mesh (n = 18) had 0% recurrence ($P = .04$). Elevated body mass index was a significant risk factor predicting hernia recurrence ($P = .003$).Contamination ($P = .04$) and enterocutaneous fistula ($P = .02$) at the time of surgery were associated with increased major complications, whereas body mass index ($P = .01$) and diabetes mellitus ($P = .04$) were associated with increased minor complications.

Conclusions.—Large complex hernias can be reliably repaired using the components separation technique despite the presence of open wounds, the need for bowel surgery, and numerous comorbidities. The long-term strength of the hernia repair is not augmented by acellular cadaveric dermis but seems to be improved with soft polypropylene mesh.

▶ Ko et al report a single surgeon's experience with the components separation technique for ventral incisional hernia repairs in 200 patients. This large series provides an in-depth personal analysis of the technique of repair and relays the evolution of the procedure in this surgeon's hands. Of the 200 patients, 158 had primary components separation repairs without a mesh or biologic adjunct. In addition, 6 patients had a polypropylene reinforcement, 18 had placement of a biologic mesh, and 18 patients had "soft" polypropylene mesh placed primarily in the underlay position; the recurrence rates for these procedures were 22.8%, 16.7%, 33.3%, and 0%, respectively. The complication rate was 17% to 25% in the various groups. This article is notable for an excellent description of the operative technique and the development of a technique to prevent skin loss. Furthermore, the body mass index was 30 to 35 in each of the subgroups, and, not surprisingly, obesity was associated with an increased rate of recurrence. This article is important for several reasons: (1) it is a large series by a single surgeon, (2) the evolution of the surgeon's technique is described in detail, and (3) the patients were closely followed with meticulous documentation of results. The results suggest that components separation should be in the armamentarium of all surgeons performing ventral hernia repairs. Although this study is well documented, some of the the subgroup analysis findings should be interpreted with caution because of a low number of patients in each group. Finally, although not detailed in this study, it is important that general surgery trainees learn and propagate this valuable technique, which is a valuable option in the arsenal of a surgeon performing ventral hernia repair.

K. E. Behrns, MD

Acute lower gastrointestinal bleeding in 1,112 patients admitted to an urban emergency medical center

Gayer C, Chino A, Lucas C, et al (Wayne State Univ, Detroit, MI)

Surgery 146:600-607, 2009

Background.—This study was performed to elucidate the etiology, effectiveness of diagnostic and therapeutic modalities, and outcomes in patients with acute lower gastrointestinal bleeding.

Methods.—A retrospective review of the medical records of 1,112 consecutive patients admitted to the surgical service of a single urban emergency hospital with lower gastrointestinal bleeding from 1988 to 2006. Two groups were compared: 1988–1997 and 1998–2006.

Results.—All patients underwent colonoscopy, 33.2% within 24 h of admission. Hematochezia was the most frequent presentation (55.5%), followed by maroon stool (16.7%) and melena (11.0%). Most patients, 690 (62.1%) also had upper endoscopy. Sixty-six patients subsequently had barium enemas. Eleven of 27 nuclide scans were positive. Arteriography was performed on 22 patients, with 11 positive results and 2 therapeutic. No statistical difference was found in procedures performed in our 2 time periods. Diverticulosis (33.5%), hemorrhoids (22.5%), and carcinoma (12.7%) were the most common etiologies with the diagnosis of diverticulosis more common in the 1998–2006 time period. The small bowel was the source in 14 total patients. Spontaneous cessation of the bleeding occurred in 863 (77.6%) patients. Endoscopic control increased from 1% in 1997–1998 to 4.4% in 1998–2006 ($P < .05$) with a corresponding decrease in the need for operative control from 22.6% to 16.6% in this same time period ($P < .05$). Furthermore, among elective operations, there was a decrease in right hemicolectomies from 31.6%

of total elective cases to 13.9% ($P < .05$). Emergent operations were needed in 3.4% and 4.8% of patients. The readmission rate did not change over time and was 5.2% overall with >50% because of diverticular bleeding.

Conclusion.—In this urban setting, diverticulosis, hemorrhoids, and carcinoma were the most common causes of severe acute lower gastrointestinal bleeding (LGIB) with diverticular bleed causing the highest recurrence. Colonoscopy allows for diagnosis in most patients with severe acute LGIB requiring hospitalization. Furthermore, it is now being used more effectively for hemostasis resulting in less operative intervention to control bleeding.

► Gayer et al report on a large series of patients with lower gastrointestinal (GI) bleeding that were examined, evaluated, and treated by a team of surgical endoscopists. The article compared the presentation and treatment of patients from 2 time periods, 1988-1997 ($N = 504$) versus 1998-2006 ($N = 608$). The results showed that diverticulosis, hemorrhoids, and cancer were the most frequent etiologies of bleeding, and that diverticulosis was more common in the later time period compared with the earlier evaluation period. Noticeably, vascular ectasia was an uncommon cause of bleeding, whereas the incidence of colitis was more common in the recent time period. All patients underwent a proscriptive bowel preparation followed by colonoscopy within 24 hours. Other imaging techniques were used infrequently. Three-quarters (75%) of the patients had spontaneous cessation of bleeding, but endoscopic control of bleeding increased from 1% to 4% over the time periods. Operative management decreased over time from 23% to nearly 17% with the number of elective operations decreasing considerably. The operative mortality was 3%, but emergency operations had a 10% mortality. The readmission rate for rebleeding was about 4% during both time periods. These findings are informative for 2 major reasons: (1) this is an extremely large collection of patients that were compared over 2 time periods, and (2) the systematic care of these patients was performed by a surgical team that appeared to be responsible for the patients' care from start to finish. The large retrospective nature of this study permits an evaluation over time and provides a look at relatively subtle changes that have occurred—ie, vascular ectasia is uncommon! Furthermore, the use of nuclear scans and angiography was infrequent and apparently not necessary. Finally, patients with GI bleeds too frequently receive fragmented care from medical teams, surgical teams, or GI bleed teams, but these patients had well-defined care by a surgical team. What a wonderful experience for the surgical residents and the patients!

K. E. Behrns, MD

Anal fistula plug and fibrin glue versus conventional treatment in repair of complex anal fistulas

Chung W, Kazemi P, Ko D, et al (Univ of British Columbia, Vancouver, Canada)
Am J Surg 197:604-608, 2009

Introduction.—High transsphincteric fistulas are difficult to treat because fistulotomy of involved sphincter muscle results in incontinence. We compare our outcomes for anal fistula plug, fibrin glue, advancement flap closure, and seton drain insertion.

Methods.—This is a retrospective study of patients treated for high transsphincteric anal fistulas. The primary outcome was full healing at 12 weeks postoperatively.

Results.—Between 1997 and 2008, 232 patients with anal fistula were identified in the St. Paul's Hospital Anal Fistula Database. Postoperative healing rates at the 12-week follow-up for the fistula plug, fibrin glue, flap advancement, and seton drain groups were 59.3%, 39.1%, 60.4%, and 32.6%, respectively ($P < .0001$).

Conclusions.—Closure of the primary fistula opening using a biological anal fistula plug and anal flap advancement result in similar fistula healing rates in patients with high transsphincteric fistulae. These 2 strategies are superior to seton placement and fibrin glue. Given the low morbidity and relative simplicity of the procedure, the anal fistula plug is a viable alternative treatment for patients with high transsphincteric anal fistulas.

▶ Chung and colleagues report retrospective results of treating 232 patients with high complex anal fistula with an anal plug (n = 27), fibrin glue (n = 23), seton placement (n = 86), or advancement flap (n = 96). Follow-up was complete at 12 weeks and revealed healing rates of 59%, 39%, 33%, and 60% in patients treated with a plug, fibrin glue, seton placement, and advancement flaps, respectively. Thus, patients treated with an anal plug or advancement flap had equivalent results. Many of the plug failures were related to extrusion, which has been reported frequently. The authors discuss sewing a button to the internal portion of the plug as a method to curtail extrusion. This article addresses the troublesome and often persistent problem of difficult-to-heal anal fistula. Healing of treated anal fistulas is a slow process that is highlighted by noting that the 12-week follow-up is insufficient to determine long-term healing. Furthermore, only 60% of patients, at best, had healed anal fistulas at this time point. These 2 simple notations reflect the magnitude of this nuisance problem. Because of the persistent nature of anal fistula, further investigation with the anal plug and/or advancement flap is warranted and underway in Europe. United States and Canadian centers likewise should construct trials that examine the treatment options for anal fistula. The discomfort, drainage, and valuable patient time lost dealing with an anal fistula mandate that we investigate alternative treatments that result in more rapid and complete healing.

K. E. Behrns, MD

Bariatric Surgery Outcomes at Designated Centers of Excellence vs Nondesignated Programs

Livingston EH (Univ of Texas Southwestern School of Medicine, Dallas)

Arch Surg 144:319-325, 2009

Objective.—To compare outcomes of patients undergoing bariatric procedures in hospitals designated as centers of excellence compared with nondesignated hospitals.

Design.—The 2005 National Inpatient Survey was used to compare outcomes at designated vs nondesignated hospitals. In addition to conventional null-hypothesis statistical testing to assess differences, effect sizes were calculated to estimate the clinical significance for observed differences.

Results.—Centers of excellence performed substantially more operations than nondesignated centers. Despite this, outcomes were equivalent at centers of excellence and hospitals without this designation. Volume-outcome modeling attempting to identify the optimal number for a minimum volume threshold for bariatric operations revealed that annual procedure volume has a weak effect on outcomes. Similarly, many variables that were statistically significantly different between centers and non-centers proved to be clinically unimportant by effect size analysis. Risk adjustment was effectively achieved by using the Agency for Healthcare Research and Quality–supplied variables all-payer severity-adjusted diagnostic related group expected charges and deaths.

Conclusions.—Designation as a bariatric surgery center of excellence does not ensure better outcomes. Neither does high annual procedure volume. Extra expenses associated with center of excellence designation may not be warranted.

▶ This article by Livingston addresses the important and burgeoning topic of the use of databases and centers of excellence designation as a model for programmatic quality improvement. Bariatric surgery outcomes from programs designated as centers of excellence by the American College of Surgeons or the American Society for Metabolic and Bariatric Surgery were retrieved from the National Inpatient Survey (NIS) database and compared with nondesignated program results. This comparison demonstrated that centers of excellence did more bariatric surgery; however, the outcomes were equivalent between the centers. Complex statistical modeling showed that annual operative volume has a weak effect on outcomes. Thus, high volume and a designation as a center of excellence do not ensure a better outcome. This raises the question of whether center of excellence designation and the mandated complex system improvements provide the value in truly enhancing patient outcome. The accompanying invited critique is enlightening and stresses many important points. However, in addition to these instructive comments, we must recognize that by its very patient population bariatric surgery programs of any size require a systematic approach. Therefore, differences between centers of excellence and nondesignated centers may be small because most nondesignated programs that report data to the NIS, in fact, have a system in place to monitor bariatric processes and outcomes, although the outcomes may not be the traditional outcomes reported in these databases. Hence, when examining outcomes of a procedure, we need to examine not only volume and outcome relationships but also the underlying systems in play that permit excellent outcomes. Improving surgical care will require an integrated systems approach that addresses the variations in complex surgical practices.

K. E. Behrns, MD

Bowel Obstruction Following Appendectomy: What is the True Incidence?

Leung TTW, Dixon E, Gill M, et al (Univ of Calgary, Alberta, Canada)

Ann Surg 250:51-53, 2009

Introduction.—Appendicitis is a common problem that is typically treated with an appendectomy. Following abdominal surgery, adhesions may form and may cause a subsequent small bowel obstruction (SBO). The purpose of our study was to determine the rate of post-appendectomy SBO in an adult population, and to observe any difference in SBO rates between open versus laparoscopic appendectomies.

Methods.—All patients who underwent an appendectomy at an adult hospital in the Calgary Health Region between 1999 and 2002 were identified by using the administrative discharge database. Pathology and operative technique (laparoscopic, McBurney incision, midline laparotomy) were reviewed. Using those regional health numbers, any further admissions with a diagnostic code for bowel obstruction were identified. Medical charts (n = 1777) were reviewed to confirm the rate of post-appendectomy SBO. A logistic regression was performed to identify risk factors of post-appendectomy SBO and expressed as odds ratios (95% confidence interval).

Results.—The overall SBO rate was 2.8% over an average 4.1-year follow-up period. The risk factors for developing SBO following appendectomy for appendicitis included perforated appendicitis (odds ratio [OR] = 3.1, 95% confidence interval [CI]: 1.5–6.6), and midline incisions (OR = 5.4, 95% CI: 2.8–10.4). Those with pathology of cancer or chronic appendicitis conferred the greatest overall risk of SBO (OR = 7.4, 95% CI: 2.7–20.3).

Conclusions.—The rate of SBO following appendectomy in adults was 2.8%, or 0.0069 cases per person-year. The greatest risk factors for developing SBO were midline incision and nonappendicitis pathology. There is no statistically significant difference in SBO rates following laparoscopic appendectomy compared with open approaches.

▶ Leung et al answered the question, what is the true incidence of bowel obstruction following appendectomy? After reviewing 1777 medical charts the authors found that 2.8% of patients developed a bowel obstruction following appendectomy. Patients most likely to develop a small bowel obstruction include those that had a midline celiotomy approach and a pathologic diagnosis of cancer or fibrosis. Interestingly, a laparoscopic appendectomy did not confer a decreased risk of small bowel obstruction. A normal appendix or perforated appendix resulted in increased risk of bowel obstruction compared with suppurative appendicitis. Notably, only 20 patients required an operation for bowel obstruction. Furthermore, it is likely that most patients who develop a bowel obstruction can be treated with nonoperative therapy. The findings presented here suggest that a midline incision should not be performed for appendicitis and that the laparoscopic approach, although not associated with a decreased incidence of bowel obstruction, is not associated with an increased risk and offers the advantage of a low likelihood of abdominal wall herniation. In summary, the topic of bowel obstruction following appendectomy appears to have received more attention than there are operative cases for obstruction. Although we need to consider bowel obstruction in the differential diagnosis of abdominal pain after appendectomy, it is uncommon and rarely requires operative therapy.

K. E. Behrns, MD

Branch duct intraductal papillary mucinous neoplasms in a retrospective series of 190 patients

Woo SM, Ryu JK, Lee SH, et al (Seoul Natl Univ College of Medicine, Yeongeon-dong, Jongno-gu, Korea)
Br J Surg 96:405-411, 2009

Background.—A consensus conference has recommended close observation of branch duct intraductal papillary mucinous neoplasms (BD-IPMNs) smaller than 30 mm, without symptoms or mural nodules. This study investigated whether these recommendations could be validated in a single-centre experience of BD-IPMNs.

Methods.—Some 190 patients with radiological imaging or histological findings consistent with BD-IPMN were enrolled between 1998 and 2005. Those with less than 6 months' follow-up and no histological confirmation were excluded.

Results.—BD-IPMN was diagnosed by computed tomography and pancreatography in 105 patients and pathologically in 85. Eighteen patients had adenoma, 53 borderline malignancy, five carcinoma *in situ* and nine invasive carcinoma. Findings associated with malignancy were the presence of radiologically suspicious features ($P < 0 \cdot 001$) and a cyst size of at least 30 mm ($P = 0 \cdot 001$). Had consensus guidelines been applied, 54 patients would have undergone pancreatic resection, whereas only 28 of these patients actually had a resection; 12 of the latter patients had a malignancy compared with none of the 26 patients who were treated conservatively.

Conclusion.—A simple increase in cyst size is not a reliable predictor of malignancy. Observation is recommended for patients with a BD-IPMN smaller than 30 mm showing no suspicious features on imaging.

▶ Woo et al reviewed a single-center experience with the management of 190 patients with branch duct intraductal papillary mucinous neoplasm (BD-IPMN) of the pancreas. The characteristics of malignant or premalignant BD-IPMN that warrant resection have been elusive. Cyst size has been the most widely used characteristic, but recent evidence shows that size alone does not accurately predict malignant transformation. The presence of mural nodules and a thickened cyst wall are important to note, and, in this study, predictive of malignancy. Heretofore, resection was performed primarily for BD-IPMN lesions that reached 2.5 to 3.0 cm; however, of those patients who had surgery with an established pathologic diagnosis, this study shows that the likelihood of malignancy is nearly 4% in lesions less than 3 cm without suspicious imaging features, 20% for lesions greater than 3 cm without suspicious findings, 38% for lesions less than 3 cm with suspicious features, and 100% for lesions greater than 3 cm with suspicious features. Thus, identification of suspicious cyst features may be critical. Importantly, though not discussed in detail in this article, this may lead to a change in the diagnostic evaluation of these cysts. Even though morphologic cyst characteristics can be identified on typical cross-sectional imaging, endoscopic ultrasonography (EUS) typically provides enhanced analysis of morphologic changes. Because cysts are routinely followed on a 3- to 6-month basis, this raises the question of the need for surveillance EUS. Indeed, this would be an invasive and costly proposition, and, therefore, careful additional studies are needed to determine the optimal balance of surveillance versus resection in this curable premalignant cyst.

K. E. Behrns, MD

Caspofungin for prevention of intra-abdominal candidiasis in high-risk surgical patients

Senn L, Eggimann P, Ksontini R, et al (Univ of Lausanne (UNIL), Switzerland)
Intensive Care Med 35:903-908, 2009

Purpose.—Thirty to forty percent of patients with recurrent gastrointestinal perforation/anastomotic leakage or acute necrotizing pancreatitis develop intra-abdominal invasive candidiasis (IC). A corrected *Candida* colonization index (CCI) $\geq$0.4 is a powerful predictor of IC. Fluconazole prevents intra-abdominal IC in this setting, but azole-resistant *Candida* species are emerging. The aim of this study was to explore the efficacy and safety of caspofungin for prevention of intra-abdominal IC in high-risk surgical patients.

Methods.—Prospective non-comparative single-center study in consecutive adult surgical patients with recurrent gastrointestinal perforation/anastomotic leakage or acute necrotizing pancreatitis. Preventive caspofungin therapy (70 mg, then 50 mg/day) was given until resolution of the surgical condition. *Candida* colonization index and CCI, occurrence of intra-abdominal IC and adverse events were monitored.

Results.—Nineteen patients were studied: 16 (84%) had recurrent gastrointestinal perforation/anastomotic leakage and 3 (16%) acute necrotizing pancreatitis. The median duration of preventive caspofungin therapy was 16 days (range 4–46). The colonization index decreased significantly during study therapy, and the CCI remained <0.4 in all patients. Caspofungin was successful for prevention of intra-abdominal IC in 18/19 patients (95%, 1 breakthrough IC 5 days after inclusion). No drug-related adverse event requiring caspofungin discontinuation occurred.

Conclusion.—Caspofungin may be efficacious and safe for prevention of intra-abdominal candidiasis in high-risk surgical patients. This needs to be further investigated in randomized trials.

▶ Advances in critical care medicine have translated to improved survival for many surgical patients. However, the improved survival may be offset by increased complications, including resistant infections. Notably, fungal infections are seen with increasing frequency and complicate the care of patients with intra-abdominal perforations. This study by Senn et al examines the use of caspofungin in a select group of patients—those with intra-abdominal perforations and high likelihood invasive candidiasis (IC). Although fluconazole is an effective agent against IC, resistant strains are emerging with increasing frequency. This is a relatively small study of 19 patients at high risk for the development of IC infection who were treated with caspofungin with excellent results, ie, only 1 patient developed IC. While the results of this industry-sponsored study are quite intriguing, the study design raises many questions. First, the population consists of patients with recurrent gastrointestinal perforation—what are the recurrences? Few patients survive recurrent intestinal perforation, yet the overall survival in this group was 74%. Second, why did the trial not include an arm in which fluconazole was administered? The results may have been similar. Are we to assume that all patients had resistant candidiasis? Finally, in a clinical study in which the endpoint is prevention of infection, 19 patients are too few to draw conclusions. Even though the authors suggest that the data are compelling and that a randomized trial should be performed, the study design limits the conclusions and, therefore, these results should be carefully interpreted before widespread use in patients with invasive fungal infections, and perhaps even before performing an expensive randomized trial.

K. E. Behrns, MD

Combined endoscopic and percutaneous drainage of organized pancreatic necrosis

Ross A, Gluck M, Irani S, et al (Virginia Mason Med Ctr, Seattle, WA)
Gastrointest Endosc 71:79-84, 2010

Background.—Severe acute pancreatitis is often complicated by organized necrosis, which can lead to abscess formation and clinical deterioration. We sought to devise a combined endoscopic and percutaneous approach to drainage of organized pancreatic necrosis, with the primary goal of preventing the formation of chronic pancreaticocutaneous fistulae, and secondary goals of avoiding the need for surgical necrosectomy and reducing endoscopic resource utilization.

Design.—Retrospective review of an institutional review board–approved database.

Setting.—Single North American tertiary referral center.

Patients.—Patients with severe acute pancreatitis complicated by organized necrosis requiring drainage.

Interventions.—CT-guided percutaneous drain, followed immediately by endoscopic transenteric drainage.

Main Outcome Measurements.—Development of chronic pancreaticocutaneous fistulae, number of endoscopic procedures requiring follow-up drainage, need for surgical necrosectomy, procedure-related morbidity, and mortality.

Results.—Fifteen patients (12 males, 3 females; mean age, 58 years) underwent combined modality drainage. All procedures were technically successful. Immediate complications included fever and hypotension ($n = 2$); late complications included parenchymal infection after drain removal ($n = 1$). Twenty-five total endoscopies (4 for drain manipulation) were performed in the cohort subsequent to the initial drainage. After a median duration of follow-up of 189 days, percutaneous drains were removed in all 13 patients in whom this was attempted; no patients had development of chronic pancreaticocutaneous fistulae. There were no deaths, and no patients required surgery.

Limitations.—Highly selected patient population, lack of comparison group, single-center experience.

Conclusions.—In some highly selected patients with infected or symptomatic organized pancreatic necrosis, combined modality drainage results in favorable clinical outcomes with low associated, procedure-related morbidity. Pancreaticocutaneous fistulae and surgical necrosectomy were avoided with minimal endoscopic resource utilization.

▶ The management of severe necrotizing pancreatitis requires multidisciplinary treatment approaches that are challenging to even the most experienced pancreatic experts, regardless of their discipline. Ross et al describe the multimodal approach using endoscopic and percutaneous drainage techniques in the treatment of organized pancreatic necrosis. Fifteen highly selected patients were treated using this approach, and no patients required surgery or had a pancreatic fistula at 189 days (median) of follow-up. These early results are very encouraging, but the resources required for this approach were intensive and, on average, included 15.5 days of hospitalization, 8 CT scans, 5 percutaneous drain manipulations, and 80 days of drainage. Furthermore, 8 of the 15 patients had the disconnected pancreatic duct syndrome when pancreatography was performed. Obviously, experience in choosing the appropriate patient for this management approach is critical. The necrosis must be well demarcated, and the approach must be appropriately timed in the course of the disease. Furthermore, how many patients are candidates for this approach? What criteria should be used to determine the appropriate patients? Finally, what is the long-term outcome of patients who have the disconnected pancreatic duct syndrome that is characterized by the late (7 months) presentation of a pancreatic pseudocyst? The authors suggest that stent placement via the gastrointestinal tract into the collection will result in a long-term fistula from the pancreas to the bowel, but, historically, even surgically created anastomoses to a pseudocyst have low long-term patency that is dependent on epithelial-to-epithelial apposition. Thus, although these results are encouraging, long-term follow-up is encouraged to determine the potentially important consequences of the treatment approach and the natural history of the disconnected pancreatic duct.

K. E. Behrns, MD

Early Endoscopic Retrograde Cholangiopancreatography in Predicted Severe Acute Biliary Pancreatitis: A Prospective Multicenter Study

van Santvoort HC, the members of the Dutch Acute Pancreatitis Study Group (Univ Med Ctr Utrecht, The Netherlands; et al)

Ann Surg 250:68-75, 2009

Summary Background Data.—The role of early endoscopic retrograde cholangiopancreatography (ERCP) in acute biliary pancreatitis (ABP) remains controversial. Previous studies have included only a relatively small number of patients with predicted severe ABP. We investigated the clinical effects of early ERCP in these patients.

Methods.—We performed a prospective, observational multicenter study in 8 university medical centers and 7 major teaching hospitals. One hundred fifty-three patients with predicted severe ABP without cholangitis enrolled in a randomized multicenter trial on probiotic prophylaxis in acute pancreatitis were prospectively followed. Conservative treatment or ERCP within 72 hours after symptom onset (at discretion of the treating physician) were compared for complications and mortality. Patients without and with cholestasis (bilirubin: >2.3 mg/dL [40 μmol/L] and/or dilated common bile duct) were analyzed separately.

Results.—Of the 153 patients, 81 (53%) underwent ERCP and 72 (47%) conservative treatment. Groups were highly comparable at baseline. Seventy-eight patients (51%) had cholestasis. In patients with cholestasis, ERCP (52/78 patients: 67%), as compared with conservative treatment, was associated with fewer complications (25% vs. 54%,

$P = 0.020$, multivariate adjusted odds ratio [OR]: 0.35, 95% confidence interval [CI]: 0.13–0.99, $P = 0.049$). This included fewer patients with >30% pancreatic necrosis (8% vs. 31%, $P = 0.010$). Mortality was nonsignificantly lower after ERCP (6% vs. 15%, $P = 0.213$, multivariate adjusted OR: 0.44, 95% CI: 0.08–2.28, $P = 0.330$). In patients without cholestasis, ERCP (29/75 patients: 39%) was not associated with reduced complications (45% vs. 41%, $P = 0.814$, multivariate adjusted OR: 1.36; 95% CI: 0.49–3.76; $P = 0.554$) or mortality (14% vs. 17%, $P = 0.754$, multivariate adjusted OR: 0.78; 95% CI: 0.19–3.12, $P = 0.734$).

Conclusions.—Early ERCP is associated with fewer complications in predicted severe ABP if cholestasis is present.

▶ This prospective, nonrandomized trial addresses yet again the use of early endoscopic retrograde cholangiopancreatography (ERCP) in patients with gallstone-induced pancreatitis. No fewer than 4 randomized trials have been published examining whether patients with acute biliary pancreatitis should have an early (< 72 hours) ERCP. Collectively, the studies have suggested that ERCP should be performed in patients with predicted severe pancreatitis and in those in whom cholestasis, but not cholangitis, is present. This study by van Santvoort et al essentially confirms this finding. They noted that complications were reduced in patients who underwent early ERCP in the face of cholestasis. Seemingly, no further studies on this topic are required because the findings of several studies are in agreement. However, the difficult clinical question is what defines cholestasis? These authors had excellent rigorous criteria that nicely categorized the patients with cholestasis, but in several previous trials gallstones were not present in up to 40% of the patients. Wide adoption of strict criteria for cholestasis will ensure that appropriate patients are selected for ERCP. Another conundrum is present in this study because although ERCP was beneficial in patients with cholestasis, presumably because of extracted stone material, there was no difference in the presence of stone material in the common bile duct in those patients with or without cholestasis. This raises the possibility that some patients without cholestasis will have common bile duct stones and potentially have aggravated pancreatitis. How should these patients be identified? Magnetic resonance cholangiopancreatography may be useful in these patients. All told, the multiple studies examining ERCP in gallstone pancreatitis are providing incremental knowledge and refining our research question.

K. E. Behrns, MD

Endoscopic and Surgical Treatment of Mucosal (T1a) Esophageal Adenocarcinoma in Barrett's Esophagus

Prasad GA, Wu TT, Wigle DA, et al (Mayo Clinic College of Medicine, Rochester, MN)

Gastroenterology 137:815-823, 2009

Background & Aims.—Endoscopic therapy is emerging as an alternative to surgical therapy in patients with mucosal (T1a) esophageal adenocarcinoma (EAC) given the low likelihood of lymph node metastases. Long-term outcomes of patients treated endoscopically and surgically for mucosal EAC are unknown. We compared long-term outcomes of patients with mucosal EAC treated endoscopically and surgically.

Methods.—Patients treated for mucosal EAC between 1998 and 2007 were included. Patients were divided into an endoscopically treated group (ENDO group) and a surgically treated group (SURG group). Vital status information was queried using an institutionally approved internet research and location service. Statistical analysis was performed using Kaplan–Meier curves and Cox proportional hazard ratios.

Results.—A total of 178 patients were included, of whom 132 (74%) were in the ENDO group and 46 (26%) were in the SURG group. The mean follow-up period was 64 months (standard error of the mean, 4.8 mo) in the SURG group and 43 months (standard error of the mean, 2.8 mo) in the ENDO group. Cumulative mortality in the ENDO group (17%) was comparable with the SURG group (20%) ($P = .75$). Overall survival also was comparable using the Kaplan–Meier method. Treatment modality was not a significant predictor of survival on multivariable analysis. Recurrent carcinoma was detected in 12% of patients in the ENDO group, all successfully re-treated without impact on overall survival.

Conclusions.—Overall survival in patients with mucosal EAC when treated endoscopically appears to be comparable with that of patients treated surgically. Recurrent carcinoma occurs in a limited proportion of patients, but can be managed endoscopically.

▶ Recent advances in the endoscopic treatment of mucosal esophageal adenocarcinoma provide reasonable alternatives to esophagectomy for these patients. This study by Prasad et al retrospectively reviews the Mayo Clinic experience treating patients with T1a esophageal adenocarcinoma. Because of the retrospective nature of this investigation, the authors appropriately recognize several potential biases that may be introduced into the study, and they conclude that endoscopic therapy is a viable alternative to esophagectomy for patients with these cancers. Although it is likely an alternative to esophagectomy, any notion of equivalence should be dismissed. This study was not designed to test equivalence, and the patients in both the endoscopic group and surgery group were highly selected. Furthermore, some of the variables that likely determined selection were not discussed—what was the size of the cancer in the surgery group? Moreover, the surgery group had an open esophagectomy, which should not be the standard for esophagectomy for T1a lesions—these patients should have a laparoscopic esophagectomy. Most importantly, endoscopic therapy does not address the underlying Barrett's mucosa that remains and, thus, provides an environment for a high rate of recurrence. Although the recurrence rate in this study is noted to be 12% and amenable to repeat endoscopic therapy, surgery is curative. Should we not be trying to cure all the patients who are surgical candidates? Finally, limited data exist regarding long-term follow-up patients with recurrent disease. How often do they have endoscopic surveillance, and how many treatments are required? Endoscopic therapy is a viable alternative to esophagectomy, but selection criteria are of paramount importance, and the tendency to relax strict treatment criteria over time may permit the costly recurrence of esophageal cancer that could have been cured.

K. E. Behrns, MD

Esophagectomy Compared With Chemoradiation for Early Stage Esophageal Cancer in the Elderly

Abrams JA, Buono DL, Strauss J, et al (Columbia Univ College of Physicians and Surgeons, NY; Columbia Univ, NY; Albert Einstein College of Medicine, NY)

Cancer 115:4924-4933, 2009

Background.—Esophagectomy has been the traditional treatment of choice for early stage esophageal cancer. However, esophagectomy is associated with high mortality and morbidity in the elderly, and these patients often receive chemoradiation instead. The authors of this report compared outcomes of esophagectomy versus chemoradiation in a population-based sample of elderly patients with early stage esophageal cancer.

Methods.—The Surveillance, Epidemiology, and End Results Medicare database was used to identify patients aged ≥65 years who were diagnosed with stage I or II esophageal cancer from 1991 to 2002. The associations of treatment with esophagectomy or chemoradiation were assessed along with demographic and clinical variables. A survival analysis was performed to compare outcomes with treatment modality and was adjusted for potential confounders.

Results.—Seven hundred thirty patients with stage I or II esophageal cancer were identified who underwent esophagectomy (n = 341; 46.7%) or chemoradiation (n = 389; 53.3%). Older age, squamous cell histology, and lower socioeconomic status were associated with increased odds of receiving chemoradiation. In multivariate analyses, chemoradiation was associated with worse disease-specific survival (hazard ratio [HR], 2.08; 95% confidence interval [CI], 1.64-2.64) and overall survival (HR, 1.92; 95%CI, 1.58-2.34). The receipt of chemoradiation was associated with worse survival for patients with adenocarcinoma (HR, 3.01; 95%CI, 2.24-4.04), but there was no significant difference for patients with squamous cell carcinoma (HR, 1.33; 95%CI, 0.98-1.80).

Conclusions.—Compared with chemoradiation, esophagectomy may be associated with improved survival for early stage esophageal cancer in the elderly. The current results suggest that there also may be a subset of patients with squamous cell carcinoma for whom chemoradiation is adequate therapy. A randomized trial would be useful to determine the optimal treatment for elderly patients with early stage esophageal cancer.

► Esophageal resection for stage I and II disease is the preferred method of treatment of this highly lethal malignancy, but recent studies have shown that some elderly patients may be treated by chemoradiation therapy alone. The article by Abrams et al cautions that nonoperative treatment may lead to decreased survival compared with treatment, including esophagectomy. The authors used the Surveillance, Epidemiology, and End Results (SEER) database to determine outcomes of elderly patients who were treated for either squamous cell carcinoma or adenocarcinoma of the esophagus. The data are convincing in suggesting that incorporation of esophagectomy into a treatment plan leads to improved outcomes. However, we must be careful of the interpretation of these data because they are derived from a large database that does not easily permit assessment of comorbidities, and thus, selection bias in the treatment groups is highly likely. Nonetheless, as surgeons it is our responsibility to decrease mortality and morbidity associated with complex operations like esophagectomy. The relatively recent employment of laparoscopic and/or thoracoscopic esophagectomy has led to major improvements in pulmonary-related complications following esophageal resection. In addition, high-volume centers that perform esophagectomies and have a systematic approach to the care of these patients also tend to have improved outcomes. Collectively, these findings suggest that we need to train surgeons in minimally invasive approaches for these complex upper gastrointestinal cancers, and that the care of these patients should be in centers with a well-organized multidisciplinary approach.

K. E. Behrns, MD

Fast-track surgery after laparoscopic colorectal surgery: Is it feasible in a general surgery unit?

Scatizzi M, Kröning KC, Boddi V, et al (Misericordia e Dolce Hosp, Prato, Florence; Univ of Florence, Prato; et al)

Surgery 147:219-226, 2010

Background.—The aim of the "fast-track surgery" program is to decrease the peri-operative stress response to surgical trauma and thus to a decrease in complication rates after elective surgery. Critics of fast-track (FT) rehabilitation may argue that all reports of successful programs came from major specialized hospital units and that implementation in smaller or less specialized units may be difficult if not impossible.

Methods.—We retrospectively studied 101 patients who, from November 2004 to October 2007, underwent laparoscopic colorectal surgery in our institute. A detailed FT surgery protocol had been prepared and given to patients, physicians and nurses, with the aim to create a standard treatment. Data about demographics, ASA score, pre-operative complicating diseases, diagnosis, type of surgery, and postoperative clinical data were analyzed. Univariate analysis of the relationship between all factors (patient characteristics, intervention characteristics, protocol compliance and presence of complications) described here and length of hospital stay was performed.

Results.—We compared our results to published major trials and observed no substantial differences in morbidity, mortality and length of postoperative hospital stay between the 2. Univariate analysis showed that compliance to the elements of the FT protocol influences the length of postoperative period more significantly than patient characteristics or surgical procedure.

Conclusion.—Based on 6 comparative single-center studies, the FT program was found to reduce length of hospital stay, and was deemed safe for major abdominal surgeries. Present study shows that enhanced recovery or FT program can also be implemented safely in a general surgery unit.

▶ The introduction of laparoscopic surgery has encouraged many providers and groups to assess the hospital length of stay following abdominal surgery, be it open or laparoscopic surgery. One of the products of these investigations has been the evidence-based clinical pathway that outlines a typical patient's preoperative and postoperative course. Scatizzi et al present essentially an evidence-based clinical pathway or a fast-track surgery following laparoscopic colorectal surgery in a general surgery unit. Heretofore, many providers have been skeptical of the ability to accomplish an evidenced-based pathway in the setting of a general surgical unit. This study nicely demonstrates that a well-outlined protocol that is instituted with sound education to the clinical providers and nursing staff can reduce the length of stay and be associated with good outcomes. The authors show that hospital length of stay was 4.7 days with zero mortality and 12% morbidity for 101 patients. The readmission rate, however, was nearly 22%. These results compare favorably with 6 other series that the article highlights. This study is important because of the focus on standardization of care that is aimed at reducing the variability and thereby improving the quality of care. This is a topic of considerable interest in quality improvement circles, and, if accomplished properly, not only should care be improved but also costs should be reduced. With the prospect of bundled payments for patient care, standardization of procedures as well as preoperative and postoperative care should result in improved value (better outcomes with less cost) for surgical care.

K. E. Behrns, MD

Flat Adenomas of the Large Bowel: A Single Endoscopist Study

Gorgun E, Church J (Digestive Diseases Inst, Cleveland, OH)

Dis Colon Rectum 52:972-977, 2009

Purpose.—Flat colorectal adenomas may not be recognized or they may be seen and dismissed as normal mucosa. As a result, the "true" incidence of flat lesions is unknown. The aim of this study was to report the incidence and character of flat adenomas in a large series of patients in the United States.

Methods.—Details of colorectal polyps seen during colonoscopy are entered into a prospective database that was queried for flat adenomas. No magnification or dye spray was used. The colonoscopy completion rate was 96.8 percent. The flat adenoma detection rate of the senior author is in line with that of Japanese colonoscopists.

Results.—During 2,659 colonoscopies, 5,749 colorectal lesions were seen in 2,003 patients. Of these patients, 1,125 were men and 878 were women, with a mean age of 65 years (± 12 years). There were 3,115 adenomas (54 percent of lesions); 315 were flat (10.1 percent), 23 (0.8 percent) were depressed, 2,575 were sessile (82.7 percent), and 200 were pedunculated (6.4 percent). Two hundred twelve patients had flat adenomas (10.6 percent of patients); 172 patients had one and 40 had multiple (2 to 8) flat adenomas. Eight patients with flat adenomas had more flat adenomas on follow-up.

Conclusions.—Colonoscopists in the United States must be aware of the existence of flat adenomas and sensitive to their appearance.

▶ Colorectal polyps are common, and detection of these lesions has become a recent quality marker for colonoscopists. It appears, however, that the benchmarks for polyp detection have not been well described, and variability between the West and Japan exists. Furthermore, the morphologically described "flat adenomas" have received particular attention because they are difficult to identify, and missed lesions may be associated with the development of interval (between colonoscopies) cancer. Gorgun and Church addressed this important topic and demonstrated the results of an experienced senior colonoscopist. It would appear that like a Meckel's diverticulum, the "rule of tens" applies to flat adenomas. About 10% of patients harbor these lesions, and 10% of all adenomas will be flat. Most of these lesions are located proximal to the splenic flexure. Importantly, this study shows that, albeit in a small number of patients, the risk of severe dysplasia when corrected for size is increased in relatively small (6-10 mm) flat adenomas. This study shows superior results largely because of what we know with other procedures like esophagectomy and pancreatectomy—clinicians with substantial experience and expertise have superior results. However, experience is gained over time and, thus, new techniques or a change in the interval for colonscopy may be necessary to properly survey high-risk patients. Chromoendoscopy offers the promise of a new technique that may assist in the diagnosis of flat adenomas. Furthermore, a longitudinal multicenter study with a large number of patients with flat adenomas may assist with defining the interval of colonoscopy and the risk of cancer. This study highlights the importance of quality benchmarks, the experience of a senior investigator, and the benefits of a longitudinal database in which all patients are entered.

K. E. Behrns, MD

Fundamentals of Laparoscopic Surgery simulator training to proficiency improves laparoscopic performance in the operating room—a randomized controlled trial

Sroka G, Feldman LS, Vassiliou MC, et al (McGill Univ, Montreal, Canada)
Am J Surg 199:115-120, 2010

Background.—The purpose of this study was to assess whether training to proficiency with the Fundamentals of Laparoscopic Surgery (FLS) simulator would result in improved performance in the operating room (OR).

Methods.—Nineteen junior residents underwent baseline FLS testing and were assessed in the OR using a validated global rating scale (GOALS) during elective laparoscopic cholecystectomy. Those with GOALS scores ≤15 were randomly assigned to training (n = 9) or control (n = 8) groups. An FLS proficiency-based curriculum was used in the training group. Scoring on FLS and in the OR was repeated after the study period. Evaluators were blinded to randomization status.

Results.—Sixteen residents completed the study. There were no differences in baseline simulator (49.1 ± 17 vs 39.5 ± 16, $P = .27$) or OR scores (11.3 ± 2.0 vs 12.0 ± 1.8; $P = .47$). After training, simulator scores were higher in the trained group (95.1 ± 4 vs 60.5 ± 23, $P = .004$). OR performance improved in the control group by 1.8 to 13.8 ± 2.2 ($P = .04$), whereas the trained group improved by 6.1 to 17.4 ± 1.9 ($P = .0005$ vs control; $P < .0001$ vs baseline).

Conclusions.—This study clearly demonstrates the educational value of FLS simulator training in surgical residency curricula.

▶ Several competing forces are interacting on surgical resident training: duty hour restrictions, more stringent supervision by the teaching surgeon versus the need for trainee autonomy, a desire for an enhanced skill set on entry into the operating room, ethical considerations for the patient, and the introduction of new knowledge, technologies, and perhaps, competencies all challenge trainees and teachers alike. Resolution of these challenges will require an integrated, thoughtful effort by multiple constituencies. One component of this effort is the introduction of simulation training as a surrogate for operative experience. Sroka et al showed that a well-defined and supervised program of simulator training can improve the intraoperative performance of less-experienced trainees using the standardized Fundamentals of Laparoscopic Surgery (FLS) training program. They showed that with a relatively small time investment (7.5 hours), the intraoperative performance of surgical residents trained via FLS improved markedly. This is an important finding because many simulator skills can readily be learned by trainees, but often the transference to the operating room is nil, and the enthusiasm for such training sessions is diminished. Obviously, these results suggest that a structured program that incorporates these training sessions is a must. Although we must include these educational sessions that teach technical competence, we must also establish a culture whereby surgical trainees spend their "free time" practicing technical skills. This expectation could be established at the outset of their training by conducting a "boot camp" that includes skills assessment and evaluation. The technical skills of surgery are as important as the cognitive skills, and only practice and repetition by the trainees will make them more skilled surgeons.

K. E. Behrns, MD

Identification of Specific Quality Improvement Opportunities for the Elderly Undergoing Gastrointestinal Surgery

Bentrem DJ, Cohen ME, Hynes DM, et al (Northwestern Univ; Univ of Illinois at Chicago)

Arch Surg 144:1013-1020, 2009

Hypothesis.—Specific complications occur more frequently in elderly patients undergoing major gastrointestinal (GI) tract operations that may represent opportunities for quality improvement.

Design.—Retrospective cohort study.

Setting.—One hundred twenty-one hospitals participating in American College of Surgeons National Surgical Quality Improvement Program (ACS-NSQIP).

Patients.—Using the ACS-NSQIP participant use file (2005-2006), patients undergoing upper gastrointestinal tract (n = 4115), hepatobiliary or pancreatic (n = 3364), and colorectal (n = 17 268) operations at 121 hospitals were examined.

Main Outcome Measures.—Risk-adjusted 30-day outcomes were assessed using regression modeling adjusting for patient characteristics, comorbidities, and surgical procedures. The elderly were defined as those older than 75 years.

Results.—Between January 1, 2005, and December 31, 2006, a total of 54 747 patients who underwent major GI tract operations were identified from the ACSNSQIP data file. In the elderly, overall perioperative morbidity was 1.2 to 2 times higher and mortality was 2.9 to 6.7 times higher than in younger patients after adjusting for differences in preoperative comorbidities. Irrespective of procedure type, the elderly were significantly more likely to experience cardiac (acute myocardial infarction and cardiac arrest), pulmonary (pneumonia, pulmonary embolism, and respiratory failure), and urologic (urinary tract infection and renal failure) complications. However, surgical site infections, postoperative bleeding events, deep venous thromboses, and rates of return to the operating room did not differ significantly by age.

Conclusions.—Morbidity and mortality are markedly higher in older patients. Quality measures for the elderly currently address only myocardial infarction, surgical site infection, and deep venous thrombosis. If care for the elderly is to be improved, quality improvement initiatives need to be expanded to include postoperative pulmonary and renal complications.

▶ Bentrem et al address the important topic of performing major abdominal surgery in elderly patients. Many studies have demonstrated institution-specific results demonstrating the safety of major abdominal operations in the elderly. Often, these institutions are highly specialized in the treatment of a medical condition and the surgical results exceed the norm. This article uses the American College of Surgeons National Surgical Quality Improvement Program (ACS-NSQIP) data to examine outcomes after upper gastrointestinal surgery, hepatobiliary or pancreatic surgery, and colorectal surgery. Examination of the data is focused on patients greater than 75 years of age, the definition of elderly in this study. The data convincingly demonstrate that the elderly have a morbidity rate that is 1.2 to 2 times higher and mortality rate that is 2.9 to 6.7 times higher than younger patients. The organ systems associated with these outcomes are cardiopulmonary and renal. Our current national outcome measures are focused on cardiac, wound, and venous thrombosis, but pulmonary and renal complications are not regularly measured parameters. This study highlights the need to more broadly examine the outcomes in the elderly population because this will be an increasing surgical patient population. In addition, outcome parameters that are specific for these patients should be measured. More importantly, we should develop systems and clinical care pathways that attempt to decrease the known risks in this patient population. For example, perhaps these patients should have an indwelling urinary catheter for only a short period of time and then, if needed, intermittent urinary catheterization should be used to decrease the risk of urinary tract infection. As a surgical community, we must become more proactive in the treatment of elderly patients because this is clearly a unique group of patients with different outcomes and specific needs.

K. E. Behrns, MD

Improvement in Glucose Metabolism After Bariatric Surgery: Comparison of Laparoscopic Roux-en-Y Gastric Bypass and Laparoscopic Sleeve Gastrectomy: A Prospective Randomized Trial

Peterli R, Wölnerhanssen B, Peters T, et al (St Claraspital, Basel, Switzerland; Univ Hosp, Basel, Switzerland)

Ann Surg 250:234-241, 2009

Background.—The exclusion of the proximal small intestine is thought to play a major role in the rapid improvement in the metabolic control of diabetes after gastric bypass.

Objective.—In this randomized, prospective, parallel group study, we sought to evaluate and compare the effects of laparoscopic Roux-en-Y gastric bypass (LRYGB) with those of laparoscopic sleeve gastrectomy (LSG) on fasting, and meal-stimulated insulin, glucose, and glucagon-like peptide-1 (GLP-1) levels.

Methods.—Thirteen patients were randomized to LRYGB and 14 patients to LSG. The mostly nondiabetic patients were evaluated before, and 1 week and 3 months after surgery. A standard test meal was given after an overnight fast, and blood samples were collected before and after food intake in both groups for insulin, GLP-1, glucose, PYY, and ghrelin concentrations. This trial was registered in www.clinicaltrials.gov (NCT00356213) before the first patient was randomized.

Results.—Body weight and body mass index decreased markedly ($P < 0.002$) and comparably after either procedure. Excess BMI loss was similar at 3 months (43.3 ± 12.1% vs. 39.4 ± 9.4%, $P > 0.36$). After surgery, patients had markedly increased postprandial plasma insulin and GLP-1 levels, respectively ($P < 0.01$) after both of these urgical procedures, which favor improved glucose homeostasis. Compared with LSG, LRYGB patients had early and augmented insulin responses as early as 1-week postoperative; potentially mediating improved early glycemic control. After 3 months, no significant difference was observed with respect to insulin and GLP-1 secretion between the 2 procedures.

Conclusion.—Both procedures markedly improved glucose homeostasis: insulin, GLP-1, and PYY levels increased similarly after either procedure. Our results do not support the idea that the proximal small intestine mediates the improvement in glucose homeostasis.

▶ Peterli et al conducted a randomized, prospective trial aimed at determining the mechanism(s) of improved glucose homeostasis following bariatric surgery. Obese, primarily nondiabetic patients were randomized to either laparoscopic Roux-en-Y gastric bypass (LRYGB; $N = 13$) or laparoscopic sleeve gastrectomy (LSG; $N = 14$), and parameters of glucose metabolism were studied preoperatively and at 1 week and 3 months postoperatively. The authors hypothesized that a principal component of improved glucose metabolism would include diversion of nutrients from the proximal small bowel; thus, the LRYGB patients would have improved glucose metabolism, whereas the LSG patients would not experience these metabolic benefits. Following bariatric surgery, both groups of patients lost an equivalent amount of excess weight; however, to the authors' surprise, both groups of patients also experienced improved glucose homeostasis before significant weight loss occurred. Therefore, these authors, along with many other investigators, thought the diversion from the small bowel was critical for glucose metabolism. This study does not support that conclusion. This important study essentially waves the white flag about our understanding of the complex mechanisms involved in glucose homeostasis following bariatric surgery. Despite a carefully designed trial (though the target patient population could have been solely diabetic patients) including assessment of multiple hormonal mediators at various time points, the mechanisms underlying gastrointestinal hormone function and glucose control remain somewhat mysterious. Even though large, multicenter trials that examine the effect of bariatric surgery on glucose metabolism are underway, this study provides a cautionary note that broad application of bariatric surgery to treat the complex and poorly understood glucose metabolic pathway may result in disappointing findings and unintended consequences. This study is a call for further investigation of the surgical physiology of bariatric surgery and glucose metabolism before broad surgical application.

K. E. Behrns, MD

Improving the Management of Acute Adhesive Small Bowel Obstruction with CT-Scan and Water-Soluble Contrast Medium: A Prospective Study

Trésallet C, Lebreton N, Royer B, et al (Université Pierre et Marie Curie, Paris, France)

Dis Colon Rectum 52:1869-1876, 2009

Purpose.—Adhesive small bowel obstruction is usually managed nonoperatively, but there is still debate over the optimal duration of nonoperative management and the factors that predict failure of medical treatment. The aim of this study was to evaluate an algorithm using CT-scans and Gastrografin® in the management of small bowel obstruction.

Methods.—In a prospective study, each patient admitted for small bowel obstruction underwent a physical examination, a plain film, and a CT-scan evaluation. Patients underwent emergency surgical exploration when bowel ischemia was suspected. Other patients received oral Gastrografin®, and a second plain abdominal radiograph was done after 12 hours. In patients with clinical improvement, the nasogastric tube was removed and an immediate liquid diet was resumed. Other patients were referred for surgery.

Results.—In total, 118 patients with 123 episodes of small bowel obstruction were included. Thirty-six (29%) required immediate surgery because they presented clinical characteristics of bowel ischemia (36/36; 100%) or a defect in vascularization of the small bowel on CT-scan (5/36; 14%). The 87 remaining patients were managed nonoperatively, of which 28 deteriorated and were referred for surgery. The 59 other patients showed clinical improvement.

Conclusion.—This study demonstrated the diagnostic role of Gastrografin® in discriminating between partial and complete small bowel obstruction. CT-scans were disappointing in their ability to predict the necessity of emergent laparotomies. We therefore recommend the use of Gastrografin® in adhesive small bowel obstruction patients who do not have clinical evidence of bowel ischemia. CT-scans should not be routinely performed in the decision-making process except when clinical history, physical examination, and plain film are not conclusive for small bowel obstruction diagnosis.

▶ The conundrum in the management of small bowel obstruction is the time to surgically intervene to relieve an obstruction that is not associated with obvious signs of bowel compromise but, conversely, is unlikely to resolve without operation. Trésallet et al examined the role of Gastrografin enterography in relieving bowel obstruction or predicting the need for surgical management. The results suggest that the lack of transit of water-soluble contrast into the colon within 12 hours predicts the need for operative relief of an adhesive obstruction. Importantly, the study also shows that CT scan is not reliable in the diagnosis of partial obstruction. Thus, the use of CT demonstrates marked overuse of this imaging modality that does not reliably distinguish between complete obstruction and partial small bowel obstruction. This work represents a reasonable alternative to the "wait-and-see approach" in which patients are hospitalized with a nasogastric tube in place and awaiting the return of bowel function. If bowel function does not resume or patients are unable to eat, then an operation is required; however, this approach necessitates several days in the hospital. Thus, a study that attempts to decrease the length of hospitalization has significant potential, especially when the examination can be performed shortly after patient admission. This study examines an everyday question and provides a practical answer with good results. This is the type of practical clinical research question that should be studied regularly because it results in immediate positive changes in patient care.

K. E. Behrns, MD

In-Hospital Mortality after Pancreatic Resection for Chronic Pancreatitis: Population-Based Estimates from the Nationwide Inpatient Sample

Hill JS, McPhee JT, Whalen GF, et al (Univ of Massachusetts Med School, Worcester; et al)

J Am Coll Surg 209:468-476, 2009

Background.—Pancreatic resection can be performed to ameliorate the sequelae of chronic pancreatitis in selected patients. The perceived risk of pancreatectomy may limit its use. Using a national database, this study compared mortality after pancreatic resections for chronic pancreatitis with those performed for neoplasm.

Study Design.—Patient discharges with chronic pancreatitis or pancreatic neoplasm were queried from the Nationwide Inpatient Sample, 1998 to 2006. To account for the Nationwide Inpatient Sample weighting schema, design-adjusted analyses were used.

Results.—There were 11,048 pancreatic resections. Malignant neoplasms represented 64.2% of the sample; benign neoplasms and pancreatitis comprised 17.1% and 18.7%, respectively. In-hospital mortality rates were 2.2% and 1.7% for the pancreatitis and benign tumor cohorts, respectively, compared with 5.9% for the malignancy cohort (overall $p < 0.01$). A multivariable logistic regression examined differences in mortality among diagnoses while adjusting for patient and hospital characteristics; covariates included patient gender, race, age, comorbidities, type of pancreatectomy, payor, hospital teaching status, hospital size, and hospital volume. After adjustment, patients undergoing resection for pancreatitis were at a significantly lower risk of in-hospital mortality when compared with those with malignant neoplasm (odds ratio, 0.43; 95% CI, 0.28 to 0.67).

Conclusions.—Pancreatectomies for chronic pancreatitis have lower in-hospital mortality than those performed for malignancy and similar rates as resection for benign tumors. Pancreatic resection, which can improve quality of life in chronic pancreatitis patients, can be performed with moderate mortality rates and should be considered in appropriate patients.

▶ Surgery for chronic pancreatitis is often not considered in a timely fashion because many clinicians deem operative therapy too morbid, associated with a high mortality rate, and unlikely to result in long-term pain relief or improvement in nutritional status. Hence, when patients are referred for pancreatic surgery they typically have exhausted all other medical options, are in disabling pain, and have a poor nutritional status that mandates preoperative nutritional therapy. Nonetheless, as demonstrated by Tseng and colleagues, appropriate selection of operative candidates and a surgical procedure performed in the setting of a high-volume hospital frequently results in a relatively low risk of mortality for patients with chronic pancreatitis. Using the Nationwide Inpatient Sample (NIS) administrative database, this study shows that patients with chronic pancreatitis have lower mortality rates than patients with pancreatic resection for malignant disease. This finding is especially poignant for patients undergoing pancreatic head resection, which tended to be performed at teaching hospitals. This study confirms what others have shown for pancreatic surgery in general: mortality is lower if the surgery is performed in a teaching hospital that does a relatively high volume. Although not proven by the NIS dataset, the surrogate for lower mortality is that a patient is treated by a surgeon, or more likely, a team of experts specifically trained or with significant experience in pancreatic disease. Thus, although the authors' conclusion is based on sound data suggesting that pancreatic resection for chronic pancreatitis is safe, these operations may be quite difficult and demanding, and require a significant amount of experience and expertise.

K. E. Behrns, MD

Laparoscopic Adjustable Gastric Banding in Severely Obese Adolescents: A Randomized Trial

O'Brien PE, Sawyer SM, Laurie C, et al (Ctr for Obesity Res and Education, Melbourne, Australia; Univ of Melbourne, Australia)

JAMA 303:519-526, 2010

Context.—Adolescent obesity is a common and serious health problem affecting more than 5 million young people in the United States alone. Bariatric surgery is being evaluated as a possible treatment option. Laparoscopic adjustable gastric banding (gastric banding) has the potential to provide a safe and effective treatment.

Objective.—To compare the outcomes of gastric banding with an optimal lifestyle program on adolescent obesity.

Design, Setting, and Patients.—A prospective, randomized controlled trial of 50 adolescents between 14 and 18 years with a body mass index (BMI) higher than 35, recruited from the Melbourne, Australia, community, assigned either to a supervised lifestyle intervention or to undergo gastric banding, and followed up for 2 years. The study was performed between May 2005 and September 2008.

Main Outcome Measures.—Weight loss. Secondary outcomes included change in metabolic syndrome, insulin resistance, quality of life, and adverse outcomes.

Results.—Twenty-four of 25 patients in the gastric banding group and 18 of 25 in lifestyle group completed the study. Twenty-one (84%) in the gastric banding and 3 (12%) in the lifestyle groups lost more than 50% of excess weight, corrected for age. Overall, the mean changes in the gastric banding group were a weight loss of 34.6 kg (95% CI, 30.2-39.0), representing an excess weight loss of 78.8% (95% CI, 66.6%-91.0%), 12.7 BMI units (95% CI, 11.3-14.2), and a BMI z score change from 2.39 (95% CI, 2.05-2.73) to 1.32 (95% CI, 0.98-1.66). The mean losses in the lifestyle group were 3.0 kg (95% CI, 2.1-8.1), representing excess weight loss of 13.2% (95% CI, 2.6%-21.0%), 1.3 BMI units (95% CI, 0.4-2.9), and a BMI z score change from 2.41 (95% CI, 2.21-2.66) to 2.26 (95% CI, 1.91-2.43). At entry, 9 participants (36%) in the gastric banding group and 10 (40%) in the lifestyle group had the metabolic syndrome. At 24 months, none of the gastric banding group had the metabolic syndrome ($P = .008$; McNemar χ^2) compared with 4 of the 18 completers (22%) in the lifestyle group ($P = .13$). The gastric banding group experienced improved quality of life with no perioperative adverse events. However, 8 operations (33%) were required in 7 patients for revisional procedures either for proximal pouch dilatation or tubing injury during follow-up.

Conclusions.—Among obese adolescent participants, use of gastric banding compared with lifestyle intervention resulted in a greater percentage achieving a loss of 50% of excess weight, corrected for age. There were associated benefits to health and quality of life.

Trial Registration.—ANZCTR Identifier: 12605000160639.

▶ Obesity is one of the top, if not the top, health care condition of concern in the United States and other countries like Australia. This disabling disease gives rise to diabetes mellitus, osteoarthritis, cardiac issues, sleep apnea, and long-lasting emotional and psychologic dysfunctions. It is particularly troubling that obesity is not only a disease of adults but has drifted into the younger age groups, including adolescents. For years we have known that medical therapies aimed at lifestyle changes have been ineffective in the adult population, and now, thanks to O'Brien et al, we realize that gastric banding is superior to lifestyle modifications in adolescents. They definitively show that gastric banding is advantageous in losing greater than 50% of excess weight, eliminating the metabolic syndrome, and improving the quality of life. Perioperative complications were nil; however, 7 of 25 patients required reoperation at a later date. These data demonstrate quite convincingly that gastric bypass is an effective treatment for adolescent obesity, provided the risks are acceptable. In this study, perioperative risks were not an issue, but, as a surgical community, we must aim for a lower rate of reoperation than the 28% demonstrated herein. Over the last several years, many of the operations we perform have seen decreased mortality; however, the new frontiers are decreased morbidity, reoperations, and readmissions. Even though decreasing the mortality was difficult, reducing the morbidity will require a system-based approach because, as one can see from this study, some of the reoperations were due to system, and not surgeon, issues. Collectively, this will require teamwork and surgeon leaders to continually look for opportunities to decrease morbidity.

K. E. Behrns, MD

Laparoscopic Liver Resection for Malignant and Benign Lesions: Ten-Year Norwegian Single-Center Experience

Kazaryan AM, Marangos IP, Rosseland AR, et al (Rikshospitalet Univ Hosp, Oslo, Norway; et al)

Arch Surg 145:34-40, 2010

Background.—The introduction of laparoscopic liver resection has been challenging because new and safe surgical techniques have had to be developed, and skepticism remains about the use of laparoscopy for malignant neoplasms. We present herein a large-volume single-center experience with laparoscopic liver resection.

Design.—Retrospective study.

Setting.—Rikshospitalet University Hospital.

Patients.—One hundred thirty-nine patients who underwent 177 laparoscopic liver resections in 149 procedures from August 18, 1998, through October 14, 2008. One hundred thirteen patients had malignant lesions, of whom 96 had colorectal metastases.

Intervention.—Laparoscopic liver resection for malignant and benign lesions.

Main Outcome Measures.—Perioperative and oncologic outcomes and survival.

Results.—Five procedures (3.4%) were converted to laparotomy and 1 (0.7%) to laparoscopic radiofrequency ablation. The remaining 143 procedures were completed laparoscopically, during which 177 liver resections were undertaken, including 131 nonanatomic and 46 anatomic resections. The median operative time and blood loss were 164 (50-488) minutes and 350 (<50-4000) mL, respectively. There were 10 intraoperative (6.7%) and 18 post-operative (12.6%) complications. One patient (0.7%) died. The median postoperative stay and opioid requirement were 3 (1-42) and 1 (0-11) days, respectively. Tumor-free resection margins determined by histopathologic evaluation were achieved in 140 of 149 malignant specimens (94.0%). The 5-year actuarial survival for patients undergoing procedures for colorectal metastases was 46%.

Conclusions.—In experienced hands, laparoscopic liver resection is a favorable alternative to open resection. Perioperative morbidity and mortality and long-term survival after laparoscopic resection of colorectal metastases appear to be comparable to those after open resections.

▶ Hepatic resection has long been considered one of the more technically demanding operations because of the risk of catastrophic blood loss. In recent years, blood loss from major hepatic resections has decreased markedly because of improved preoperative and intraoperative localization of the tumor in relationship to major vascular structures in the liver and early ligation of the vascular pedicle supplying the liver segment(s) occupied by the tumor. These same principles have been adopted and extended to laparoscopic liver resections, which are being performed with increasing frequency. The work by Kazaryan et al demonstrates the feasibility and safety of laparoscopic liver resection in 139 patients with benign and malignant disease. The complication rate, oncologic results, and mortality compare favorably with open procedures. Furthermore, the length of stay was considerably less (~3 days) than historical results for open hepatic resection. Given these excellent results, what limits the number of laparoscopic hepatectomies? This procedure remains very technically demanding and requires a substantial knowledge of open liver surgery and laparoscopic skills. Furthermore, even though the blood loss in this series was relatively low (~350 ml), this represents a significant amount of blood loss in a laparoscopic procedure. Evacuation of this blood is time consuming, limits visibility, and requires patience and perspective about the progress of the laparoscopic resection. In addition, the laparoscopic approach requires substantial preoperative planning and intraoperative skill with laparoscopic ultrasound to identify the tumor and surrounding vascular structures. This article demonstrates the feasibility and effectiveness of laparoscopic hepatectomy, and with continued improvements and dispersion of knowledge this operation will become more commonplace.

K. E. Behrns, MD

Latest Results (12–21 Years) of a Prospective Randomized Study Comparing Billroth II and Roux-en-Y Anastomosis After a Partial Gastrectomy Plus Vagotomy in Patients With Duodenal Ulcers

Csendes A, Burgos AM, Smok G, et al (Univ of Chile, Santiago)

Ann Surg 249:189-194, 2009

Introduction.—After a partial resection of the stomach, the continuity of the gastrointestinal tract can be restored either by a Billroth II gastrojejunal anastomosis or a Roux-en-Y gastrojejunostomy. Each procedure has its advantages and disadvantages.

Objective.—To determine through a prospective and random clinical trial, the clinical outcome and the endoscopic and histologic alterations of the distal esophagus and the gastric remnant in patients who received a partial distal gastrectomy due to duodenal ulcers and a Billroth II or Roux-en-Y reconstruction.

Material and Methods.—In this prospective random trial, a total of 75 patients with duodenal ulcers were included. A bilateral selective vagotomy and partial distal gastrectomy were performed in all patients. A Billroth II or Roux-en-Y 60-cm-long loop was randomly used for reconstruction of the gastrointestinal tract. During the latest follow-up clinical evaluation, upper endoscopy and biopsy samples from the distal esophagus and gastric remnant were obtained.

Results.—There was 1 operative mortality and 6 patients had some morbidity. The average follow-up period was 15.5 years (range, 11–21). Patients with Roux-en-Y gastrojejunostomy were significantly more asymptomatic and had greater Visick I grading than patients with Billroth II reconstruction ($P < 0.001$). In the distal esophagus, endoscopic findings were normal in 90% of the Roux-en-Y group, but only in 51% of the Billroth II group ($P < 0.0009$). Nearly 25% of the latter group had the appearance of a short-segment Barrett esophagus compared with 3% of the Roux-en-Y group ($P < 0.0001$). The gastric remnant endoscopic findings were normal in 100% of the Roux-en-Y group and in 18% of the Billroth II group ($P < 0.02$). Histologic analyses showed similar proportions of normal fundic mucosa and chronic active fundic gastritis. However, chronic atrophic fundic gastritis and intestinal metaplasia were significantly more frequent after Billroth II reconstruction ($P < 0.008$). *Helicobacter pylorus* was present in a similar proportion of patients.

Conclusions.—This prospective and random study showed that Roux-en-Y gastrojejunostomy is significantly better than a Billroth II reconstruction in patients with duodenal ulcers, through subjective and objective endoscopic and histologic evaluations during the latest follow-up evaluation.

► Since the introduction of histamine antagonists in the 1970s and the subsequent introduction of proton pump inhibitors, surgery for peptic ulcer disease has become increasingly uncommon. When surgery is performed it is generally for ulcer disease that is recalcitrant or complicated by bleeding, perforation, or obstruction. For decades the dilemmas for ulcer surgery have been whether to perform a vagotomy (or not) and how to establish intestinal continuity (Billroth I vs Billroth II vs Roux-en-Y). The article by Csendes et al sheds light on the latter question and provides data that definitively advocate for Roux-en-Y reconstruction. The results were obtained over a long period of time, and the randomized trial was halted before achieving the goal of 80 patients because of accrual issues. Nonetheless, 75 patients were randomized and long-term follow-up demonstrated that Roux-en-Y reconstruction was associated with fewer symptoms and less esophageal and gastric injury. For years, we have been taught that the Billroth II reconstruction was favorable because the alkaline secretion that bathed the gastrojejunostomy was protective—apparently not, because the rate of recurrent ulcer disease was similar. This is a bit bothersome because the Roux limb was created as an ulcerogenic experimental procedure. In addition, the Roux limb has been associated with a stasis syndrome that results in pain, nausea, vomiting, and delayed gastric emptying, yet the rate of gastric atony was exceedingly low, and the authors state that they just do not see this complication. However, scores of well-documented articles have reported both the clinical findings and pathophysiologic consequences of this syndrome. So, does this article provide definitive answers? The data are convincing, but are the results widely applicable or dependent on a select group of patients who had the reconstruction for duodenal ulcers only? Likely, this will go unanswered because too few patients will be available for study, but for now, a Roux-en-Y gastrojejunostomy appears to be the favored operation.

K. E. Behrns, MD

Management of Nonparasitic Hepatic Cysts

Mazza OM, Fernandez DL, Pekolj J, et al (Hosp Italiano, Buenos Aires, Argentina)

J Am Coll Surg 209:733-739, 2009

Background.—The optimal management of nonparasitic hepatic cysts (NPHC) is a topic of debate. The purpose of this study was to evaluate our 17-year experience with NPHC.

Study Design.—From January 1990 to August 2007, 131 consecutive patients with NPHC were evaluated and treated at our institution. Seventy-eight patients (60%) had simple hepatic cysts (SHC). The remaining 53 (40%) had polycystic liver disease (PLD). Morbidity, mortality, and recurrence rates for each of the two groups were evaluated.

Results.—Thirty-seven patients underwent open deroofing (SHC, 24; PLD,13), 66 had laparoscopic deroofing (SHC, 46; PLD, 20), 19 had percutaneous drainage (SHC, 4; PLD, 15), 3 had major hepatic resections (PLD, 3), 4 had cystojejunostomy (SHC, 4), and 2 had combined hepatorenal transplantation (PLD, 2). Corresponding morbidity, mortality, and recurrence rates were, respectively: conventional deroofing: SHC, 29%, 0%, 8%; PLD, 8%, 0%, 0%; laparoscopic deroofing: SHC, 2%, 0%, 2%; PLD, 25%, 0%, 5%; percutaneous drainage: SHC, 0%, 0%, 75%;

PLD, 0%, 0%, 20%; cystojejunostomy: SHC, 75%, 0%, 25%; major hepatic resections: PLD, 66%, 0%, 0%; and hepatorenal transplantation: PLD, 50%, 50%, 0%.

Conclusions.—Laparoscopic deroofing provided complete relief of symptoms for both SHC and PLD. Percutaneous drainage was our procedure of choice for infected liver cysts and potentially for patients who cannot tolerate general anesthesia. Liver and liver-kidney transplantations were reserved for patients with end-stage PLD alone and in association with end-stage renal disease, respectively.

▶ Hepatic cysts are frequently detected on cross-sectional imaging and are rarely the cause of symptoms. However, some large hepatic cysts may be associated with symptoms that range from troublesome, such as early satiety and bloating, to frankly disabling with profound weight loss, and failure to thrive. These later larger cysts require treatment, but before initiating therapy, these cysts should be identified as simple cysts or as a component of polycystic liver disease. Mazza et al summarized the treatment of 131 patients with simple or complex hepatic cysts over 17 years. A few patients with these cysts will present with infected cysts that should be treated with percutaneous drainage to relieve the symptoms of sepsis, but patients should be forewarned that definitive treatment would likely be needed after the infected cyst is drained because recurrence is nearly universal. The authors aptly incorporated laparoscopic unroofing and drainage into their management scheme for simple cysts or dominant cysts in polycystic liver disease. For complex cysts associated with polycystic liver disease, resection or transplantation may be the most appropriate treatment, but these patients are not frequently encountered. The recurrence rates for the various procedures were low in this series, indicating appropriate selection of patients matched to an appropriate procedure. However, for clinicians who perform these operations infrequently, a recurrent cyst may be quite troublesome. Too frequently, patients with recurrent cysts are subjected to multiple percutaneous drains with or without sclerosis. As the data in this study indicate, percutaneous drainage is rarely definitive treatment and, therefore, recurrent cysts should be managed by drainage, a cyst-enteric anastomosis, or resection. Because surgical treatment of recurrent cysts is uncommon, management by a surgeon with experience in the treatment of this condition may be appropriate.

K. E. Behrns, MD

Management of the hernial sac in inguinal hernia repair

Stylianidis G, Haapamäki MM, Sund M, et al (Umeå Univ Hosp, Sweden; et al)

Br J Surg 97:415-419, 2010

Background.—There is no consensus on the best management of the indirect hernial sac in groin hernia surgery. The aim of this study was to investigate to what extent different management options are associated with reoperation for recurrence.

Methods.—This study used data from the Swedish Hernia Register. Surgeons registered whether the indirect hernial sac was managed by division (leaving the distal part in place), excision or invagination.

Results.—An indirect hernia was found in 48 433 operations; the sac was excised in 49·5 per cent, invaginated in 37·6 per cent and divided in 12·9 per cent of operations. The 5-year cumulative reoperation incidence was 1·7 per cent for hernial sac excision, 1·7 per cent for division and 2·7 per cent for invagination. For indirect hernia repair, the relative risk of reoperation for recurrence was 0·63 (95 per cent confidence interval 0·51 to 0·79) for excision of the sac and 0·72 (0·53 to 0·99) for division compared with invagination. Lichtenstein repair combined with hernial sac excision had a 5-year cumulative reoperation incidence of only 1·0 per cent.

Conclusion.—Excision of the indirect hernial sac in inguinal hernia repair is associated with a lower risk of hernia recurrence than division or invagination.

▶ Over the last few decades, inguinal hernia surgery has continued to evolve such that we are no longer focused solely on recurrence rates. The benchmark recurrence rate of 1% or less has been set by a few hernia specialist centers. Although not all the techniques and care pathways of these centers have been widely promulgated, these low recurrence rates definitively demonstrated how inguinal hernia surgery should be performed. In addition to recurrence rates, the practice of inguinal hernia surgery is now focused on a minimal post-operative pain experience. Thus, the question arises about the role of hernia sac management and how this may be related to recurrence or pain. The study by Stylianidis et al uses the large Swedish Hernia Register (SHR) to examine the role of sac excision, division, and invagination in the recurrence of inguinal hernias. They found that excision of an indirect inguinal hernia sac was associated with a lower risk of recurrence than division or invagination. This was especially true when a Lichtenstein repair was performed with a reoperation rate of 1%. These data are remarkable because they do not represent results from a hernia specialist center but from nationwide results submitted to a registry. Furthermore, approximately 98% of all hernia surgeries are reported to this registry. Thus, it would appear that careful monitoring of outcomes leads to better results. This article is an excellent example of the competency (practice-based learning) that we are trying to inculcate in our trainees. It is obviously applicable to all surgeons. As we continue to refine surgical care by carefully monitoring results, as demonstrated in this study, our patients will have better care and the surgical experience will be improved.

K. E. Behrns, MD

Midline Versus Transverse Incision in Major Abdominal Surgery: A Randomized, Double-Blind Equivalence Trial (POVATI: ISRCTN60734227)

Seiler CM, Deckert A, Diener MK, et al (Univ of Heidelberg, Germany)

Ann Surg 249:913-920, 2009

Objective.—There are 2 main types of access for patients requiring major open, elective abdominal surgery: the midline or the transverse approach. The aim of this study is to compare both approaches by focusing on postoperative pain, complications, and frequency of incisional hernias.

Summary Background Data.—A recent Cochrane review suggested that transverse incisions may be less painful but incisional hernia rates do not differ.

Methods.—Randomized, patient- and observer-blinded, monocentric, equivalence clinical trial. Patients were scheduled for elective primary abdominal incisions. Composite primary end point measured 48 hours after surgery was the total amount of analgesics (piritramide) required in the last 24 hours and pain (Visual Analogue Scale). Secondary end points were early-onset and late complications. This study is registered in the ISRCTN registry and has the ID number ISRCTN60734227.

Results.—Two hundred patients (101 midline and 99 transverse) were randomized. Both incision types resulted in similar amounts of required analgesics (95% confidence interval [−0.38; −0.33] was included in the equivalence level). For the Visual Analogue Scale, both the 95% and 90% CI (0–10) were neither within the equivalence levels nor were their differences significant at the 5% level. No relevant differences between midline and transverse incisions were observed for 30-day mortality (2 vs. 2, $P = 0.99$), mortality after one year (15 vs. 23, $P = 0.15$), pulmonary complications (13 vs. 17, $P = 0.43$), median length of hospital stay (11 vs. 12 days, $P = 0.08$), median time to tolerance of solid food (12 vs. 14 days, $P = 0.30$), and incisional hernias after one year (13 vs. 8, $P = 0.48$). More wound infections occurred in the transverse group (15 vs. 5, $P = 0.02$).

Conclusion.—The decision about the incision should be driven by surgeon preference with respect to the patient's disease and anatomy.

► The debate over which abdominal incision provides the best operative exposure with the least pain and the lowest likelihood of an incisional hernia has raged on for decades. Many of the trials have shown a small benefit of a longitudinal incision compared with a transverse incision and vice versa. The study by Seiler et al is unique because of the design and execution of the trial and the meticulous and rigorous statistical analysis. Despite the elegant experimental design and analysis, this trial proves equivalency of the 2 incisions and concludes that the decision for the type of incision should be driven by the surgeon's preference in the context of the patient's disease and anatomy. Although this study was brilliantly conceived and superbly conducted, does it and other potentially confirmatory studies like it advance surgical science? As a surgical research community, would we be better served performing basic science studies investigating adjuvants to wound healing and the molecular mechanisms that underlie improved wound healing in the face of additional therapy? This is a difficult question to answer, but we need to move surgical science forward with bold experimental therapeutics and innovative approaches to surgical diseases. In recent years, relatively high-risk surgical science has been discouraged by poor funding levels, impediments to patient enrollment by highly restrictive review boards, and perhaps most importantly, the need to provide an ever-increasing volume of clinical surgery for financial solvency. These constraints do not permit out-of-the-box thinking with innovative approaches, but as a surgical research community, we need to continue to advocate for surgical research and be involved in the process by volunteering for study sections, review boards, article reviews, and so forth. Although the pressure for clinical care is significant, we must continue to advance a surgical scientific culture to continue to promote our discipline.

K. E. Behrns, MD

Operative Results and Quality of Life After Gracilis Muscle Transposition for Recurrent Rectovaginal Fistula

Lefèvre JH, Bretagnol F, Maggiori L, et al (Beaujon Hosp (AP-HP), Clichy, France)

Dis Colon Rectum 52:1290-1295, 2009

Purpose.—The aim of this study was to assess the efficacy of gracilis muscle transposition for recurrent rectovaginal fistula.

Methods.—Gracilis muscle transposition for recurrent rectovaginal fistula was performed in eight patients. Causes of fistulas included Crohn's disease (n = 5), perineal surgery (n = 2), and obstetrical injury (n = 1). All patients underwent a mean of three (range, 1–6) previous repairs. Fecal diversion was performed in all cases.

Results.—Six of eight patients (75%) healed after gracilis muscle transposition alone. The other two patients required a second gracilis. These two patients failed with another recurrence and one of them underwent laparotomy with successful omental interposition. Thus, after a median follow-up of 28 (range, 4–55) months, the per-gracilis muscle transposition healing rate was 60% (6/10) and the overall healing success rate after gracilis muscle transposition and other procedures was 88% (7/8). For patients with Crohn's disease, four of five (80%) presented no recurrent rectovaginal fistula. Seven of eight patients underwent ileostomy closure after gracilis, but two required subsequent stomas, one for a late recurrence. Overall, five of eight patients are stoma-free. Despite healing, postoperative quality of life and sexual activity remained significantly altered.

Conclusion.—Gracilis muscle transposition can be proposed in cases of recurrent rectovaginal fistula. The procedure has a good success rate, especially in Crohn's disease patients.

▶ Definitive treatment of rectovaginal fistulae has long challenged surgeons because of a high recurrence rate and relatively poor quality of life after repair. Lefèvre et al report on a small group of 8 patients who underwent gracilis muscle transposition to treat multiple recurrent rectovaginal fistulae. These patients, on average, had 3 previous attempts at repair—a testament to the difficulty of adequately treating this problem surgically. The results of treatment are within the range of previous reports, in that 50% of the patients were adequately treated with a single operation and an additional 25% of patients had relief with a stoma or total abdominal colectomy and proctectomy. Two patients developed recurrent rectovaginal fistulae. This study is important because despite admirable results, the quality-of-life outcomes demonstrate that, although they may have obviated passage of stool or gas per vagina, their physical, emotional, and sexual well-being were far from normal. Too infrequently outcome studies assess how our patients fare physically and emotionally following surgical treatment. As a surgical community, we tend to be focused on the relatively hard or measurable outcomes of death, morbidity, survival, etc. Importantly, to advance surgical care we also need to assess patients' physical and psychosocial well-being. Can our patients return to full or part-time employment? Do they feel well enough to exercise regularly? Do they have meaningful relationships with their spouse and family? The authors should be commended for examining quality of life; future surgical outcome studies should address these issues so that refinements in surgical care can progress.

K. E. Behrns, MD

Outcomes after a decade of laparoscopic giant paraesophageal hernia repair

Luketich JD, Nason KS, Christie NA, et al (Univ of Pittsburgh, PA)
J Thorac Cardiovasc Surg 139:395-404, 2010

Objective.—Laparoscopic repair of giant paraesophageal hernia is a complex operation requiring significant laparoscopic expertise. Our objective was to compare our current approach and outcomes for laparoscopic repair of giant paraesophageal hernia with our previous experience.

Methods.—A retrospective review of patients undergoing nonemergency laparoscopic repair of giant paraesophageal hernia, stratified by early versus current era (January 1997–June 2003 and July 2003–June 2008), was performed. We evaluated clinical outcomes, barium esophagogram, and quality of life.

Results.—Laparoscopic repair of giant paraesophageal hernia was performed in 662 patients (median age 70 years, range 19–92 years) with a median percentage of herniated stomach of 70% (range 30%–100%). With time, use of Collis gastroplasty decreased (86% to 53%), as did crural mesh reinforcement (17% to 12%). Current era patients were 50% more likely to have a Charlson comorbidity index score greater than 3. Thirty-day mortality was 1.7% (11/662). Mortality and complication rates were stable with time, despite increasing comorbid disease in current era. Postoperative gastroesophageal reflux disease health-related quality of life scores were available for 489 patients (30-month median follow-up), with good to excellent results in 90% (438/489). Radiographic recurrence (15.7%) was not associated with symptom recurrence. Reoperation occurred in 3.2% (21/662).

Conclusions.—With time, we have obtained significant minimally invasive experience and refined our approach to laparoscopic repair of giant paraesophageal hernia. Perioperative morbidity and mortality remain low, despite increased comorbid disease in the current era. Laparoscopic repair provided excellent patient satisfaction and symptom improvement, even with small radiographic recurrences. Reoperation rates were comparable to the best open series.

▶ For the past 2 decades, laparoscopic approaches to upper gastrointestinal diseases have been evaluated and have generally resulted in improved patient outcomes. However, laparoscopic treatment of giant paraesophageal hernias has proven to be the most difficult in which to obtain durable, outstanding outcomes. In fact, in the past, some authors have even suggested that the laparoscopic approach be reconsidered because of the high recurrence rate. The article by Luketich et al reports a large series of patients accumulated over 10 years. Their results are excellent, with a radiographic recurrence rate of nearly 16%. However, this study notes that many of these radiographic recurrences are not associated with symptoms. Therefore, these patients likely do require reoperation, an event that occurred in about 3% of patients in this study. Early in this series, Collis gastroplasty and mesh crural repair were liberally used, while in more recent years they focused on esophageal lengthening and primary crural repair with an intact overlying peritoneum. The observations and changes in techniques that resulted from this attention to detail have produced excellent results and an improvement in the quality of care. This article is a superb example of developing a technique, recording pertinent intraoperative details, and correlating these findings with patient outcomes. This article defines practice-based learning and should be used as an instructional tool for surgical trainees.

K. E. Behrns, MD

Outcomes From 3144 Adrenalectomies in the United States: Which Matters More, Surgeon Volume or Specialty?

Park HS, Roman SA, Sosa JA (Yale Univ School of Medicine, New Haven, CT)

Arch Surg 144:1060-1067, 2009

Objective.—To assess the effect of surgeon volume and specialty on clinical and economic outcomes after adrenalectomy.

Design.—Population-based retrospective cohort analysis.

Setting.—Healthcare Cost and Utilization Project Nationwide Inpatient Sample.

Participants.—Adults (≥18 years) undergoing adrenalectomy in the United States (1999-2005). Patient demographic and clinical characteristics, surgeon specialty (general vs urologist), surgeon adrenalectomy volume, and hospital factors were assessed. Main Outcome Measures: The χ^2 test, analysis of variance, and multivariate linear and logistic regression were used to assess in-hospital complications, mean hospital length of stay (LOS), and total inpatient hospital costs.

Results.—A total of 3144 adrenalectomies were included. Mean patient age was 53.7 years; 58.8% were women and 77.4% white. A higher proportion of general surgeons were high-volume surgeons compared with urologists (34.1% vs 18.2%, $P < .001$). Low-volume surgeons had more complications (18.2% vs 11.3%, $P < .001$) and their patients had longer LOS (5.5 vs 3.9 days, $P < .001$) than did high-volume surgeons; urologists had more complications (18.4% vs 15.2%, $P = .03$) and higher costs ($13 168 vs $11 732, $P = .02$) than did general surgeons. After adjustment for patient and provider characteristics in multivariate analyses, surgeon volume, but not specialty, was an independent predictor of complications (odds ratio = 1.5, $P < .002$) and LOS (1.0-day difference, $P < .001$). Hospital volume was associated only with LOS (0.8-day difference, $P < .007$). Surgeon volume, specialty, and hospital volume were not predictors of costs.

Conclusion.—To optimize outcomes, patients with adrenal disease should be referred to surgeons based on adrenal volume and laparoscopic expertise irrespective of specialty practice.

► Adrenalectomy had been a relatively uncommon surgical procedure because exposure of the deep retroperitoneal organ required a large incision for an anterior approach or a posterior approach in which visualization may be limited. A laparoscopic approach to adrenalectomy has eliminated the large incisions and improved visual inspection of the organ and surrounding structures. Park et al demonstrated that, indeed, the rate of adrenalectomy has increased. An increased incidence of an operation must be accompanied by low risks, and assessment of complications using the National Inpatient Sample database showed that the complication rate was 11% for high-volume surgeons and 18% for low-volume surgeons—a relatively low rate of complications. Notably, the analysis showed that high-volume surgeons had a lower complication rate and a shorter length of stay. Specialty training, general surgery versus urology, had no bearing on the outcome, whereas higher hospital volume was associated with a shorter length of stay. The authors recommend a referral pattern to high-volume surgeons with expertise in laparoscopy. However, is this possible across the United States? For adrenalectomy, regionalization of care may be possible because of the relatively low number of required operations per year. However, regionalization of more common yet highly specialized procedures could be problematic because access to a high-volume laparoscopic surgeon may be difficult. These data suggest that our training programs must address these highly specialized programs, but that continuing education following training is critically important in obtaining excellent results.

K. E. Behrns, MD

Outcomes in Patients with Ulcerative Colitis Undergoing Partial or Complete Reconstructive Surgery for Failing Ileal Pouch-Anal Anastomosis

Mathis KL, Dozois EJ, Larson DW, et al (Mayo Clinic, Rochester, MN)

Ann Surg 249:409-413, 2009

Objective.—Evaluate outcomes of patients with an original diagnosis of ulcerative colitis (UC) who required partial or complete ileal pouch reconstruction due to poor function or infectious complications.

Methods.—A prospectively collected ileal pouch-anal anastomosis (IPAA) database was reviewed retrospectively to identify UC patients undergoing major reconstructive revisions of their IPAA at our institution between 1981 and 2005. Functional results were derived from continued surveys of patients.

Results.—Fifty-one UC patients were identified but 22 subsequently proved to have Crohns disease (CD). The initial IPAA was constructed at our institution in 32 patients and elsewhere in 19 patients. Indications for revision included infectious/inflammatory complications (65%) and mechanical difficulties (35%). Pouch revision was partial in 57% of patients and complete in 43%. There were no postoperative deaths. Following reconstruction, patients reported on average 5 daytime and 1 nighttime bowel movements. Daytime incontinence was occasional in 43% and frequent in 4%. Nighttime incontinence was occasional in 54% and frequent in 7%. The probability of pouch survival after reconstruction was 93% at 1 year and 89% at 5 years. Of the pouches that subsequently failed, 75% occurred in patients with a later diagnosis of CD. Postreconstruction abscess was a significant risk factor for ultimate pouch failure.

Conclusions.—In UC patients with failing IPAA, partial or complete pouch reconstruction can be done safely with good functional results, and may avoid pouch excision and permanent ileostomy in carefully selected patients, especially those with definite UC.

▶ Salvage surgery after intervention for gastrointestinal disorders is challenging, and often the results are presumed to be dismal. However, Mathis et al demonstrate that following the creation of ileal pouch-anal anastomosis (IPAA), a failing pouch can be saved with careful patient selection and judicious use of either partial or complete pouch reconstruction. However, it should be noted that this is a relatively small series gathered over 3 decades by one of the groups most experienced with this operation. Thus, these results may not be transferable, and, as noted by their various choices of procedures, one type of pouch fix is not applicable. While there has been much discussion and controversy about regionalization of care and select procedures performed at specialist centers or by super-specialists, salvage surgery in patients who had an initial complex operation is highly desirable. These difficult postsurgical problems frequently give us pause to ask the question, "When should I refer this patient to an individual with more experience?" This decision, of course, must come after thorough discussion with the patient because any transfer of care will result in significant inconvenience for the patient. Furthermore, on the receiving end, the expectations for care must be clear; that is, can this problem be corrected by further surgical intervention? All too frequently, patients are transferred with difficult problems but are disgruntled because they do not understand the reason for transfer, and, furthermore, the expectation that they have arrived at the ultimate destination for definitive care is not a realistic expectation. Obviously, a discussion between the referring physician and the accepting physician is required, as is a clear discussion with the patient. Communication with our patients must remain our highest priority so that the expectations of outcomes are clearly understood.

K. E. Behrns, MD

Pancreatic Cyst Fluid Protein Expression Profiling for Discriminating Between Serous Cystadenoma and Intraductal Papillary Mucinous Neoplasm

Allen PJ, Qin L-X, Tang L, et al (Memorial Sloan-Kettering Cancer Ctr, New York; et al)

Ann Surg 250:754-760, 2009

Background.—Many patients with benign serous cystadenoma (SCA) of the pancreas will undergo resection because of the inability to reliably discriminate between SCA and premalignant mucinous cysts (intraductal papillary mucinous neoplasm [IPMN], mucinous cystic neoplasm [MCN]).

Methods.—Cyst fluid from patients with SCA (n = 15), non main-duct and noninvasive IPMN (n = 32), and noninvasive MCN (n = 12) was aspirated at the time of operative resection and analyzed. Commercially available and custom designed multiplex assays (Luminex) were performed using a biomarker panel developed for pancreatic cancer. Differential protein expression (fluorescence intensity, FI) was compared between the 3 groups for each protein (Wilcoxon rank sum test). Unsupervised sample clustering (hierarchical clustering) and supervised sample classification (prediction analysis for microarrays [PAM]) was then performed.

Results.—Differential protein expression ($P < 0.05$) was identified between SCA and IPMN (34/51 proteins, 67%) and between SCA and MCN (13/51 proteins, 25%). The majority of proteins were down-regulated in IPMN and MCN compared with SCA. The only proteins significantly overexpressed in the cyst fluid of patients with mucinous cysts were CEA (median FI: IPMN 11.4, MCN 13.0, SCA 5.3; $P < 0.001$, IPMN vs. SCA) and CA72.4 (median FI: IPMN 10.4, MCN 10.5, SCA 9.9; $P = 0.003$, IPMN vs. SCA). Unsupervised cluster analysis demonstrated distinct clustering of SCA and IPMN with some cross-over between MCN. Supervised sample classification with 14 proteins had an overall accuracy rate of 92% between SCA and IPMN.

Conclusions.—In this study differential cyst fluid protein expression was observed between SCA and IPMN for the majority of proteins assessed and multimarker sample classification accurately discriminated between SCA and IPMN in 92% of patients.

▶ Cross-sectional imaging for a variety of abdominal symptoms has resulted in the diagnosis of many incidentally discovered cystic lesions of the pancreas. Many of these lesions are small (< 3 cm), and it is difficult to distinguish histologically benign serous cystadenomas (SCA) from mucinous, and potentially malignant, neoplasms. SCAs are nearly always benign, and when the SCAs are small, they do not require resection. As a result, identifying these lesions in comparison with mucinous cystic neoplasms (MCN) and intraductal papillary mucinous neoplasms (IPMN) would spare patients a potentially morbid operation. Currently, the best predictor of a mucinous neoplasm is cystic CEA concentration with 80% accuracy. Allen and colleagues further tested the hypothesis that intracystic protein concentrations could reliably distinguish SCA from mucinous neoplasms. In this study, the lesions were aspirated post-resection and the fluid was subjected to a protein array that contained 51 proteins. Not surprisingly, CEA was the most differentially expressed protein, and if analyzed solely, correctly predicted 86% of mucinous lesions. When analyzed in the context of the other proteins the diagnosis was correct in 92% of patients. Thus, this study confirms the previous work on CEA and provides incremental improvement in diagnostic capabilities when CEA is assessed in the context of other proteins. Even though this investigation was well-designed and performed, an improved diagnostic accuracy from 80% to 92% will not substantially affect the few numbers of patients with small cystic lesions that cannot be reliably distinguished by imaging methods. However, this work represents a step in the right direction of identifying protein markers, which will be the signature of future diagnostic tests.

K. E. Behrns, MD

Pancreatic Necrosectomy: North American Mortality Is Much Lower than Expected

Parikh PY, Pitt HA, Kilbane M, et al (Indiana Univ, Indianapolis)

J Am Coll Surg 209:712-719, 2009

Background.—The aim of this analysis was to explore the American College of Surgeons National Surgical Quality Improvement Program (ACS-NSQIP) database to determine outcomes of patients undergoing debridement for pancreatic and peripancreatic necrosis. Single-institution series suggest that the mortality of patients undergoing pancreatic necrosectomy has improved but remains at 15% to 20%. But no national data have been available for patients with necrotizing pancreatitis. In 2007, a CPT code specific for debridement of pancreatic necrosis became available.

Study Design.—The ACS-NSQIP Participant Use File was queried for all patients who had debridement of pancreatic and peripancreatic necrosis (CPT code 48105) from January 1, 2007, through December 31, 2007. Patient demographics, observed (O) and expected (E) morbidity and mortality, and indices (O/E) were evaluated. A multivariate stepwise logistic regression was performed to determine predictors of mortality.

Results.—During this 12-month period, data were accumulated on 161 patients. The mean age was 54 years; 71% were male; and 75% were Caucasian. The mean body mass index was 30.3 kg/m^2; 29% had diabetes; and 11% abused alcohol. Forty-two percent were transferred to NSQIP hospitals from other facilities. Overall morbidity was 62%, and 30-day mortality was 6.8%, but morbidity and mortality indices were 0.86 and 0.33, respectively. Increased age and blood urea nitrogen were independent predictors of mortality.

Conclusions.—These data suggest that patients undergoing debridement for pancreatic and peripancreatic necrosis at ACS-NSQIP hospitals provide a new North American sample and have better than predicted outcomes. We concluded that ACS-NSQIP is a powerful tool to assess contemporary outcomes of uncommon, high-risk procedures.

▶ Traditionally, necrotizing pancreatitis has been associated with mortality rates of approximately 20% and morbidity rates that exceed 50%, making it one of the most lethal and devastating diseases that a general surgeon can treat. This article by Parikh et al used the American College of Surgeons National Surgical Quality Improvement Program (ACS-NSQIP) database to retrospectively review the prospectively collected outcome data on 161 patients. The results showed that at 30 days the mortality rate was 6.8% and the morbidity rate was 62%, both much lower than the expected rates. These data were collected from 173 hospitals participating in NSQIP and, of note, the authors' institution contributed 25 patients, suggesting that many of these patients came from tertiary referral centers. Likely, these excellent results are not representative of care across a wide spectrum of health care institutions because many of the NSQIP participating centers are academic and have a keen interest in diseases like necrotizing pancreatitis. Although, as the authors suggest, these data are encouraging, the results must be put into perspective. First, NSQIP data capture occurs on an 8-day cycle, and thus, the number of patients entered is only representative. Furthermore, data are typically obtained for only 30 days, and patients with acute pancreatitis generally have long recovery periods so that the surgical care may not be complete by 30 days. Also, NSQIP currently does not permit collection of disease-specific complications like pancreatic fistula, pseudocyst development, and disconnected pancreatic duct syndrome. Although it is encouraging to know that patients undergoing pancreatic necrosectomy have better outcomes than expected, to truly improve care we need data collection systems that permit disease-specific data that can be used to re-engineer disease-specific treatment approaches.

K. E. Behrns, MD

Poly(glycerol sebacate) films prevent postoperative adhesions and allow laparoscopic placement

Pryor HI II, O'Doherty E, Hart A, et al (MassGeneral Hosp for Children, Boston, MA)

Surgery 146:490-497, 2009

Background.—The objectives of this study were to evaluate the efficacy of poly(glycerol) sebacate (PGS) films for the prevention of visceroparietal peritoneal (VP) adhesions and demonstrate the ease of laparoscopic PGS film placement. Peritoneal adhesions occur in nearly 95% of all abdominal operations. VP adhesions can cause serious postoperative complications. The interposition of a barrier between damaged peritoneal areas during re-epithelialization has been shown to prevent adhesion formation. Current barrier products have serious drawbacks, including poor degradability, variable efficacy, and difficult handling characteristics.

Methods.—The efficacy of PGS films to prevent VP adhesions was evaluated in a rat peritoneal adhesion model. The animals were evaluated for the presence of VP adhesions at 3, 5, and 8 weeks. The laparoscopic applicability of PGS films was demonstrated by placement into a juvenile porcine abdomen using standard laparoscopic equipment and techniques.

Results.—A statistically significant 94% reduction in VP adhesion formation rate was observed between control animals (75%) and animals with a PGS film barrier (4.8%). PGS films were easily placed in the juvenile porcine abdomen and could be readily repositioned without material loss or tissue damage.

Conclusion.—PGS films possess a unique combination of properties, including biocompatibility, resorbability, and ease of handling. PGS barrier films were shown to be efficacious in reducing VP adhesions in the rat model. They also can be placed using standard laparoscopic techniques. These promising results suggest that PGS films will be effective barriers to adhesion formation for patients undergoing open and laparoscopic abdominal operations.

▶ Intra-abdominal adhesion formation represents a significant clinical problem for the general surgeon. On a daily basis, we evaluate patients with problems potentially related to adhesion formation. Whether on rounds evaluating a post-operative patient who has delayed return of bowel function that may be due to adhesions or seeing patients in the clinic with abdominal pain of an unclear etiology, but potentially related to adhesions, we are confronted by difficult decisions. An adjunctive treatment to decrease or abolish adhesion formation would represent a major advance in clinical care and result in substantial cost savings. Many products have been developed, and some are even in widespread clinical use, but their effectiveness and handling remain major drawbacks. This study by Pryor et al demonstrates that polyglycerol sebacate films largely prevent adhesions in a rat model and that the handling is sufficient to permit laparoscopic placement of this material. This investigation is an outstanding example of translational science that may have a relatively quick clinical impact. These simple, yet elegant, animal studies have impressive results, and a clinical trial should be initiated in the near future. This study highlights the importance of the impact of translational research. The research question is straightforward and the methodology is simple. However, the impact of the research question, in terms of patient outcomes and costs, may be of enormous magnitude. In addition to the importance of the impact of the research question, we, as a surgical research community, need to convince funding agencies that work such as this is meritorious and may have a significant clinical impact.

K. E. Behrns, MD

Post-operative antibiotic use in nonperforated appendicitis

Le D, Rusin W, Hill B, et al (Univ of Utah Health Sciences Ctr, Salt Lake City)
Am J Surg 198:748-752, 2009

Background.—The appropriate use of preoperative antibiotics in patients undergoing appendectomy for acute appendicitis has been shown to decrease the rate of surgical site infections (SSIs). The benefits of postoperative courses of antibiotics in these patients, however, remain unclear.

Methods.—The authors retrospectively reviewed all cases of nonperforated appendicitis performed at their institution over a 10-year period from 1997 to 2007. Patient outcomes were evaluated to include the post-operative development of SSIs, urinary tract infections, diarrhea, and *Clostridium difficile* infections.

Results.—A total of 763 patients who underwent appendectomy for nonperforated appendicitis during the study period were identified. Five hundred seven of these patients had appropriate follow-up data and were the subjects of this study. Comparing patients who did and did not receive postoperative antibiotics, no significant differences in the rates of all SSIs (10% vs 9%, $P = .64$), superficial SSIs (9.3% vs 5.4%, $P = .13$), deep SSIs (.3% vs .5%, $P = 1.0$), organ space SSIs (2.8% vs 2.7%, $P = .87$), urinary tract infections (.6% vs .5%, $P = 1.0$), and diarrhea (2.5% vs 1.1%, $P = .34$) were found between groups.

Conclusions.—The use of postoperative antibiotics in patients with nonperforated appendicitis does not decrease the rate of SSIs, while it may increase the cost of care.

▶ Despite several decades of studies that include many randomized trials assessing the need for perioperative antibiotics, many questions remain unanswered. This study addresses the role of postoperative antibiotics in patients who had surgery for nonperforated appendicitis. Heretofore, most of the studies have addressed the role and timing of administration of preoperative antibiotics, but few have investigated the need for postoperative doses of antimicrobials. Le et al found in 763 patients (follow-up complete in 507) that whether the patient received postoperative antibiotics or not made no difference in superficial or deep surgical site infections, organ space infections, postoperative diarrhea, or urinary tract infections. Frequently, the decision to place the patient on postoperative antibiotics is determined by the surgeon's intraoperative assessment of the appendix—is it gangrenous or perforated? This study found no correlation between the surgeon's assessment and the pathologic analysis; thus, an intuitive decision of whether the patient may benefit from antibiotics seems ill advised. Although this study is retrospective and has self-described limitations, it identifies an important area for future study. Does the use of postoperative antibiotics decrease the rate of wound infection, not only in appendicitis but many other surgical cases? Are postoperative antibiotics necessary just because a chest tube remains in place after cardiothoracic surgery? Likewise, does postoperative antibiotic use definitively lower the risk of graft infection in vascular surgery? No doubt industry will not step up to fund these studies, but for the safety of our patients and potentially a reduction in cost, we should critically examine this issue so that we have improved value for the surgical care we deliver.

K. E. Behrns, MD

Prospective randomized controlled trial comparing V-Y advancement flap with primary suture methods in pilonidal disease

Nursal TZ, Ezer A, Çalişkan K, et al (Başkent Univ, Adana, Turkey)

Am J Surg 199:170-177, 2010

Background.—An ideal treatment method for the widely prevalent pilonidal sinus disease is not yet available. The most commonly practiced technique is simple closure following resection of the affected tissue. However, high recurrence rates in some series have led to the search for other methods. One of these methods is the V–Y advancement flap (VYAF), which in theory results in the flattening of the natal cleft without tension in the suture line.

Methods.—In this prospective randomized controlled study, the VYAF method was compared to 2 simple primary closure techniques. In 238 patients, following resection, in the AL (all layers) group, all layers were closed with polypropylene sutures. In the SS (subcutaneous suture) group, polyglactin subcutaneous sutures were used to approximate the wound edges. Skin was closed separately in the SS group. In addition, demographic variables, past history, physical examination findings, defect dimensions, and wound tension were recorded.

Results.—Surgical site infection was observed in 23.9%, 17.4%, and 10.2% of the patients in AL, SS, and VYAF groups, respectively ($P=.129$). Early wound dehiscence without infection was detected in 11.9%, 7.4%, and 10.2% of the patients in groups AL, SS, and VYAF, respectively ($P=.665$). Mean follow-up was 29.7 ± 15.6 months. Survival (time without recurrence) was not significantly different between groups ($P=.648$). In the whole group, independent predictors of recurrence according to logistic regression analysis were younger age, recurrent disease, presence of discharge on physical examination, and development of postoperative surgical site infection.

Conclusions.—VYAF is not superior to simple primary closure techniques in terms of postoperative complications, recurrence, and patient satisfaction. For most cases, simple primary closure would suffice. Patients should be informed of the increased risk of recurrence if any of the independent predictors (being a recurrent case, presence of discharge, development of postoperative infection) are present.

▶ Although in theory surgical treatment of pilonidal disease is a straightforward resection with closure of the wound, this operation is often delayed because of wound healing problems that may be chronic and quite bothersome to the patient. Because of the difficulties with wound healing, several methods of closure or treating an open wound have been used. No randomized trial has definitively shown that one method of wound care is superior to a comparator. This study by Nursal et al is prospective and randomized and shows that a V-Y advancement flap has no advantage over the 2 methods of simple closure. This result is a bit at odds with other smaller nonrandomized series that show some advantage for a V-Y advancement flap. However, the results generated in this report appear to come from a well-designed trial and, therefore, are convincing. Essentially, this leaves the surgeon with the anticipation that 10% to 16% of patients will develop a recurrence, so perhaps the best we can do is appropriately excise the entirety of the lesion, close the defect primarily, and if a wound infection develops, open the wound early and manage with the best available wound care, likely a vacuum-assisted wound closure. This solution may appear less than ideal, but applying large operations with more risk appears to do little for the patient.

K. E. Behrns, MD

Quality of Life After Iatrogenic Bile Duct Injury: A Case Control Study

Hogan AM, Hoti E, Winter DC, et al (St. Vincent's Univ Hosp, Dublin, Ireland)

Ann Surg 249:292-295, 2009

Objective.—To compare quality of life (QOL) of patients following iatrogenic bile duct injuries (BDI) to matched controls.

Summary Background Data.—BDI complicate approximately 0.3% of all cholecystectomy procedures. The literature regarding impact on quality of life is conflicted as assessment using clinical determinants alone is insufficient.

Methods.—The medical outcomes study short form 36 (SF-36), a sensitive tool for quantification of life quality outcome, was used. The study group of iatrogenic BDI was compared with an age- and sex-matched group who underwent uncomplicated cholecystectomy. Telephone questionnaire using the SF-36 quality of life tool was administered to both groups at a median postoperative time of 12 years 8 months (range, 2 months –20 years).

Results.—Seventy-eight patients were referred with BDI but due to mortality (n = 10) and unavailability (n = 6) 62 participated. The age- and sex-matched control cohort had undergone uncomplicated cholecystectomy (n = 62). Comparison between groups revealed that 7 of 8 variables examined were statistically similar to those of the control group (physical functioning, role physical, bodily pain, general health perceptions, vitality and social functioning, and mental health index). Mean role emotional scores were slightly worse in the BDI group (46 vs. 50) but the significance was borderline ($P = 0.045$). Subgroup analysis by method of intervention for BDI did not demonstrate significant differences.

Conclusion.—Quality of life of surviving patients following BDI compares favorably to that after uncomplicated laparoscopic cholecystectomy.

▶ Quality-of-life measures following potentially devastating surgical outcomes are too rarely examined. The article by Hogan et al addresses the important question of quality of life in patients who had a significant bile duct injury requiring primarily operative management following open or laparoscopic cholecystectomy. Sixty-two patients who sustained a bile duct injury were examined with the short form 36 (SF-36) quality measurement tool about 12 years following treatment and were compared with patients who had an uncomplicated cholecystectomy. The results demonstrated equivalence between the bile duct injury and cholecystectomy groups with the exception of a possible difference in emotional scores being lower in the bile duct injury group ($P = .045$). Bile duct injury is obviously a potentially devastating injury both for the patient and for the operating surgeon. The patient anticipates a relatively straightforward, uncomplicated cholecystectomy that will be performed on an outpatient basis, yet many times these patients will have both interventional and operative procedures over a period of months. Thus, it is quite notable that over time these patients have an excellent quality-of-life outcome and are able to overcome the physical, mental, and emotional trauma associated with bile duct injury. These outcomes are particularly noteworthy in that many patients who have a bile duct injury will also be involved in litigation. Although this was not addressed in this article, if these patients were involved in a legal case, they recovered remarkably well. These data, however, may be biased because they come from a single center that addresses nearly all the significant bile duct injuries in Ireland, and, thus, the outcomes are likely better than might be expected if the salvage surgery was performed at a center with less experience.

K. E. Behrns, MD

Radiofrequency Ablation in Barrett's Esophagus with Dysplasia

Shaheen NJ, Sharma P, Overholt BF, et al (Univ of North Carolina at Chapel Hill; Veterans Affairs Med Ctr and Univ of Kansas School of Medicine; Gastrointestinal Associates, Knoxville, TN; et al)

N Engl J Med 360:2277-2288, 2009

Background.—Barrett's esophagus, a condition of intestinal metaplasia of the esophagus, is associated with an increased risk of esophageal adenocarcinoma. We assessed whether endoscopic radiofrequency ablation could eradicate dysplastic Barrett's esophagus and decrease the rate of neoplastic progression.

Methods.—In a multicenter, sham-controlled trial, we randomly assigned 127 patients with dysplastic Barrett's esophagus in a 2:1 ratio to receive either radiofrequency ablation (ablation group) or a sham procedure (control group). Randomization was stratified according to the grade of dysplasia and the length of Barrett's esophagus. Primary outcomes at 12 months included the complete eradication of dysplasia and intestinal metaplasia.

Results.—In the intention-to-treat analyses, among patients with low-grade dysplasia, complete eradication of dysplasia occurred in 90.5% of those in the ablation group, as compared with 22.7% of those in the control group ($P<0.001$). Among patients with high-grade dysplasia, complete eradication occurred in 81.0% of those in the ablation group, as compared with 19.0% of those in the control group ($P<0.001$). Overall, 77.4% of patients in the ablation group had complete eradication of intestinal metaplasia, as compared with 2.3% of those in the control group ($P<0.001$). Patients in the ablation group had less disease progression (3.6% vs. 16.3%, $P=0.03$) and fewer cancers (1.2% vs. 9.3%, $P=0.045$). Patients reported having more chest pain after the ablation procedure than after the sham procedure. In the ablation group, one patient had upper gastrointestinal hemorrhage, and five patients (6.0%) had esophageal stricture.

Conclusions.—In patients with dysplastic Barrett's esophagus, radiofrequency ablation was associated with a high rate of complete eradication of both dysplasia and intestinal metaplasia and a reduced risk of disease progression. (ClinicalTrials.gov number, NCT00282672.)

▶ The treatment of Barrett's esophagus has vexed esophagologists and esophageal surgeons because response to either medical therapy or surgical treatment has been disappointing. For several years, the primary debate has been whether patients are more effectively treated with proton pump inhibitors or fundoplication. No study has provided a definitive answer to this dilemma. This randomized trial of radiofrequency ablation versus sham procedure is convincing in that it overwhelmingly demonstrates that ablation results in eradication of dysplasia and metaplasia, and decreases the risk of disease progression. However, these data must be viewed carefully because of the 755 patients that were screened only 84 patients had ablation; thus, a number of patients are not eligible for treatment. Furthermore, the results in the control group are so abysmal that it raises the question of whether this was the appropriate control. Should one arm of treatment have included fundoplication? In addition, multivariate analysis failed to reveal predictors of response to therapy, and therefore, selection of the appropriate patients for ablation may be challenging. Obviously, longer follow-up is needed to ensure the completeness of ablation and the potential for delayed stricture formation. Furthermore, ablation treats the complication of reflux but does not adequately address the underlying altered physiology. So the question remains: What is the role of fundoplication in patients with Barrett's esophagus? Should patients that have successful ablation of the esophageal mucosa subsequently undergo fundoplication, or is medical therapy sufficient? Certainly, surgeons must play a significant role in addressing these questions.

K. E. Behrns, MD

Randomized clinical trial of symptom control after stapled anopexy or diathermy excision for haemorrhoid prolapse

Nyström P-O, Qvist N, Raahave D, et al (Karolinska Univ Hosp Huddinge, Stockholm, Sweden; Univ Hosp, Odense; North Sealand Hosp, Helsingor, Denmark; et al)

Br J Surg 97:167-176, 2010

Background.—This multicentre randomized clinical trial studied how symptoms improved after either stapled anopexy or diathermy excision of haemorrhoids.

Methods.—The study involved 18 hospitals in Sweden, Denmark and the UK. Some 207 patients were randomized to either anopexy or Milligan–Morgan haemorrhoidectomy, of whom 90 in each group were operated on. Patients reported symptoms before surgery and after 1 year. Daily postoperative pain scores were recorded in a patient diary. Surgeons evaluated the anal anatomy before surgery and after 1 year.

Results.—Correction of prolapse in the anopexy and haemorrhoidectomy groups was similar at 1 year (88 and 90 per cent respectively; $P = 0{\cdot}80$). Freedom from symptoms was obtained in 44 and 69 per cent respectively ($P = 0{\cdot}002$). Stapled anopexy was associated with less post-operative pain, which resolved more quickly ($P = 0{\cdot}004$). Significant improvements were noted in anal continence and well-being 1 year after both operations ($P < 0{\cdot}001$). Excessive pain was the most common complication after diathermy excision and disturbed bowel function after stapled anopexy.

Conclusion.—Haemorrhoidal prolapse was corrected equally by either operation. Diathermy haemorrhoidectomy gave better symptom relief but was more painful. Neither operation provided complete cure but well-being was greatly improved. Registration number: ISRCTN68315343 (http://www.controlled-trials.com).

▶ Mucosal prolapse of the distal rectum is a bothersome condition that is characterized by significant pain, incontinence, and disruption of daily living. Operative therapy for hemorrhoidal prolapse is often delayed because of the significant pain associated with sometimes extensive hemorrhoidectomy to correct the defect. The advent of the stapled anopexy was hailed as the procedure to relieve mucosal prolapse with little pain. Obviously, this would be a major advance in the care of patients with mucosal prolapse. However, the results presented in this randomized multicenter trial of anopexy versus hemorrhoidectomy show that stapled anopexy is most appropriate for simple mucosal prolapse and that only 29% of patients could be "cured." However, hemorrhoidectomy did not fare much better because only 43% of these patients were "cured." The findings of this study suggest that neither of the operations correct the underlying defect and, therefore, innovative therapy must be developed to improve operative outcome. The etiologic factors associated with prolapse are obviously not correct to a sufficient extent to return patients to normal living, and thus, reinvigorated analysis of the underlying pathophysiology should be undertaken to yield new therapies with improved results.

K. E. Behrns, MD

Rigorous Histopathological Assessment of the Colectomy Specimen in Patients With Inflammatory Bowel Disease Unclassified Does Not Predict Outcome After Ileal Pouch–Anal Anastomosis

Nasseri Y, Melmed G, Wang HL, et al (Cedars-Sinai Med Ctr, Los Angeles, CA; et al)

Am J Gastroenterol 105:155-161, 2010

Objectives.—Abdominal colectomy has been used in patients with inflammatory bowel disease unclassified (IBDU), requiring surgery to allow histopathological evaluation of the colectomy specimen to rule out Crohn's disease (CD). We evaluated whether any histopathological feature was associated with an adverse postoperative outcome.

Methods.—Patients with ulcerative colitis (UC) or IBDU undergoing ileal pouch–anal anastomosis (IPAA) were prospectively examined. A checklist of 17 histopathological features atypical for UC was developed. Outcomes of acute pouchitis (AP), chronic pouchitis (CP), and *de novo* CD were assessed.

Results.—The 153 study patients included 119 (78%) UC and 34 (22%) IBDU patients. The following atypical features were identified (n; %): broad-based ulcer (99; 65%), appendiceal involvement (78; 51%), V-shaped ulcer (48; 31%), crypt-associated granuloma (42; 27%), isolated giant cells (39; 25%), discontinuous active inflammation (36; 24%), slit-like fissure (32; 21%), discontinuous chronic inflammation (16; 10%), ileal villous architectural distortion (12; 8%), neural hypertrophy (10; 7%), backwash ileitis (10; 7%), transmural inflammation (8; 5%), discontinuous ileitis (8; 5%), muscle hypertrophy (5; 3%), ileal ulcer (4; 3%), and ileal pyloric metaplasia (1; 1%). A total of 29 patients (19%) developed AP, 17 (11%) developed CP, and 13 patients (8%) developed *de novo* CD. On univariate analysis, *de novo* CD developed in 3 of the 10 patients (30%) with neural hypertrophy compared with only 10 of the 143 patients (7%) without neural hypertrophy ($P = 0.01$). Multivariate regression did not show a single atypical histopathological feature, which predicted a worse outcome after IPAA.

Conclusions.—No single atypical histopathological feature of UC, or combination of features, was associated with any adverse pouch outcome after IPAA. There seems to be no value in performing a staged IPAA in IBDU patients.

▶ In about 80% of patients with inflammatory bowel disease involving the colon, the diagnosis of ulcerative colitis is readily apparent and colectomy, proctectomy, and ileal pouch-anal anastomosis (IPAA) are performed with good results and a functional outcome. However, in the remaining 20% of patients the diagnosis of ulcerative colitis, Crohn's disease, or unclassified inflammatory bowel disease may be in play. Of course, the fear is that the surgeon would perform IPAA in a patient with Crohn's disease and a poor outcome would ensue. To circumvent this situation, subtotal colectomy is performed to permit histologic analysis and to markedly decrease the possibility of performing IPAA in a patient with Crohn's disease. This study demonstrates that this strategy, unfortunately, has not resulted in the appropriate diagnosis and operation. Although Nasseri et al critically examined 17 histologic variables that may predict the diagnosis of ulcerative colitis versus Crohn's disease, multivariate logistic regression analysis failed to identify any significant parameter. This study highlights the difficulty in distinguishing ulcerative colitis from Crohn's disease not only histologically but also clinically. In addition, serum biomarkers have not proven to be diagnostic, and even genomic analysis will not clearly distinguish between these diseases. It would appear that surgeons will perform IPAA in some patients who will have a delayed diagnosis of

Crohn's disease. So what are the consequences? Patients with indeterminate colitis who undergo IPAA may develop chronic pouchitis that may be complicated by perineal fistulae, abscess, and pouch failure. Although this concern is appropriate, the incidence of pouch failure does not appear to be appreciably different among patients with ulcerative colitis versus indeterminate colitis. Therefore, IPAA is appropriate in patients with unclassified inflammatory bowel disease in whom overt signs of Crohn's disease are not evident clinically or histologically.

K. E. Behrns, MD

Single-Incision Laparoscopic Cholecystectomy Using Conventional Instruments: Early Experience in Comparison with the Gold Standard

Philipp SR, Miedema BW, Thaler K (Univ Hosps and Clinics, Columbia, MO)

J Am Coll Surg 209:632-637, 2009

Background.—The aim of this pilot study was to describe our initial experience with single-incision laparoscopic cholecystectomy (SILC) using conventional laparoscopic equipment in comparison with concurrent patients undergoing conventional multiincision laparoscopic cholecystectomy.

Study Design.—During the 7-month study period, data from all consecutive patients undergoing SILC by two surgeons were retrospectively analyzed and compared with data from patients undergoing conventional laparoscopic cholecystectomy by the same surgeons during the same time period. Outcomes measures included completion rate of attempted SILC, operative time, length of hospital stay, postoperative pain, and assessment of complications.

Results.—From 51 laparoscopic cholecystectomies performed during the study period, 29 were attempted using single-incision technique and 22 were performed using the conventional four incisions. Of the attempted SILC cases, 14 (48%) were successfully completed, with the remainder requiring one to three additional skin incisions. There were no conversions to open in either group. Operative time was significantly longer in SILC cases compared with conventional laparoscopic cholecystectomy (85 versus 67 minutes; $p = 0.01$). There was a tendency toward greater postoperative pain in the SILC group. No substantial difference in complications was identified.

Conclusions.—SILC using conventional laparoscopic instrumentation is an effective alternative to standard four-incision laparoscopic cholecystectomy in selected patients. Development of a standardized technique and additional experience is needed for more consistent success. Additional studies of SILC are needed to demonstrate safety, define selection criteria, and determine any benefits over conventional laparoscopic cholecystectomy.

▶ The advent of new technologies such as natural orifice transluminal endoscopic surgery (NOTES) is often accompanied by a new generation of techniques in existing surgical procedures. In this case, the development of NOTES has resulted in attempts to improve on laparoscopic cholecystectomy by the introduction of single-incision laparoscopic cholecystectomy (SILC). The purported advantage of SILC is one periumbilical incision that permits safe cholecystectomy that heals with a nearly imperceptible scar. The cosmetic outcome of this procedure should compete favorably with NOTES in the eyes of the patient. From the surgeon's perspective, this procedure would likely be preferable to NOTES because it uses the already learned techniques of laparoscopic cholecystectomy, whereas NOTES requires several skill sets that may not be in the domain of the practicing general surgeon, and it violates the enteric lumen. Therefore, SILC would appear to be a better alternative than NOTES, but is it a major advance over conventional laparoscopic cholecystectomy? Philipp et al compared SILC with conventional lap cholecystectomy in 29 patients in the SILC arm of the nonrandomized study. They found that SILC resulted in longer operative time, increased postoperative pain, and more local wound complications, and it was technically more difficult to perform. Although these data do not bode well for the rapid introduction of SILC, it should be noted that these procedures were performed by the introduction of 3 standard trocars through an umbilical incision—an operative configuration that is difficult to manipulate. The recent development of single-port working platforms will ease these constraints and likely provide higher surgeon satisfaction with the operation. Nonetheless, with the introduction of new techniques such as SILC come new challenges that must be balanced by the question: Is this a safer operation for the patient?

K. E. Behrns, MD

The Association Between Cholecystectomy and Gastroesophageal Reflux Symptoms: A Prospective Controlled Study

Lin OS, Kozarek RA, Arai A, et al (Virginia Mason Med Ctr, Seattle, WA; et al)
Ann Surg 251:40-45, 2010

Objective.—A large controlled prospective observational study to compare pre-and postsurgery changes in reflux symptoms between cholecystectomy and hernia repair surgery patients.

Summary Background Data.—Six studies have suggested that gastroesophageal reflux worsens after cholecystectomy. However, all these studies had design limitations.

Methods.—We recruited 302 patients scheduled to undergo elective cholecystectomy (study group) or hernia repair (controls) at 2 hospitals. Both groups filled out the validated Reflux Symptom Score (RSS) and

Gastrointestinal Symptom Rating Scale (GSRS) questionnaires 1 to 15 days prior to and 4 to 12 weeks after the operation. Changes in symptom scores between the pre and postsurgery assessments were measured, and compared between the 2 groups.

Results.—Baseline RSS and GSRS reflux subscores were higher in the study group than controls (1.44 vs. 1.02 and 1.91 vs. 1.43, respectively; $P < 0.05$). There were no significant differences in any of the symptom score changes between the 2 groups except for the GSRS pain subscore, which decreased more in the study group than the control group (−0.59 vs.−0.10; $P < 0.001$). With regard to reflux, the RSS decreased by −0.34 in the study group and −0.14 in controls ($P = 0.27$), while the GSRS reflux subscore decreased by −0.32 in the study group and −0.05 in controls ($P = 0.12$). GSRS diarrhea and constipation subscores decreased slightly after surgery, to the same extent in both groups.

Conclusions.—This large prospective controlled study, the only one using validated reflux symptom questionnaires, shows that cholecystectomy does not lead to an increase in reflux symptoms. As expected, GSRS pain subscores were decreased in the cholecystectomy group but not the controls.

▶ Upper gastrointestinal symptoms are frequently nonspecific, and identification of the cause of the symptoms often requires an extensive evaluation. Not surprisingly, these nonspecific symptoms can result in an incorrect diagnosis based on symptoms alone. As Lin et al note, the diagnosis of gastroesophageal reflux is purportedly increased following cholecystectomy. To specifically address this question, they performed a prospective study using patients as their own control before and after cholecystectomy. However, surprisingly, no association between cholecystectomy and the development of reflux was evident in this carefully controlled study. Although previous studies have suggested that cholecystectomy may be followed by reflux, the hard evidence of this is lacking. Furthermore, the diagnosis of reflux alone requires a significant evaluation that may include esophagogastroduodenoscopy, esophageal manometry, upper gastrointestinal barium radiography, a 24-hour pH probe, and a gastric emptying study. If 4 or 5 diagnostic studies are required to diagnose reflux in isolation, the diagnosis in combination with symptoms reflective of gallbladder-associated diseases will not be any easier. This study highlights the specificity required for various upper gastrointestinal diagnoses and how confusing the various combinations of symptoms may be. Therefore, it is not surprising that some patients will undergo operative treatment for a proximal gut condition and have persistent symptoms. Operative treatment for "functional" upper gastrointestinal diseases may result in this outcome and, thus, this possibility should be discussed with patients. In summary, patients with upper gastrointestinal symptoms should undergo a directed specific workup and understand that some operative therapies may be accompanied by persistent symptoms.

K. E. Behrns, MD

Transanal Endoscopic Microsurgery Is Feasible for Adenomas Throughout the Entire Rectum: A Prospective Study

de Graaf EJR, Doornebosch PG, Tetteroo GWM, et al (IJsselland Hosp, Capelle aan den IJssel, The Netherlands; Leiden Univ Medical Ctr, The Netherlands)

Dis Colon Rectum 52:1107-1113, 2009

Introduction.—Transanal endoscopic microsurgery for rectal adenomas is safe and has low recurrence rates. However, the feasibility of the procedure for all rectal adenomas is unclear. This issue was investigated prospectively.

Methods.—From 1996 to 2007, 353 consecutive rectal adenomas were evaluated according to a standard protocol. Transanal endoscopic microsurgery was intended in all rectal adenomas.

Results.—The median diameter was 3 cm and median distance was 8 cm. The peritoneum was opened peroperatively without any adverse effects in 8.7 percent. The conversion rate was 9.6 percent, with an alternative local procedure performed in 4.2 percent and a transabdominal procedure performed in 5.4 percent. Conversion rate correlated with the distance of the tumor ($P = 0.007$) and the operating surgeon's level of experience ($P = 0.004$). The median operation time was 45 minutes. Operation time correlated with specimen area, experience, and operating surgeon (all $P < 0.001$). All rectal adenomas were excised in one piece. Complete margins were observed in 85 percent. Rectal adenomas with incomplete margins were larger ($P < 0.001$) and were located more proximally ($P < 0.001$). Morbidity was 7.8 percent and mortality 0.6 percent. The median hospital stay was four days. The median follow-up was 27 months. The recurrence rate at three years was 9.1 percent. The median time from operation to recurrence was 12 (range, 4–54) months. Resection margin status was a predictor of recurrence, with 6.1 percent recurrence in cases of complete margins and 25.2 percent in cases of incomplete margins ($P < 0.001$).

Conclusions.—For nearly all rectal adenomas, transanal endoscopic microsurgery is safe, feasible, and has excellent results.

▶ Is transanal endoscopic microsurgery (TEM) the new laparoscopy for anorectal surgery? Adoption of this technique has been relatively slow, but, increasingly, published reports on the feasibility and outcomes for excision of rectal adenomas and early stage cancers show promise. The study by de Graaf et al is notable because of the number of patients (N = 342) treated for rectal adenomas (N = 353). This represents the largest series with excellent outcomes. The conversion rate was just shy of 10% with nearly 9% of cases associated with opening of the peritoneum, which did not appear to be a significant technical problem. Importantly, all the adenomas were removed in 1 piece, a less frequent occurrence in transanal excision. In addition, the margins were complete in 85% and the recurrence rate was about 9%. These results show that this technique is no longer a gimmick, but, in skilled hands, this technology results in excellent outcomes. As the authors point out, a few issues should be addressed before widespread adoption. First, the equipment can be finicky, and meticulous care is required. The manufacturer can address these issues with improved design, service, and education. Most important, however, is the need for excellent training for surgeons performing anorectal surgery. This should come not only through colorectal surgery training programs but also general surgery training. Will the technique proliferate to the thousands of already trained surgeons? Likely not, because only those surgeons with a relatively large anorectal practice will find a regular use for TEM. However, patients seeking care for anorectal adenomas or early stage cancers should consider seeking surgeons highly trained in this technique.

K. E. Behrns, MD

Trends and Outcomes of Hospitalizations for Peptic Ulcer Disease in the United States, 1993 to 2006

Wang YR, Richter JE, Dempsey DT (Temple Univ School of Medicine, Philadelphia, PA)

Ann Surg 251:51-58, 2010

Objectives.—Despite progress in diagnosis and treatment, peptic ulcer disease (PUD) remains a common reason for hospitalization and operation. The purpose of this study was to quantify the time trends of hospitalizations and operations for PUD in the United States (US) since 1993.

Data and Methods.—The Healthcare Cost and Utilization Project Nationwide Inpatient Sample is a 20% stratified sample of all hospitalizations in the United States. It was used to study hospitalizations with PUD as the principal diagnosis during 1993 to 2006, including details on ulcer site, complications, procedures, and mortality. Statistical methods included the χ^2 test and multivariate logistic regression.

Results.—The national estimate of hospitalizations for PUD decreased significantly from 222,601 in 1993 to 156,108 in 2006 (−29.9%), with a larger reduction in duodenal ulcers (95,552 in 1993 vs. 60,029 in 2006, −37.2%) than gastric ulcers (106,987 in 1993 vs. 86,064 in 2006, −19.6%). The inpatient mortality rate of PUD decreased from 3.8% to 2.7% during 1993 to 2006 ($P < 0.001$). Hemorrhage remained the most common complication (71.6% in 1993; 73.3% in 2006) but perforation had the highest mortality (15.1% in 1993; 10.6% in 2006). In comparison to 1993, patients hospitalized for PUD in 2006 more frequently had endoscopic treatment to control bleeding (12.9% vs. 22.2%, $P < 0.001$), similar use of surgical oversewing of ulcer (7.6% vs. 7.4%), less use of gastrectomy (4.4% vs. 2.1%, $P < 0.001$), and less use of vagotomy (5.7% vs. 1.7%, $P < 0.001$). In multivariate logistic regressions, the determinants of mortality were similar in 1993 and 2006.

Conclusions.—Hospitalizations for PUD decreased in the United States from 1993 to 2006, suggesting a decrease in the prevalence and/or severity of ulcer complications over this recent time period. Despite increased patient age and comorbidities, there has been a significant decrease in

PUD mortality, a significant increase in the use of therapeutic endoscopy for bleeding ulcer, and a significant decrease in the use of definitive surgery (vagotomy or resection) for ulcer complications.

▶ Since the introduction of histamine antagonists in the 1970s, followed by the use of proton pump inhibitors, the elective surgical treatment of peptic ulcer disease (PUD) has decreased. Furthermore, identification of the causal agent, *Helicobacter pylori*, has changed the type of operations performed. Wang et al used the Nationwide Inpatient Sample (NIS) database to look at trends (1993-2006) in the incidence, treatment, and outcome of patients with PUD. They found that the hospital admission rate decreased and mortality decreased, but the rate of death from perforation remained high, endoscopic treatment was used more frequently to control bleeding, and the performance of vagotomy and gastric resection decreased. This study is an excellent example of the use of the NIS to show treatment trends over time. Likely, no single institutional study would have enough patients to identify the trends noted in this work. Furthermore, the reduction in mortality is the most impressive statistic because the commonly held belief is that although treatment of PUD may have been refined over the last few decades, this change was not accompanied by decreased mortality. In fact, although not necessarily causal, as the authors surmise, the reduction in mortality could be due to increased use of endoscopic treatment of bleeding and decreased performance of definitive ulcer operations. Since we know the infectious cause of PUD, when, if ever, should we perform vagotomy or gastric resection? Because of the risk of postgastrectomy complications, these operations should only be performed in *H pylori*-negative patients with complications that mandate resection. This is an infrequent finding with very few of these operations performed annually even in large teaching hospitals.

K. E. Behrns, MD

A Single-Center Surgical Experience of 122 Patients With Single and Multiple Hepatocellular Adenomas

Dokmak S, Paradis V, Vilgrain V, et al (Univ of Paris and Beaujon Hosp, Clichy, France)

Gastroenterology 137:1698-1705, 2009

Background & Aims.—Hepatocellular adenoma (HA) is associated with risk of bleeding and malignancy, justifying resection. Patients with multiple forms of HA are difficult to manage. We evaluated the characteristics and outcome of 122 patients with single and multiple HAs after surgery.

Methods.—From 1990 to 2004, 122 patients (14 male) underwent surgical resection. Complications (hemorrhage and malignancy) were assessed according to size, number, and histologic subtype (steatotic, telangiectatic, and unclassified), with a mean follow-up period of 70 months.

Results.—Hemorrhagic HA occurred in 21% of cases and malignant HA occurred in 8%. Risk of complications was not related to the number of HAs but was associated with size (>5 cm), especially of telangiectatic and unclassified subtypes. Patients with steatotic HA had a low risk of complications. Malignant HA was more frequent in men (43%); all patients treated by partial resection survived, without recurrent malignancy, after a mean follow-up period of 78 months. After surgery, 109 patients with benign HA revealed recurrence or progression of HA in 8% and regression in 9% of cases. No complications were observed in 11 women who became pregnant during the follow-up period.

Conclusions.—Patients with HAs greater than 5 cm, telangiectatic or unclassified subtypes, and men have an increased risk of complicated disease; resection should be restricted to these patients. The risk of complications was not related to the number of HAs, so patients with multiple HAs do not need liver transplantation.

▶ The very experienced and high-functioning liver surgery group from Beaujon Hospital in Clichy, France, presents a contemporary and thorough analysis of patients with single and multiple hepatic adenomas. This article serves as the current landmark article in the surgical treatment of this uncommon disease. The authors used a well-established database to prospectively collect data, which allowed them to identify subtypes of hepatic adenomas and to establish similarities and differences between patients with single and multiple adenomas. Importantly, they identified the pathologic characteristics of steatotic adenomas, telangiectatic adenomas, and otherwise unclassified adenomas. They also noted that patients with numerous adenomas (2-10 adenomas) and liver adenomatosis (LA; > 10 adenomas) had more similarities than differences, and that the designation of LA probably added little to diagnostic and therapeutic decision-making processes. Importantly, they found that size (especially those > 5 cm) of the adenoma was the best predictor of complications, especially bleeding. They recommend surgical resection for patients with hepatic adenomas that have the following characteristics: men with hepatocellular adenoma (HA), adenomas 5 cm or greater in size, telangiectatic adenomas, and otherwise undesignated adenomas. This report likely represents the current definitive article on the surgical management of hepatic adenoma, which is a relatively rare disease. This publication demonstrates the value of prospectively collected data over a long period of time, and how expert groups, focused on organ-specific surgery, can interpret these data to advance care of the surgical patient.

K. E. Behrns, MD

Emergent embolization of the gastroduodenal artery in the treatment of upper gastrointestinal bleeding. The experience from a surgeon-initiated interventional program

Burris JM, Lin PH, Johnston WF, et al (Michael E. DeBakey VA Med Ctr, Houston, TX)

Am J Surg 198:59-63, 2009

Background.—Intractable nonvariceal upper gastrointestinal bleeding (UGIB) is associated with significant morbidity and mortality. Endovascular therapy is an alternative to surgery for high-risk patients.

Materials and Methods.—Review of prospectively collected data from patients who underwent emergent gastroduodenal artery embolization for UGIB.

Results.—Eight patients (mean age 68.5 years) were identified. They all had significant comorbidities and were deemed to be at high risk for surgical intervention. Endoscopy was performed in 7 patients. Active extravasation was present at the time of embolization in 5 (62.5%) patients. The technical success and clinical response rates were each 100%. The 30-day mortality rate was 8%. There were no procedure-related complications. During mean follow-up of 9 months, 1 patient developed recurrent bleeding that was managed conservatively.

Comments.—Endovascular embolization is a safe alternative to open surgical intervention after failed endoscopic treatment for UGIB. Surgeons with endovascular skills can perform this procedure with superior results.

▶ This case series addresses the important topic of endovascular treatment of recalcitrant upper gastrointestinal bleeding (UGIB) from a duodenal ulcer. The mortality of UGIB has remained 15% to 20% for several decades despite advances in endoscopic and endovascular therapies. The article by Burris et al highlights the fact that timely embolization of the gastroduodenal artery was performed by endovascular surgeons. The mean time to embolization was approximately 4.5 hours with prompt correction of coagulation deficits. The results are quite remarkable in that 100% of the patients had both technical and clinical successes with only 3 units of blood transfused postembolization in the 8 patients. The mortality rate was 8%—half of the traditionally reported mortality! Even more impressive was the fact that these results are stellar, albeit in 8 patients, compared with the summary results of the 10 series shown in Table 2 in the original article. The data in Table 2 suggest that 1 in 3 patients will not be adequately treated by endovascular therapy and thus operative intervention is required. Is time to intervention the key to success? Too frequently patients with UGIB undergo 1 to 3 endoscopic procedures before embolization or surgery is considered in these high-risk patients. Furthermore, in some institutions, angiography may not be performed without obtaining a tagged red blood cell scan that demonstrates active bleeding—a further delay of therapeutic intervention. Thus, the time-honored dictum of performing definitive therapy before the time of transfusion of 6 units of blood appears appropriate.

The key to success is likely limiting the bleeding as soon as possible with definitive therapy. The authors should prove this with a larger, follow-up study.

K. E. Behrns, MD

Prospective Clinical Trial of Factors Predicting the Early Development of Incisional Hernia after Midline Laparotomy

Veljkovic R, Protic M, Gluhovic A, et al (Clinical Ctr Vojvodina, Novi Sad, Serbia; et al)

J Am Coll Surg 210:210-219, 2010

Background.—Information-based scoring systems predictive of outcomes of midline laparotomy are needed; these systems can support surgical decisions with the aim of improving patient outcomes and quality of life, and reducing the risk of secondary surgical procedures.

Study Design.—All study subjects were followed for a minimum of 6 months after operation. Numerous demographic, clinical, treatment, and outcomes-related perioperative factors were recorded to determine statistical association with the primary end point: incisional hernia development. The first analysis was designed to establish the statistical model (scoring system) for estimating the risk of incisional hernia within 6 months of midline laparotomy. Univariate and multivariate analyses were performed. A simple additive model was constructed using stepwise logistic and linear regression. The second part of the study analysis was validation of the scoring systems developed initially.

Results.—A logistic linear minimum regression model was developed based on four covariates independently predictive of incisional hernia: Body mass index (BMI) > 24.4 kg/m^2; fascial suture to incision ratio (SIR) < 4.2; deep surgical site, deep space, or organ infection (SSI); and time to suture removal or complete epithelialization > 16 days (TIME). The hernia risk scoring system equation $[p(\%) = 32(SIR) + 30(SSI) + 9(TIME) + 2(BMI)]$ provided accurate estimates of incisional hernia according to stratified risk groups based on total score: low (0 to 5 points), 1.0%; moderate (6 to 15 points), 9.7%; increased (16 to 50 points), 30.2%; and markedly increased (>50 points), 73.1%.

Conclusions.—A statistically valid, straightforward, and clinically useful predictive model was developed for estimating the risk of incisional hernia within 6 months of midline laparotomy. Prospective independent validation of this model appears indicated.

▶ Veljkovic et al prospectively developed a model that predicts incisional hernia development following a midline laparotomy. Four independent covariates were used in the development of this model: body mass index, fascial suture-to-incision ratio, deep surgical site infection, and time to suture removal. Most of these factors make intuitive sense, especially because body mass index, suture-to-incision ratio, and deep organ space infection have previously been identified as factors associated with incisional hernia development. These factors can largely be modified by the patient or surgeon. The patient can lose weight under the direction of a care provider. The surgeon should select the appropriate suture length and remove sutures in a timely fashion. Although deep space organ infection cannot necessarily be eliminated, it can be recognized early and appropriately treated. Whether this would curtail the development of an incisional hernia is unknown. So if these factors have been previously known to be associated with hernia formation and they are modifiable, why do up to 15% of midline abdominal incisions result in hernia formation? Clearly, not all factors are included in the authors' model, and likely many factors are not recognized, especially the pathobiology of hernia repair. Wound healing depends on adequate activation of the inflammatory response with recruitment of first neutrophils followed by fibroblasts that produced adequate amounts of cross-linked collagen. This process is balanced by the production of matrix metalloproteinases, the biology and activation of which is incompletely understood. This article identifies clearly modifiable factors; however, suspicion abounds that even meticulous attention to these factors will not result in a significant reduction in hernia formation and that further investigation of the underlying pathophysiologic factors will be necessary.

K. E. Behrns, MD

The Effect of Mesh Removal and Selective Neurectomy on Persistent Postherniotomy Pain

Aasvang EK, Kehlet H (Copenhagen Univ, Denmark)
Ann Surg 249:327-334, 2009

Summary Background Data and Objective.—Persistent pain affects everyday activities in 5% to 8% of patients after groin hernia repair. Because previous reports on the effect of neurectomy and/or mesh removal suffer from methodological problems we performed a detailed prospective trial of the effect of neurectomy and mesh removal on persistent postherniotomy pain.

Methods.—Twenty-one patients with postherniotomy pain >1 year, pain-related impairment of daily activities and a well-defined maximum pain localization where included. Inserted mesh was removed and a selective neurectomy was done in case of macroscopic nerve injury. The primary end point was changes in pain-related impairment of everyday activities assessed by the validated activities assessment scale before surgery and 6 months postoperatively. Quantitative sensory testing was used to evaluate sensory functions pre and postoperatively.

Results.—All patients completed the 6-month follow-up. There was a significant improvement in the activities assessment scale score for the whole group (preoperative vs. 6 months = 27 vs. 13 points, $P = 0.004$), despite 3 patients worsening. Quantitative sensory testing showed a significant postoperative increase in pressure pain detection threshold ($P = 0.045$) and cutaneous detection and pain thresholds (mechanical and warmth) ($P < 0.03$).

Conclusions.—Selective neurectomy and mesh removal may improve pain-related activity impairment in patients with persistent postherniotomy pain. Detailed neurophysiologic assessment is recommended to identify patients who may or may not benefit from reoperation and to allocate patients to specific surgical and/or medical intervention.

▶ Aasvang and Kehlet report on the important finding and treatment of persistent pain following inguinal hernia pain, a finding that complicates 5% to 8% of all hernia repairs. Although the number of patients was small at 21, the function assessment was extensive and the data complete. The results show that patients who had mesh removal or neurectomy fared well with decreased pain in most patients. Only 3 patients did not experience pain relief. Of note, the symptoms were not related to depression or anxiety. Furthermore, follow-up at 6 months demonstrated that some patients had more pain at 6-month follow-up compared with pain at 3 months. Recurrent hernias were noted in only 2 patients. These findings highlight an important, disabling condition that complicates hernia repair, especially repair with mesh. Too frequently, these patients are dismissed from clinic as malingerers who do not wish to return to work. However, this study shows that properly selected patients benefit from mesh removal or neurectomy. Furthermore, their work shows that meticulous technique is required because in many cases mesh was incorporated in the cord structures or the sutures trapped nerves. Therefore, careful attention to operative detail is required and of great potential consequence. Furthermore, this work highlights the importance of detailed and thorough training in hernia repair. These operations can and do have major morbidity that significantly disrupts daily activities.

K. E. Behrns, MD

11 Oncology

Introduction

This year has seen a number of important clinical trials and clinical contributions that should have impact on the surgeon who practices cancer surgery. Here are synopses of the articles I reviewed this year.

In the area of breast cancer, a study by Smith et al from MD Anderson Cancer Center looked at breast-conserving surgery in older patients and geographic variation. While a substantial portion of women in the United States with early breast cancer were treated with breast conservation, there is substantial geographic variation that appears to be related to socioeconomic advantages. Adequately evaluating margins in patients who received breast-conserving surgery remains a challenge.

A very novel paper in cancer research is studying a new technology—optical coherence tomography. While this is in early stages of development, and has some limitations, this type of technology should help the surgeon intraoperatively to determine margin status.

In the paper by Blair et al, they show there is not yet uniform consensus among surgeons regarding an "acceptable" margin status for either invasive breast cancer or DCIS.

In a paper in the *Journal of Clinical Oncology* is a large prospective multicenter study that evaluates different models of prediction of non-sentinel lymph node status. In their opinion, the Memorial Sloan-Kettering Cancer Center nanogram and Tenon score outperform other methods for all patients.

In a paper from the University Hospitals Leuven, the authors show that older patients may have a greater likelihood of axillary lymph node involvement. Whether or not this is related to the fact that screening mammography is routinely not performed after the age of 70 is unclear. Genomic information, which is rapidly being developed, will likely begin to identify tumors that are more likely to spread to lymph nodes.

In a paper from H Lee Moffitt Cancer Center, Dr Charles E. Cox and colleagues examined the indications for sentinel lymph node biopsy in the setting of prophylactic mastectomy. They concluded that sentinel lymph node biopsy is not indicated in patients undergoing bilateral prophylactic mastectomy. Also, patients undergoing mastectomy for very early stage disease on one side, but prophylaxis on the other generally have no benefit from sentinel lymph node biopsy in the contralateral prophylactic mastectomy.

In a paper from the University of Arkansas, the authors use a technique of axillary reverse mapping to demonstrate lymphatic drainage from the arm. This manuscript has some very nice photographs; however, postoperative sequelae to axillary dissection are mitigated by careful dissection of sentinel lymph nodes. Clearly, sentinel lymph node biopsy has significantly less morbidity than axillary lymph node dissection.

There is an excellent paper from David Krag and The National Surgical Adjuvant Breast and Bowel Project that looks at specific screening methods in obtaining high overall sentinel lymph node resection rates.

The Danish Breast Cancer Cooperative Group documented the prevalence of breast pain following surgery for breast cancer in a substantial portion of patients. Breast conservation and sentinel lymph node biopsies have reduced these problems but not eliminated them.

In the next few years, genomic information about breast cancer will become available. In the meantime, segregating breast cancer tumors into specific categories such as the basal type of breast cancer (triple negative breast cancer) will be helpful to select individual therapies. In a paper in the *Journal of Cancer*, the authors have long-term follow up of patients with this type of tumor. It confirms the feeling that basal-type tumors possess a different mechanism of spread when compared to ER-positive tumors. Look for new targeted therapies to impact this spread.

The National Cancer Institute's Surveillance, Epidemiology, and End Results registry provided insight into surgeon recommendations and receipt of mastectomy, which was published in JAMA. About one-fourth of mastectomy use is related to patient preference, which appears to be out of concern for disease recurrence as well as fear of radiation or the inconvenience of radiation therapy. Careful discussion by the surgeon caregiver (as documented in this study) will help select the proper surgical intervention for each individual patient.

In a related manuscript, a paper in the *Journal of the National Cancer Institute* looks specifically at the metropolitan Los Angeles and Detroit areas, examining the use of mastectomy among racially and ethnically diverse breast cancer patients. Once again, women who had concerns about recurrence and radiation therapy tended to have higher mastectomy rates.

In a paper from the Winship Cancer Institute the authors documented a substantially higher number of "non eligible" African American patients as well as "refusal" in dealing with minority patients with stage III breast cancer. Understanding their reasons for refusal will help providers to administer more appropriate and effective treatments in these patients.

Finally, a very important paper from the MD Anderson Cancer Center published in *Cancer* documents the important advancements in treatment of breast cancer patients because of clinical trial participation in that institution. Certainly, the NSABP and ACOSOG clinical trials cooperative group welcome participation of surgeons from nonacademic institutions as well as academic institutions, providing the opportunity for all surgeons to administer cutting-edge interventions for their patients with breast cancer.

In a very important paper from Henry Ford Hospital, these authors show a very nice interdependence of hospital volume, showing that higher volume predicts a higher resource count and predicts a higher health count quality score.

In a related paper from Johns Hopkins University, the authors showed that less than half the patients with pancreatic cancer were being referred to high volume centers, especially among minority patients. Clearly, high-volume centers have more accessible resources and tend to have better outcomes for tumors such as pancreatic cancer.

In a study from the National Cancer Center Hospital in Tokyo, Japan, the authors demonstrate the histologic characteristics of intraductal papillary mucinous neoplasm associated with recurrence.

In a paper published from the New South Wales Pancreatic Cancer Network in Sydney, Australia, the authors looked at patients undergoing resection for invasive pancreatic cancer, and showed that a resection margin of greater than 1.5 millimeters is important to long-term survival. This was even more important in patients who had tumors of the pancreatic head.

One of the major complications following a pancreatic resection is anastomotic leak. In a multi-institutional group, the authors display that 3 different pancreatic surgeons from 2 different institutions were able to obtain excellent results utilizing a specific type of duct-to-mucosa anastomosis, which is well detailed in the figures in the manuscript.

There were some important papers in the area of colorectal surgery. For example, the paper from the Mayo Clinic examined a group of patients receiving neoadjuvant treatment for rectal cancer. Anastomotic leak was associated with high ASA class and cardiovascular disease as well as age. While it requires a second procedure, ileostomy will certainly minimize the risk of morbidity in these patients following neoadjuvant treatment.

In a paper from Basel, Switzerland, the authors show that tumor border configuration, in addition to TMN staging, better stratifies the stage II colorectal cancer patient. This feature, as well as potentially newer genomic and gene-based panels, will help to segregate patients with stage II colon cancer into prognostic groups that require further adjuvant therapies.

Patients who have malignant colorectal obstruction require intervention but frequently have a number of comorbidities. Stent placement can offer palliation. A significant study looks at quality of life and symptom control after stent placement. The authors concluded this was an excellent primary treatment even though recommendation for stent placement versus open surgical procedures is very individualized.

There are several contributions with respect to gastric cancer. A large single-institution study from Korea evaluates the accuracy of surgical diagnosis in early gastric cancer. The point of this contribution is that surgical evaluation can improve preoperative studies for evaluation of gastric cancer; however, there are a few surgeons with enough experience in the United States to have the expertise to completely use this evaluative process.

Another paper from the National Cancer Center in Korea looked at intraoperative surgical staging. Once again, the authors concluded that intraoperative staging can help predict prognosis. This requires an experienced and well-trained surgeon with expertise in gastric cancer.

A paper from MD Anderson looked at 600 consecutive patients with gastroesophageal cancer and showed that older patients had a higher likelihood of reduced survival. This was true whether patients had primary surgical intervention or preoperative therapy. This is likely due to comorbidities. The future studies should include age as a variable in prognosis.

There are several interesting papers with respect to melanoma. In a study from the John Wayne Cancer Institute, the authors look at the tumor suppressor gene RUNX3 and its impact on the development of melanoma. These studies are important because targeting this gene may result in more efficacious treatment with fewer side effects.

In a study from the Hebrew University Hospital in Jerusalem, the authors used an autologous melanoma vaccine and showed that it induced antitumor immune responses. While this vaccine may not be effective in patients with widespread metastatic disease, it may be very effective in patients with high risk of metastatic disease but only microscopic foci.

There is a preclinical paper from a group in Austria that looks at a combination of treatments using the epidermal factor receptor inhibitor erlotinib and the vascular endothelial growth factor monoclonal antibody bevacizumab. This paper demonstrates the scientific rationale for this combination, and it shows it to be quite effective. Clinical trials are currently underway using this combination.

In the miscellaneous category, there is a large series presented that uses a combined blunt clamp dissection in LigaSure ligation for hepatic parenchymal dissection. The authors demonstrate superb figures and a number of technical aspects for successful hepatic surgery.

In a paper from Memorial Sloan-Kettering, the authors study subcentimeter pulmonary nodules in patients who undergo hepatic resection for metastatic colorectal cancer. They document follow-up of these pulmonary nodules and conclude in this very large series that the presence of subcentimeter pulmonary nodules was not associated with earlier progression or decreased survival.

Appendiceal neoplasms are relatively rare. In a study from Johns Hopkins, the authors show that complete cytoreduction offers long-term survival benefit to patients.

Finally, a large randomized clinical trial from a number of Danish hospitals showed that 80% oxygen administration did not result in a difference in surgical site infection. While this paper may be regarded as a "negative study," it answers an important question regarding the need for administration of higher oxygen levels to patients and substantiates best practice for reducing surgical site infection as well as secondary pulmonary complications.

This year has seen a large number of outstanding contributions that identify better surgical practices, new technologies, and newer innovations for our surgical patients with malignant disease. Adhering to recommendations of these authors will undoubtedly improve the outcomes for our patients.

Timothy J. Eberlein, MD

Breast

Breast-Conserving Surgery in Older Patients with Invasive Breast Cancer: Current Patterns of Treatment Across the United States

Smith GL, Xu Y, Shih Y-CT, et al (Univ of Texas MD Anderson Cancer Ctr, Houston; et al)

J Am Coll Surg 209:425-433, 2009

Background.—Breast-conserving surgery (BCS) followed by radiotherapy is as effective as mastectomy for treatment of early invasive breast cancer. But earlier studies report low BCS use rates of 12% to 43% nationally, especially in older patients. We sought to determine current patterns and predictors of BCS use.

Study Design.—In a national Medicare database of all beneficiaries (age greater than 65 years) with incident invasive breast cancer treated with operation in 2003, claims codes identified BCS versus mastectomy and demographic, treatment, and geographic region covariates. The 2003 Area Resource File provided socioeconomic covariates. Logistic regression modeled predictors of BCS.

Results.—In 56,725 women, 59% were treated with BCS versus 41% with mastectomy. BCS was more likely in women who were younger than 70 years (odds ratio [OR], 1.37; 95% CI, 1.31 to 1.44; $p < 0.001$) and had lymph node-negative disease (OR, 1.60; 95% CI, 1.52 to 1.68; $p < 0.001$). Socioeconomic factors influenced use, with BCS more likely in areas with low poverty (OR, 1.05; 95% CI, 1.00 to 1.09; $p = 0.03$), high education (OR, 1.13; 95% CI, 1.08 to 1.19), high density of radiation oncologists (OR, 1.30; 95% CI, 1.06 to 1.59), and in metropolitan areas (OR, 1.20; 95% CI, 1.14 to 1.26). Significant geographic variation existed: 70% of women were treated with BCS in northeastern New England compared with only 48% to 50% in the South ($p < 0.001$).

TABLE 2.—Unadjusted and Adjusted Percent Use of Breast-Conserving Surgery Versus Mastectomy by Geographic Region

Region	States	BCS, % (n = 23,275) Overall	Adjusted*	Early Stage	Mastectomy, % (n = 33,450) Overall	Adjusted*	Early Stage
West, Pacific West	AK, CA, HI, OR, WA	62	62	71	38	38	29
West, Mountain West	AZ, CO, ID, MT, NV, NM, UT, WY	57	58	66	43	42	34
Midwest, West North Central	IA, KS, MN, MO, NE, ND, SD	50	51	58	50	49	41
Midwest, East North Central	IL, IN, MI, OH, WI	61	60	70	39	40	30
Northeast, New England	CT, MA, NH, ME, RI, VT	70	63	79	30	36	21
Northeast, Mid-Atlantic	NJ, NY, PA	67	64	78	33	35	22
South, South Atlantic	DE, DC, FL, GA, MD, NC, SC, VA, WV	59	59	68	41	41	32
South, West South Central	AK, LA, OK, TX	50	54	59	50	45	41
South, East South Central	AL, KY, MS, TN	48	51	57	52	48	43

BCS, breast-conserving surgery.
*Adjusted for covariates, including age, race, comorbidity score, axillary lymph node involvement, axillary dissection, chemotherapy, screening mammography, physician visits, surgeon density, radiation oncologist density, metropolitan area, poverty, and education.

Conclusions.—Currently, more than half of older women across the US diagnosed with nonmetastatic invasive breast cancer treated surgically receive BCS, representing a substantial increased use compared with historical data. Lack of BCS use appears in part associated with socioeconomic disadvantage, suggesting that persistent barriers to breast conservation exist.

▶ This study from the MD Anderson Cancer Center supported by the Department of Defense is a very interesting article looking at breast-conserving surgery throughout the United States in patients older than 65. As seen in Table 2, there was significant variation in the use of breast-conserving surgery in this age group with patients in Northeastern New England having the highest likelihood of having breast conservation, and patients in Alabama, Kentucky, Mississippi, and Tennessee having the lowest likelihood of breast conservation. As seen in Table 3, using a multivariate analysis, breast-conserving surgery was more likely in areas with low poverty, high education, and high density of radiation oncologists as well as patients who live in a metropolitan area.

There were some limitations to this study. First, it was a claims-based database study restricted to older breast cancer patients.

However, more than half of older women across the United States are treated with breast conservation. There exists, however, substantial variation geographically that primarily relates to socioeconomic disadvantages. Overcoming

TABLE 3.—Multivariate Logistic Model: Predictors of Use of Breast-Conserving Surgery

Covariate	Entire Sample Odds Ratio	95% CI		p Value	Early-Stage Subgroup Odds Ratio	95% CI		p Value
Age 66 to < 70 y vs ≥ 70 y	1.37	1.31	1.44	< 0.001	1.15	1.09	1.22	< 0.001
Race								
Caucasian versus African American	1.14	1.05	1.23	< 0.001	0.95	0.86	1.04	0.26
Caucasian versus other race	1.29	1.15	1.45	< 0.001	1.17	1.08	1.27	< 0.001
Charlson comorbidity score								
0 versus 1 comorbid condition	1.18	1.13	1.24	< 0.001	1.21	1.15	1.28	< 0.001
0 versus 2 or more comorbid conditions	1.38	1.29	1.47	< 0.001	1.17	1.08	1.27	< 0.001
0 versus unknown comorbid conditions	1.12	1.01	1.25	0.03	0.91	0.79	1.05	0.20
Lymph node-negative disease	1.60	1.52	1.68	< 0.001	—	—	—	—
No axillary lymph node dissection*	4.00	3.85	4.17	< 0.001	4.65	4.46	4.88	< 0.001
No chemotherapy*	1.32	1.25	1.39	< 0.001	0.63	0.57	0.69	< 0.001
Screening mammography	2.02	1.87	2.17	< 0.001	0.89	0.80	1.00	0.04
One or more visits to physician	1.43	1.22	1.68	< 0.001	1.97	1.60	2.43	< 0.001
Geographic region†								
West, Pacific West	0.86	0.78	0.95	0.008	0.81	0.72	0.92	0.001
West, Mountain West	0.71	0.63	0.80	< 0.001	0.69	0.60	0.80	< 0.001
Midwest, West North Central	0.50	0.45	0.55	< 0.001	0.45	0.40	0.51	< 0.001
Midwest, East North Central	0.80	0.73	0.88	< 0.001	0.75	0.67	0.84	< 0.001
Northeast, Mid-Atlantic	1.05	0.95	1.16	0.34	1.06	0.94	1.19	0.36
South, South Atlantic	0.76	0.69	0.83	< 0.001	0.69	0.62	0.78	< 0.001
South, West South Central	0.58	0.53	0.65	< 0.001	0.54	0.48	0.61	< 0.001
South, East South Central	0.51	0.45	0.57	< 0.001	0.45	0.39	0.52	< 0.001
Surgeon density‡	1.00	0.99	1.01	0.13	1.00	0.99	1.01	0.14
Radiation oncologist density§	1.30	1.06	1.59	0.01	1.37	1.07	1.75	0.01
Living in metropolitan area	1.20	1.14	1.26	< 0.001	1.20	1.13	1.27	< 0.001
Percent living in poverty < 11%‖	1.05	1.00	1.09	0.03	1.05	1.00	1.11	0.06
Percent with college education > 23%‖	1.13	1.08	1.19	< 0.001	1.15	1.09	1.21	< 0.001

*A model excluding axillary lymph node dissection and chemotherapy, which are treatments likely to occur concurrently or after surgery, did not affect risk estimates for other covariates.

†Compared with reference category Northeast New England. The likelihood ratio test for all strata of the variable for region was statistically significant ($p < 0.001$).

‡Increased odds per 1 surgeon per 100,000 persons (continuous variable).

§Increased odds per 1 radiation oncologist per 10,000 persons (continuous variable).

‖Continuous variables dichotomized at the median value.

these socioeconomic disadvantages should provide better, more contemporary care to all patients thoughout the United States.

T. J. Eberlein, MD

Intraoperative Evaluation of Breast Tumor Margins with Optical Coherence Tomography

Nguyen FT, Zysk AM, Chaney EJ, et al (Univ of Illinois at Urbana-Champaign; et al)

Cancer Res 69:8790-8796, 2009

As breast cancer screening rates increase, smaller and more numerous lesions are being identified earlier, leading to more breast-conserving surgical procedures. Achieving a clean surgical margin represents a technical challenge with important clinical implications. Optical coherence tomography (OCT) is introduced as an intraoperative high-resolution imaging technique that assesses surgical breast tumor margins by providing real-time microscopic images up to 2 mm beneath the tissue surface. In a study of 37 patients split between training and study groups, OCT images covering 1 cm^2 regions were acquired from surgical margins of lumpectomy specimens, registered with ink, and correlated with corresponding histologic sections. A 17-patient training set used to establish standard imaging protocols and OCT evaluation criteria showed that areas of higher scattering tissue with a heterogeneous pattern were indicative of tumor cells and tumor tissue in contrast to lower scattering adipocytes found in normal breast tissue. The remaining 20 patients were enrolled into the feasibility study. Of these lumpectomy specimens, 11 were identified with a positive or close surgical margin and 9 were identified with a negative margin under OCT. Based on histologic findings, 9 true positives, 9 true negatives, 2 false positives, and 0 false negatives were found, yielding a sensitivity of 100% and specificity of 82%. These results show the potential of OCT as a real-time method for intraoperative margin assessment in breast-conserving surgeries (Table 1).

▶ Evaluation of margin status is becoming more important as the number of lumpectomies increases. The authors present a completely new technology—optical coherence tomography (OCT). This is an intraoperative high-resolution imaging technique to assess breast tumor surgical margins by providing real-time microscopic images up to 2 mm beneath the tissue surface. As seen in Table 1, the intraoperative margin assessment using this technology had a positive predictive value of 82% and a negative predictive value of 100%.

A relatively large pool of blood or cauterized tissue can limit the penetration depth of OCT. However, saline can be used to irrigate the surface, which then

TABLE 1.—Intraoperative Tumor Margin Assessment (OCT Versus Histopathology)

	Histology (Positive)	Histology (Negative)	Total	
OCT (positive)	9 (true positive)	2 (false positive)	11	Positive predictive value = 82%
OCT (negative)	0 (false negative)	9 (true negative)	9	Negative predictive value = 100%
Total	9	11	20	
	Sensitivity = 100%	Specificity = 82%		

allows better OCT imaging depth. In the future, handheld probes will permit surgeons to ascertain not only the in situ tumor cavity but also the lumpectomy specimen margin. Future refinements to this technology are likely to make it more readily available to the surgical community.

T. J. Eberlein, MD

Attaining Negative Margins in Breast-Conservation Operations: Is There a Consensus among Breast Surgeons?

Blair SL, Thompson K, Rococco J, et al (Univ of California San Diego; State Univ of New York Health Science Ctr at Syracuse; et al)

J Am Coll Surg 209:608-613, 2009

Background.—The purpose of this survey was to ascertain the most common surgical practices for attaining negative (tumor-free) surgical margins in patients desiring breast-conservation treatment for breast cancer to see if a consensus exists for optimal treatment of patients.

Study Design.—We sent a survey to 1,000 surgeons interested in the treatment of breast cancer. Three hundred eighty-one surgeons responded to this survey and 351 were used for the analysis (response rate of 38%).

Results.—Answers showed a large variety in clinical practices among breast surgeons across the country. There was little intraoperative margin analysis; only 48% of surgeons examine the margins grossly with a pathologist and even fewer used frozen sections or imprint cytology. Decisions to reexcise specific margins varied greatly. For example, 57% of surgeons would never reexcise for a positive deep margin, but 53% would always reexcise for a positive anterior margin. Most importantly, there was a large range in answers about acceptable margins with ductal carcinoma in situ and invasive carcinoma. Fifteen percent of surgeons would accept any negative margin, 28% would accept a 1-mm negative margin, 50% would accept a 2-mm negative margin, 12% would accept a 5-mm negative margin, and 3% would accept a 10-mm negative margin.

Conclusions.—Results of this survey highlight the wide variety of practice patterns in the US for handling surgical margins in breast-conservation treatment. This issue remains controversial, with no prevailing standard of care. Consequently, additional study is needed in the modern era of multimodality treatment to examine the minimal amount of surgical treatment necessary, in conjunction with chemotherapy and radiation, to attain adequate local control rates in breast-conservation treatment.

▶ This work was supported by a Department of Defense Idea Grant and surveyed a large number of surgeons who had a focus on the treatment of breast cancer. This is an interesting article that documents the heterogeneous behavior of surgeons who focus on breast disease. For example, only 10% of surgeons always excise the whole cavity when performing a re-excision for positive margins. In another example, most surgeons (57%) responded that they would not re-excise patients for focally positive deep margins. Fig 3 is

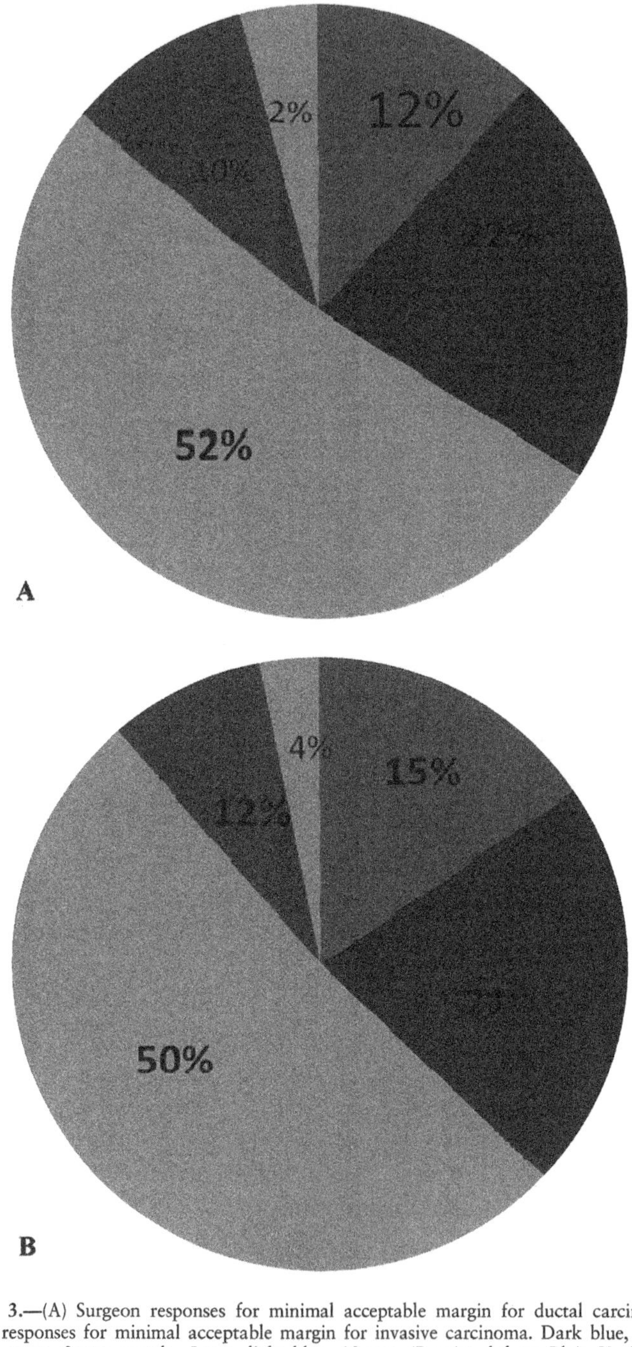

FIGURE 3.—(A) Surgeon responses for minimal acceptable margin for ductal carcinoma in situ. (B) Surgeon responses for minimal acceptable margin for invasive carcinoma. Dark blue, any negative; pink, 1 mm; green, 2 mm; purple, 5 mm; light blue, 10 mm. (Reprinted from Blair SL, Thompson K, Rococco J, et al. Attaining negative margins in breast-conservation operations: is there a consensus among breast surgeons? *J Am Coll Surg*. 2009;209:608-613, with permission from the American College of Surgeons.)

quite illuminating with regard to heterogeneity of surgeons. Part A of the figure shows margin results for ductal carcinoma in situ (DCIS), and part B shows margins for invasive breast cancer. As can be seen, there is a diversity of acceptable margin status for each of these pathology variances.

There are some limitations to this study. This is a survey that relies on self-reported data. However, the overall conclusion is there are considerable differences in the perception of a negative margin among surgeons who focus their practice on the treatment of breast cancer. A prospective, carefully controlled study would help to clarify this diversity of opinion.

T. J. Eberlein, MD

Comparison of Models to Predict Nonsentinel Lymph Node Status in Breast Cancer Patients with Metastatic Sentinel Lymph Nodes: A Prospective Multicenter Study

Coutant C, Olivier C, Lambaudie E, et al (Assistance Publique Hôpitaux de Paris and Univ Pierre et Marie Curie, France; Assistance Publique Hôpitaux de Paris, France; Institut Paoli-Calmettes, Marseille, France; et al)

J Clin Oncol 27:2800-2808, 2009

Purpose.—Several models have been developed to predict nonsentinel lymph node (non-SN) status in patients with breast cancer with sentinel lymph node (SN) metastasis. The purpose of our investigation was to compare available models in a prospective, multicenter study.

Patients and Methods.—In a cohort of 561 positive-SN patients who underwent axillary lymph node dissection, we evaluated the areas under the receiver operating characteristic curves (AUCs), calibration, rates of false negatives (FN), and number of patients in the group at low risk for non-SN calculated from nine models. We also evaluated these parameters in the subgroup of patients with micrometastasis or isolated tumor cells (ITC) in the SN.

Results.—At least one non-SN was metastatic in 147 patients (26.2%). Only two of nine models had an AUC greater than 0.75. Three models were well calibrated. Two models yielded an FN rate less than 5%. Three models were able to assign more than a third of patients in the low-risk group. Overall, the Memorial Sloan-Kettering Cancer Center nomogram and Tenon score outperform other methods for all patients, including the subgroup of patients with only SN micrometastases or ITC.

Conclusion.—Our study suggests that all models do not perform equally, especially for the subgroup of patients with only micrometastasis or ITC in the SN. We point out available evaluation methods to assess their performance and provide guidance for clinical practice (Table 3).

▶ A major question in managing patients with breast cancer is whether or not axillary lymph node dissection is required for women with positive sentinel

TABLE 3.—Prospective Validation of the Models for the 561 Positive-SN Patients With Breast Cancer and for the 246 Patients With Micrometastasis or ITC in the SN

Model	Threshold	No. of Patients*	%	AUC	95% CI	Calibration Plot: *P*	E max	E aver	FN Rate %	FN Rate 95% CI	No. of FN Rate†	Range
Overall population, N = 561												
MSKCC nomogram[12]	≤10%	201	35.8	0.78	0.76 to 0.81	$<10^{-3}$	15	6	6.5	3.9 to 10.3	13	7.8-20.7
Mayo nomogram[11]	≤10%	16	2.9	0.74	0.71 to 0.76	.08	5	5	12.5	3.5 to 35.6	2	0.6-5.7
Cambridge nomogram[15]	≤10%	126	22.5	0.73	0.7 to 0.75	.1	6	3	10.3	6.2 to 12.8	13	7.8-16.1
Stanford nomogram[14]	≤10%	101	18	0.72	0.7 to 0.74	$<10^{-3}$	58	23	4.9	2.2 to 10.7	5	2.2-10.8
Tenon score[10]	≤3.5	273	48.7	0.81	0.79 to 0.83	Not adequate			4.4	2.6 to 7.1	12	7.1-19.4
MDA score[6]	≤0	140	25	0.73	0.7 to 0.75	Not adequate			5.7	3 to 10.5	8	4.2-14.7
Saidi score[16]	≤2	140	25	0.65	0.62 to 0.67	Not adequate			15	10.3 to 21	21	14.4-29.4
RP-ROC[14]	≤10	173	30.8	0.68	0.65 to 0.7	Not adequate			5.2	2.8 to 9.2	9	4.8-15.9
CART[14]	≤10	186	33.2	0.65	0.63 to 0.67	Not adequate			6.4	3.8 to 10.5	12	7.1-19.5
OLR				0.84, 0.81‡		1	3	1.6				
Subgroup of patients with micrometastasis or ITC in the SN (n = 246)												
MSKCC nomogram[12]	≤10	143	58.1	0.72	0.66 to 0.79	.1	6	4	3.5	1.6 to 6.4	5	2.3-9.2
Mayo nomogram[11]	≤10	10	4.1	0.63	0.57 to 0.7	$<10^{-3}$	51	16	10	1.8 to 38	1	0.2-3.8
Cambridge nomogram[15]	≤10	73	29.7	0.63	0.57 to 0.69	$<10^{-3}$	5	10	4.1	1.4 to 9.6	3	1-7
Stanford nomogram[14]	≤10%	91	37	0.73	0.68 to 0.79	$<10^{-3}$	67	20	2.2	0.6 to 6.4	2	0.5-5.8
Tenon score[10]	≤3.5	209	85	0.81	0.76 to 0.87	Not adequate			2.9	1.5 to 4.8	6	3.1-10
MDA score[6]	≤0	132	53.7	0.67	0.62 to 0.73	Not adequate			3.8	1.7-7	5	2.2-9.2
Saidi score[16]	≤2	71	28.9	0.62	0.57 to 0.67	Not adequate			2.8	0.8 to 8.2	2	0.6-5.8
RP-ROC[14]	≤10%	173	70.3	0.65	0.59 to 0.71	Not adequate			5.2	3.1 to 7.5	9	5.3-13
CART[14]	≤10%	186	75.6	0.6	0.54 to 0.65	Not adequate			6.4	4.3 to 8.3	9	8-15.4

Abbreviations: SN, sentinel lymph node; ITC, isolated tumor cells; AUC, area under the receiver operating characteristic curve; E, difference in predicted and calibrated probabilities between calibration and AUC; E max, maximal error; E aver, average error; FN, false negative; MSKCC, Memorial Sloan-Kettering Cancer Center; MDA, The University of Texas M. D. Anderson Cancer Center; RP-ROC, recursive partitioning with receiver operating characteristic; CART, boosted Classification and Regression Trees; OLR, optimal logistic regression model.

Editor's Note: Please refer to original journal article for full references.

*No. of patients with score or predicted probability equal or lower than the threshold.

†Estimation of the no. of patients according to the 95% CI of the FN rate.

‡ORL by bootstrapping.

nodes on final histology. This article evaluates several tools in an independent multicenter cohort of patients with breast cancer and positive sentinel nodes.

The discussion of this article is, I think, particularly good, in that it discusses specific issues, such as using lymphovascular invasion and its impact on predicting whether or not the patient would have further positive nodes if the sentinel lymph node is positive.

The major finding of this study suggests that of the 9 models evaluated (Table 3), none conformed to fit all patients. This was especially true for the subgroup of patients with only micrometastases or isolated tumor cells in the sentinel node. The authors assess model performance and provide clinical practice guidelines. Although there are no definitive guidelines presented, the authors present a thoughtful, statistical analysis of limitations of these nomograms.

T. J. Eberlein, MD

Relationship Between Age and Axillary Lymph Node Involvement in Women With Breast Cancer

Wildiers H, Van Calster B, van de Poll-Franse LV, et al (Univ Hosps Leuven, Belgium; Katholieke Universiteit Leuven, Belgium; Eindhoven Cancer Registry, the Netherlands; et al)

J Clin Oncol 27:2931-2937, 2009

Purpose.—To study the relation between the presence of axillary lymph node (LN) involvement and age in breast cancer.

Patients and Methods.—The breast cancer database of the University Hospitals Leuven contains complete data on 2,227 patients with early breast cancer consecutively treated between 2000 and 2005. A multivariate piecewise logistic regression model was used to analyze LN involvement in relation to age at diagnosis. A similar analysis was then performed on a large, independent, population-based database from the Eindhoven Cancer Registry to investigate whether the effects of the Leuven model could be replicated.

Results.—We observed a piecewise effect of age. That is, women up to 70 years of age were less likely to have positive LNs with increasing age (odds ratio per 10-year increase, 0.87). In contrast, older women were more likely to have positive LNs with increasing age. However, for older women, the effect of age interacted with tumor size ($P = .0044$), suggesting that increasing age is associated with increased risk of LN involvement, mainly in small tumors. These findings were replicated in the Eindhoven Cancer Registry database.

Conclusion.—Axillary LN involvement varies with age at diagnosis; its probability decreases with increasing age up to the age of approximately 70 years, but increases again thereafter. However, this increase is mainly seen in smaller tumors and suggests a different behavior of small breast cancers in older adult patients. We hypothesize that decreased immune

TABLE 2.—Multivariate Logistic Regression Model for Lymph Node Involvement, with Piecewise Effect of Age and Interaction Between Age and Tumor Size for Women Older Than 70 Years

	Leuven University Hospital (n = 2,227)			Eindhoven Cancer Registry (n = 3,234)		
Variable	OR	95% CI	*P*	OR	95% CI	*P*
Age, years (for women ≤70)	0.87*	0.78 to 0.96	.0048	0.82*	0.76 to 0.90	<.0001
Age, years (for women older than 70)	2.93*	1.60 to 5.35	.0008	1.84*	1.25 to 2.71	.0023
Size, mm	1.60*	1.50 to 1.70	<.0001	1.89*	1.69 to 2.11	<.0001
Grade	1.28	1.10 to 1.48	.0009	1.19	1.03 to 1.36	.0172
Triple positive	2.09	1.43 to 3.06	.0001	1.06	0.76 to 1.46	.7373
Age · size (for women older than 70 years)	0.78*	0.66 to 0.92	.0044	0.81*	0.67 to 0.99	.0414

NOTE. Model development on data from University Hospitals Leuven; model replication on data from the Eindhoven Cancer Registry.

Abbreviation: OR, odds ratio.

*Expressed per 10-year increase in age and/or per centimeter increase in size, as applicable.

defense mechanisms, related with aging, may play a role in earlier invasion into LNs (Table 2).

▶ This is an interesting article from University Hospitals Leuven where they have complete data on thousands of patients with breast cancer. Using piecewise logistic regression models, these authors analyzed lymph node involvement in relation to age at diagnosis.

These authors showed that up to age of 70 years, patients were less likely to have positive lymph nodes. However, in women over the age of 70 years, increasing age was associated with the risk of lymph node involvement, mainly in small tumors (Fig 1 in the original article) (models are seen in Table 2). This observation may be influenced by tumor biology in older patients. Additionally, it is interesting that in these populations in Belgium and the Netherlands, the breast tumors are detected in a later stage in older patients (because systemic breast cancer screening is not done for women over the age of 70 years in Belgium). Future studies may look at tumor-infiltrating lymphocytes in breast cancers in older patients and study immunologic function (which generally decreases with age). Clearly genomic information, as it becomes available, will also complete the data from this article.

T. J. Eberlein, MD

Indications for Sentinel Lymph Node Biopsy in the Setting of Prophylactic Mastectomy

Laronga C, Lee MC, McGuire KP, et al (H LeeMoffitt Cancer Ctr & Res Inst, Tampa, FL; Magee-Womens Hosp of UPMC, Pittsburgh, PA; et al)

J Am Coll Surg 209:746-752, 2009

Background.—Bilateral/contralateral prophylactic mastectomy (PM) is offered to high-risk women to decrease their actual or perceived breast cancer risk. When an invasive occult cancer is identified, prevailing wisdom suggests that an axillary dissection be performed. This single-institution study aims to identify patients who may benefit from sentinel node biopsy (SLNB) at the time of prophylactic mastectomy.

Study Design.—We performed a retrospective review of a prospective database of patients treated at our institution with bilateral/contralateral PM between 1995 and 2006. We examined patients' clinicopathologic characteristics in comparison with their incidence of occult cancer in the contralateral breast or axilla.

Results.—There were 449 patients who underwent PM and SLNB. Twenty-eight underwent bilateral PM. Of the 28, no occult cancers were identified. Occult cancers were identified in 18 of 420 (4.3%) contralateral prophylactic specimens; they were invasive in 6 (1.4%). In cases of occult carcinoma, the primary established tumor was more likely to be of invasive lobular histology. Eight of 420 (2%) patients had a positive contralateral sentinel node, and within this subset of 8 patients the majority had locally advanced disease on the known tumor side. Other features associated with a positive contralateral sentinel node included the presence of lymphovascular involvement or skin or nipple involvement and grade 2 to 3 invasive primary established tumors.

Conclusions.—Overall, SLNB in patients undergoing bilateral PM or contralateral PM associated with early-stage disease is not indicated. But patients with locally advanced primary breast cancers have a significantly increased risk of occult cancer in the contralateral axilla, likely due to crossover metastasis; this select group of patients may benefit from SLNB at the time of surgery.

▶ This is a retrospective review of a prospective database of nearly 450 patients. As seen in Table 2, the presence of lymphovascular invasion, skin or nipple involvement, high-grade tumors, and 4 or more positive lymph nodes were clearly associated with the patient having a positive contralateral sentinel lymph node without any evidence of occult disease in the prophylactic breast specimen.

Of note, these authors found that a strong family history was not associated with a risk of occult cancer in either the contralateral breast or the contralateral axilla.

TABLE 2.—Demographic Comparisons Between the Primary Established Tumor when the Prophylactic Contralateral Sentinel Node Biopsy (Axilla) Is Benign Versus When the Contralateral Sentinel Node Biopsy (Axilla) Contains Metastatic Disease (Positive)

Variable	Contralateral Prophylactic Axilla Positive (n = 8)	Contralateral Prophylactic Axilla Negative (n = 412)	p Value
Family history, n (%)			0.740
Yes	4 (50.0)	220 (53.4)	
No	4 (50.0)	187 (45.4)	
Unknown/adopted		5 (1.2)	
Skin/nipple involvement, n (%)			0.0004
Yes	5 (71.4)	55 (13.3)	
No	3 (28.6)	333 (80.1)	
Unknown		24 (5.8)	
Lymphatic invasion, n (%)			< 0.0001
Yes	7 (87.5)	58 (14.1)	
No	1 (13.5)	326 (79.1)	
Unknown	0 (0.0)	28 (6.3)	
Multifocal, n (%)			0.077
Yes	4 (50.0)	78 (18.9)	
No	4 (50.0)	308 (74.8)	
Unknown	0 (0.0)	26 (6.3)	
Median tumor size (invasive), cm	2.23 ± 2.72	1.50 ± 1.51	0.0053
Grade of primary tumor, n (%)			< 0.0001
1	0 (0.0)	53 (12.8)	
2	2 (25.0)	150 (36.4)	
3	6 (75.0)	144 (35.0)	
Unknown	0 (0.0)	65 (15.8)	
Ipsilateral nodes positive, n (%)			< 0.0001
0	1 (12.5)	191 (46.4)	
1–3	2 (25.0)	159 (38.6)	
4 or more	5 (62.5)	62 (15.0)	
Histology, n (%)			< 0.0001
IDC	6 (75.0)	227 (55.1)	
ILC	1 (12.5)	48 (11.7)	
IDC/ILC	1 (12.5)	37 (9.0)	
DCIS	0 (0.0)	77 (18.7)	
DCIS/LCIS	0 (0.0)	3 (0.7)	
DCIS with microinvasion	0 (0.0)	10 (2.4)	
Other	0 (0.0)	10 (2.4)	

DCIS, ductal carcinoma in situ; IDC, invasive ductal carcinoma; ILC, invasive lobular carcinoma; LCIS, lobular carcinoma in situ.

Sentinel lymph node biopsy in patients undergoing bilateral prophylactic mastectomy is generally not indicated. Also, patients who have early stage disease on one side generally have little or no benefit from sentinel lymph node biopsy in the contralateral prophylactic mastectomy.

T. J. Eberlein, MD

Scientific Impact Award: Axillary reverse mapping (ARM) to identify and protect lymphatics draining the arm during axillary lymphadenectomy

Boneti C, Korourian S, Diaz Z, et al (Univ of Arkansas for Med Sciences and the Winthrop P. Rockefeller Cancer Inst, Little Rock)

Am J Surg 198:482-487, 2009

Introduction.—The axillary reverse mapping (ARM) procedure distinguishes lymphatics draining the arm from those draining the breast. The aim of this study was to assess the ability of ARM to identify and preserve lymphatics draining the arm and the impact on lymphedema.

Methods.—This study included 220 patients undergoing sentinel lymph node (SLN) biopsy (SLNB) with or without axillary lymph node dissection (ALND) from May 2006 to September 2008. After SLN localization with a radioactive tracer, blue dye was used to map ARM lymphatics. Data were collected on identification and variations in lymphatic drainage, crossover rate, the incidence of metastases, and nodal status.

Results.—Crossover (ARM = SLN) occurred in 6 patients (2.8%). ARM lymphatics were near or in the SLN field in 40.6% of patients, placing it at risk for disruption during lymphadenectomy. ARM lymphatics juxtaposed to the hot SLNB (n = 12 [5.6%]) were preserved. Fifteen ARM nodes were excised and were negative even in positive axillae. There were no cases of lymphedema at 6-month follow-up where ARM nodes were preserved.

Conclusion.—Confluence of the arm and breast drainage is rarely the SLN, and none of these nodes contained metastases. Preserving the ARM nodes may translate into a lower incidence of postoperative lymphedema.

▶ This article from the University of Arkansas uses the technique of axillary reverse mapping to demonstrate lymphatic drainage from the arm to assess lymphatics and the impact of sentinel lymph node biopsy on potential lymphedema. Confluence of arm and breast drainage is relatively rare in sentinel lymph node biopsies, which likely explains the relative low morbidity to sentinel lymph node biopsy. There are some very nice photographs associated with this article; however, the take-home message is that careful dissection of sentinel lymph nodes will likely preserve the axillary drainage of the arm and lead to a low incidence of postoperative lymphedema.

T. J. Eberlein, MD

Surgeon Training, Protocol Compliance, and Technical Outcomes From Breast Cancer Sentinel Lymph Node Randomized Trial

Krag DN, for the National Surgical Adjuvant Breast and Bowel Project (Univ of Vermont, Burlington; et al)

J Natl Cancer Inst 101:1356-1362, 2009

Background.—The National Surgical Adjuvant Breast and Bowel Project B-32 trial was designed to determine whether sentinel lymph node resection can achieve the same therapeutic outcomes as axillary lymph node resection but with fewer side effects and is one of the most carefully controlled and monitored randomized trials in the field of surgical oncology. We evaluated the relationship of surgeon trial preparation, protocol compliance audit, and technical outcomes.

Methods.—Preparation for this trial included a protocol manual, a site visit with key participants, an intraoperative session with the surgeon, and prerandomization documentation of protocol compliance. Training categories included surgeons who submitted material on five prerandomization surgeries and were trained by a core trainer (category 1) or by a site trainer (category 2). An expedited group (category 3) included surgeons with extensive experience who submitted material on one prerandomization surgery. At completion of training, surgeons could accrue patients. Two hundred twenty-four surgeons enrolled 4994 patients with breast cancer and were audited for 94 specific items in the following four categories: procedural, operative note, pathology report, and data entry. The relationship of training method; protocol compliance performance audit; and the technical outcomes of the sentinel lymph node resection rate, false-negative rate, and number of sentinel lymph nodes removed was determined. All statistical tests were two-sided.

Results.—The overall sentinel lymph node resection success rate was 96.9% (95% confidence interval [CI] = 96.4% to 97.4%), and the overall false-negative rate was 9.5% (95% CI = 7.4% to 12.0%), with no

TABLE 3.—Sentinel Lymph Node Resection Success Rates and False-Negative Rates for 224 Trained Surgeons According to Training Method*

Type of Training	No. of Surgeons	Technical Success† n	N	Rate, % (95% CI)	False-Negative Results‡ No. of Surgeons	n	N	Rate, % (95% CI)
Core trained	121	3411	3527	96.7 (96.1 to 97.3)	90	52	493	10.6 (8.0 to 13.6)
Site trained	50	514	525	97.9 (96.3 to 99.0)	31	7	64	10.9 (4.5 to 21.3)
Expedited	53	916	942	97.2 (96.0 to 98.2)	32	6	125	4.8 (1.8 to 10.2)
Overall	224	4841	4994	96.9 (96.4 to 97.4)	153	65	682	9.5 (7.4 to 12.0)

*CI = confidence interval.

†For technical success, n = number of operations in which sentinel lymph nodes were successfully resected; N = total number of operations for that category. $\chi^2 = 2.553$; $df = 2$; $P = .286$. All statistical tests were two-sided.

‡For false-negative results, n = number of operations in which sentinel lymph nodes were negative but nonsentinel lymph nodes were pathologically positive; N = total number of operations in that category with any pathologically positive lymph node. $\chi^2 = 3.983$; $df = 2$; $P = .142$. All statistical tests were two-sided.

statistical differences between training methods. Overall audit outcomes were excellent in all four categories. For all three training groups combined, a statistically significant positive association was observed between surgeons' average number of procedural errors and their false-negative rate ($\rho = +0.188$, $P = .021$).

Conclusions.—All three training methods resulted in uniform and high overall sentinel lymph node resection rates. Subgroup analyses identified some variation in false-negative rates that were related to audited outcome performance measures (Table 3).

▶ This is an evaluation of a randomized prospective trial evaluating surgeon preparation and protocol compliance. There are 3 categories of training: training by a core trainer (category 1), a site trainer (category 2), and an expedited group (category 3).

It turns out that the overall sentinel lymph node resection rate was almost 97%, and the false-negative rate was under 10%. There is no difference between the 3 methods of training. Audit outcomes were excellent in all categories.

Surgeons in the expedited group seem to remove more sentinel nodes than those in either of the 2 trained groups, and this may partially explain the false-negative rate.

As more surgically initiated clinical trials are preformed, ensuring the adequate training of surgeons will be important to ensure the quality and credibility of the outcome data.

T. J. Eberlein, MD

Prevalence of and Factors Associated With Persistent Pain Following Breast Cancer Surgery

Gätner R, Jensen M-B, Nielsen J, et al (Univ of Copenhagen, Denmark; Danish Breast Cancer Cooperative Group, Copenhagen, Denmark; et al)

JAMA 302:1985-1992, 2009

Context.—Persistent pain and sensory disturbances following surgical treatment for breast cancer is a significant clinical problem. The pathogenic mechanisms are complex and may be related to patient characteristics, surgical technique, and adjuvant therapy.

Objective.—To examine prevalence of and factors associated with persistent pain after surgical treatment for breast cancer.

Design, Setting, and Patients.—A nationwide cross-sectional questionnaire study of 3754 women aged 18 to 70 years who received surgery and adjuvant therapy (if indicated) for primary breast cancer in Denmark between January 1, 2005, and December 31, 2006. A study questionnaire was sent to the women between January and April 2008.

Main Outcome Measures.—Prevalence, location, and severity of persistent pain and sensory disturbances in 12 well-defined treatment groups assessed an average of 26 months after surgery, and adjusted odds ratio

(OR) of reported pain and sensory disturbances with respect to age, surgical technique, chemotherapy, and radiotherapy.

Results.—By June 2008, 3253 of 3754 eligible women (87%) returned the questionnaire. A total of 1543 patients (47%) reported pain, of whom 201 (13%) had severe pain, 595 (39%) had moderate pain, and 733 (48%) had light pain. Factors associated with chronic pain included young age (18-39 years: OR, 3.62; 95% confidence interval [CI], 2.25-5.82;

TABLE 2.—Pain Adjusted for Age, Type of Surgery, Radiotherapy, and Chemotherapy Among 3253 Danish Women Having Surgery for Primary Breast Cancer

	No. (%) of Women		Unadjusted		Adjusted[a]	
	With Pain	Without Pain	OR (95% CI)	*P* Value	OR (95% CI)	*P* Value
Age group, y						
18-39	96 (64)	53 (36)	2.62 (1.84-3.73)			
40-49	367 (59)	251 (41)	2.11 (1.74-2.57)	<.001		
50-59	554 (49)	580 (51)	1.38 (1.18-1.62)			
60-69	526 (41)	760 (59)	1 [Reference]			
Breast surgery by age group, y[b]						
Breast-conserving surgery						
18-39	72 (71)	29 (29)			3.62 (2.25-5.82)	
40-49	240 (60)	160 (40)			2.20 (1.68-2.89)	<.001
50-59	378 (49)	395 (51)			1.42 (1.16-1.74)	
60-69	324 (40)	489 (60)			1 [Reference]	
Mastectomy						
18-39	24 (50)	24 (50)			1.18 (0.64-2.19)	
40-49	127 (58)	91 (42)			1.72 (1.21-2.45)	.03
50-59	176 (49)	185 (51)			1.21 (0.91-1.60)	
60-69	202 (43)	271 (57)			1 [Reference]	
Breast procedure						
Mastectomy	529 (48)	571 (52)	0.98 (0.85-1.14)	.79	1.13 (0.84-1.53)	.41
Breast-conserving surgery	1014 (49)	1073 (51)	1 [Reference]		1 [Reference]	
Axillary procedure						
ALND	945 (54)	795 (46)	1.69 (1.47-1.94)	<.001	1.77 (1.43-2.19)	<.001
SLND	598 (41)	849 (59)	1 [Reference]		1 [Reference]	
Radiotherapy						
LRRT + BRT/ATRT	662 (55)	539 (45)	1.88 (1.51-2.33)		1.35 (1.04-1.76)	
BRT	697 (46)	824 (54)	1.29 (1.05-1.60)	<.001	1.50 (1.08-2.07)	.03
None	184 (40)	281 (60)	1 [Reference]		1 [Reference]	
Chemotherapy						
With	664 (54)	556 (46)	1.48 (1.28-1.71)	<.001	1.01 (0.85-1.21)	.91
Without	879 (45)	1088 (55)	1 [Reference]		1 [Reference]	
Year of surgery						
2005	716 (48)	772 (52)	0.98 (0.85-1.12)	.75		
2006	827 (49)	872 (51)	1 [Reference]			
Tumor location						
Upper lateral quadrant	608 (49)	639 (51)	1.02 (0.89-1.18)	.76		
Other parts of the breast	935 (48)	1005 (52)	1 [Reference]			

Abbreviations: ALND, axillary lymph node dissection; ATRT, anterior thoracic radiotherapy corresponding to the anterior thoracic wall; BRT, breast radiotherapy corresponding to residual breast tissue; CI, confidence interval; LRRT, locoregional radiotherapy corresponding to periclavicular, axillary level 3, and for right-side breast cancers, the internal mammary nodes; OR, odds ratio; SLND, sentinel lymph node dissection.

[a]Adjusted for age, mastectomy/breast-conserving surgery, ALND/SLND, radiotherapy, and chemotherapy.

[b]A statistically significant interaction was observed between age and type of surgery (P=.03).

$P < .001$) and adjuvant radiotherapy (OR, 1.50; 95% CI, 1.08-2.07; $P = .03$), but not chemotherapy (OR, 1.01; 95% CI, 0.85-1.21; $P = .91$). Axillary lymph node dissection (ALND) was associated with increased likelihood of pain (OR, 1.77; 95% CI, 1.43-2.19; $P < .001$) compared with sentinel lymph node dissection. Risk of sensory disturbances was associated with young age (18-39 years: OR, 5.00; 95% CI, 2.87-8.69; $P < .001$) and ALND (OR, 4.97; 95% CI, 3.92-6.30; $P < .001$). Pain complaints from other parts of the body were associated with increased risk of pain in the surgical area ($P < .001$). A total of 306 patients (20%) with pain had contacted a physician within the prior 3 months for pain complaints in the surgical area.

Conclusion.—Two to 3 years after breast cancer treatment, persistent pain and sensory disturbances remain clinically significant problems among Danish women who received surgery in 2005 and 2006 (Table 2).

▶ This is an interesting study from Copenhagen and the Danish Breast Cancer Cooperative Group. It surveyed over 3700 women who had surgery in the years of 2005 and 2006. The following can be seen in Table 2: pain was more significant in young women and type of surgery had no impact. Axillary lymph node dissection, as might be expected, was associated with an increased risk of pain and adjuvant radiotherapy also increased the risk of the patient reporting pain.

The strength of the study is its large size, high response rate, and the fact that it was a relatively uniform population in Denmark. The main limitation is that it is a cross-sectional study that provided only 1 estimate of pain prevalence and did not follow patients over a period of time.

Breast pain following surgical intervention for breast cancer is a significant problem in 25% to 50% of patients. Breast conservation and sentinel lymph node biopsies have reduced these problems but have not eliminated them.

T. J. Eberlein, MD

Time to Disease Recurrence in Basal-Type Breast Cancers: Effects of Tumor Size and Lymph Node Status

Dent R, Hanna WM, Trudeau M, et al (Sunnybrook Health Sciences Ctr, Univ of Toronto, Ontario, Canada; et al)

Cancer 115:4917-4923, 2009

Background.—Basal-like breast cancers are a subgroup of breast cancers defined by the absence of staining for estrogen-receptor (ER), progesterone receptor (PR), and human epidermal growth factor receptor 2 (HER-2/*neu*) and by positive staining for the cytokeratins (CKs) expressed in the myoepithelial cells of the ducts and lobules (CK5/CK6, CK14) and for epidermal growth factor receptor (EGFR). This class of tumors has an unusually aggressive course, and it is not clear whether conventional prognostic factors for breast cancers also predict outcome for patients who have the basal phenotype.

TABLE 2.—Association Between Tumor Size (≤2 cm Versus >2 cm) and Distant Disease Recurrence in Women with Basal and Nonbasal Breast Cancer

Variable	RR (95% CI) [*P*]			
	Univariate*	Multivariate†	Multivariate‡	Multivariate§
All patients				
Tumor size, >2 vs ≤2 cm	2.52 (1.94-3.28) [$<10^{-4}$]	2.08 (1.59-2.72) [$<10^{-4}$]	1.86 (1.42-2.44) [$<10^{-4}$]	1.85 (1.41-2.43) [$<10^{-4}$]
Age, per y		0.98 (0.97-0.99) [$<10^{-4}$]	0.98 (0.97-0.99) [.0005]	0.98 (0.97-1.00) [.008]
LN status, positive vs negative	2.65 (2.01-3.49) [$<10^{-4}$]	2.50 (1.89-3.31) [$<10^{-4}$]	2.38 (1.79-3.16) [10^{-4}]	2.30 (1.69-3.13) [$<10^{-4}$]
BR grade, trend			1.64 (1.32-2.04) [$<10^{-4}$]	1.63 (1.31-2.03) [$<10^{-4}$]
Chemo, yes/no				1.08 (0.78-1.49) [.64]
Basal breast cancer				
Tumor size, >2 cm vs ≤2 cm	1.15 (0.60-2.22) [.67]	1.00 (0.50-1.97) [.99]	0.99 (0.50-1.97) [.97]	1.15 (0.56-2.36) [.70]
Age, per y		1.00 (0.97-1.02) [.81]	1.00 (0.97-1.02) [.88]	1.00 (0.98-1.03) [.79]
LN status, positive vs negative	2.03 (1.11-3.69) [.02]	1.82 (0.95-3.47) [.07]	1.78 (0.93-3.42) [.08]	1.48 (0.75-2.94) [.26]
BR grade, trend			1.35 (0.54-3.37) [.52]	1.35 (0.54-3.39) [.52]
Chemo, yes/no				1.55 (0.72-3.36) [.26]
Nonbasal breast cancer				
Tumor size, >2 vs ≤2 cm	2.76 (2.08-3.68) [$<10^{-4}$]	2.23 (1.66-2.98) [$<10^{-4}$]	1.99 (1.48-2.68) [$<10^{-4}$]	1.99 (1.48-2.69) [$<10^{-4}$]
Age, per y		0.98 (0.97-0.99) [$<10^{-4}$]	0.98 (0.97-0.99) [.003]	0.98 (0.97-0.99) [.003]
LN status, positive vs negative	2.89 (2.11-3.96) [$<10^{-4}$]	2.74 (1.99-3.77) [$<10^{-4}$]	2.55 (1.85-3.51) [$<10^{-4}$]	2.57 (1.81-3.64) [$<10^{-4}$]
BR grade, trend			1.62 (1.28-2.04) [$<10^{-4}$]	1.62 (1.28-2.05) [$<10^{-4}$]
Chemo, yes/no				0.98 (0.68-1.40) [.90]

RR indicates relative risk; 95% CI, 95% confidence interval; LN, lymph node; BR, Bloom-Richardson; Chemo, chemotherapy.
*Adjusted by age only.
†Adjusted by age and LN status.
‡Adjusted by age, LN status, and BR grade (1/2/3).
§Adjusted by age, LN status, BR grade (1/2/3), and chemotherapy (yes/no).

TABLE 3.—Association Between Tumor Size (≤2 cm Versus >2 cm) and Death Caused by Breast Cancer in Women with Basal and Nonbasal Breast Cancer

Variable	RR (95% CI) [*P*] Univariate*	Multivariate†	Multivariate‡	Multivariate§
All patients				
Tumor size, >2 cm vs ≤2 cm	2.61 (2.00-3.40) [$<10^{-4}$]	2.25 (1.71-2.95) [$<10^{-4}$]	1.97 (1.49-2.59) [$<10^{-4}$]	1.95 (1.48-2.57) [$<10^{-4}$]
Age, trend		0.99 (0.98-1.00) [.02]	0.99 (0.98-1.00) [.09]	0.99 (0.98-1.00) [.28]
LN status, positive vs negative	2.89 (2.19-3.80) [$<10^{-4}$]	2.25 (1.70-2.99) [$<10^{-4}$]	2.11 (1.59-2.80) [$<10^{-4}$]	2.04 (1.49-2.77) [$<10^{-4}$]
BR grade, trend			1.89 (1.51-2.37) [$<10^{-4}$]	1.89 (1.50-2.37) [$<10^{-4}$]
Chemo, yes/no				1.05 (0.76-1.45) [.78]
Basal breast cancer				
Tumor size, >2 cm vs ≤2 cm	1.16 (0.62-2.19) [.64]	1.01 (0.52-1.95) [.99]	0.99 (0.51-1.92) [.97]	1.12 (0.56-2.23) [.75]
Age, trend		0.99 (0.97-1.02) [.62]	0.99 (0.97-1.02) [.64]	1.00 (0.97-1.03) [.84]
LN status, positive vs negative	2.03 (1.04-3.58) [.04]	1.92 (1.03-3.59) [.04]	1.88 (1.00-3.54) [.05]	1.66 (0.85-3.25) [.14]
BR grade, trend			1.01 (0.46-2.21) [.98]	1.02 (0.46-2.22) [.97]
Chemo, yes/no				1.31 (0.63-2.73) [.46]
Nonbasal breast cancer				
Tumor size, >2 cm vs ≤2 cm	2.88 (2.15-3.87) [$<10^{-4}$]	2.46 (1.82-3.33) [$<10^{-4}$]	2.14 (1.58-2.91) [$<10^{-4}$]	2.13 (1.56-2.89) [$<10^{-4}$]
Age, trend		0.99 (0.98-1.00) [.05]	0.99 (0.98-1.00) [.11]	0.99 (0.98-1.00) [.15]
LN status, positive vs negative	3.22 (2.36-4.40) [$<10^{-4}$]	2.44 (1.77-3.36) [$<10^{-4}$]	2.20 (1.60-3.04) [$<10^{-4}$]	2.21 (1.56-3.15) [$<10^{-4}$]
BR grade, trend			1.89 (1.48-2.40) [$<10^{-4}$]	1.89 (1.47-2.40) [$<10^{-4}$]
Chemo, yes/no				0.96 (0.67-1.37) [.96]

RR indicates relative risk; 95% CI, 95% confidence interval; LN, lymph node; BR, Bloom-Richardson; Chemo, chemotherapy.
*Adjusted by age only.
†Adjusted by age and LN status.
‡Adjusted by age, LN status, and BR grade (1/2/3).
§Adjusted by age, LN status, BR grade (1/2/3), and chemotherapy (yes/no).

Methods.—A panel of 962 breast cancers was stained for 5 markers (ER, PR, HER-2/*neu*, CK5/CK6, and EGFR). The patients were followed for clinical outcomes for up to 15 years from diagnosis, and the rates of distant disease recurrence and death were compared by tumor size (≤2 cm or >2 cm) and by lymph node status within the subgroups of women with basal and nonbasal cancers.

Results.—Of the 962 women with breast cancer, 116 cancers were basal (12%), 845 were nonbasal (88%), and 1 could not be classified as either basal or nonbasal and was excluded. In total, 426 tumors measured ≤2 cm (45%), and 530 tumors measured >2 cm (55%). Among women with nonbasal cancers, large tumor size was an adverse prognostic factor. Among women with basal cancers, a transient adverse effect of size on disease recurrence was observed; however, after 10 years, mortality rates were equal for women with small tumors and women with large tumors.

Conclusions.—Among women with basal breast cancers, the long-term prognosis was similar for women with large tumors and women with small tumors. However, women with large basal tumors appeared to develop recurrent disease sooner (Tables 2 and 3).

▶ This is a prospective study that followed clinical outcomes in patients with breast cancer for up to 15 years from diagnosis, specifically looking at comparison of basal type of breast cancer (triple-negative breast cancer) with non-basal-type. It is anticipated that at 5 years, patients with basal-like breast cancer were more likely to have distant disease recurrence. However, by 15 years there was similarity of recurrence rates for women with basal-like breast cancer and nonbasal cancers. Among nonbasal group, young age, tumor size greater than 2 centimeters, high grade, and positive lymph node status were significant variables to predict distant disease recurrence and death (Table 2, Table 3). Among women in the basal group, only lymph node status was prognostic for mortality.

This study calls into question the ability to incorporate tumor size into prediction algorithms in patients with basal-type breast cancer. The other major issue in this trial is the implication for design of future clinical trials. This trial's long follow-up period of 15 years emphasizes the importance of long follow-up so that mortality is not analyzed prematurely. This study also confirms the feeling that basal-type tumors possess a different mechanism of spread when compared with estrogen-receptor (ER)–positive cancers. New targeted therapy should be directed at exploiting this difference.

T. J. Eberlein, MD

Surgeon Recommendations and Receipt of Mastectomy for Treatment of Breast Cancer

Morrow M, Jagsi R, Alderman AK, et al (Memorial Sloan-Kettering Cancer Ctr, NY; Univ of Michigan Health System, Ann Arbor; et al)

JAMA 302:1551-1556, 2009

Context.—There is concern that mastectomy is overused in the United States.

Objectives.—To evaluate the association of patient-reported initial recommendations by surgeons and those given when a second opinion was sought with receipt of initial mastectomy; and to assess the use of mastectomy after attempted breast-conserving surgery (BCS).

Design, Setting, and Patients.—A survey of women aged 20 to 79 years with intraductal or stage I and II breast cancer diagnosed between June 2005 and February 2007 and reported to the National Cancer Institute's Surveillance, Epidemiology, and End Results registries for the metropolitan areas of Los Angeles, California, and Detroit, Michigan. Patients were identified using rapid case ascertainment, and Latinas and blacks were oversampled. Of 3133 patients sent surveys, 2290 responded (73.1%). A mailed survey was completed by 96.5% of respondents and 3.5% completed a telephone survey. The final sample included 1984 female patients (502 Latinas, 529 blacks, and 953 non-Hispanic white or other).

Main Outcome Measures.—The rate of initial mastectomy and the perceived reason for its use (surgeon recommendation, patient driven, medical contraindication) and the rate of mastectomy after attempted BCS.

Results.—Of the 1984 patients, 1468 had BCS as an initial surgical therapy (75.4%) and 460 had initial mastectomy, including 13.4% following surgeon recommendation and 8.8% based on patient preference. Approximately 20% of patients (n = 378) sought a second opinion; this was more common for those patients advised by their initial surgeon to undergo mastectomy (33.4%) than for those advised to have BCS (15.6%) or for those not receiving a recommendation for one procedure over another (21.2%) ($P < .001$). Discordance in treatment recommendations between surgeons occurred in 12.1% (n = 43) of second opinions and did not differ on the basis of patient race/ethnicity, education, or geographic site. Among the 1459 women for whom BCS was attempted, additional surgery was required in 37.9% of patients, including 358 with reexcision (26.0%) and 167 with mastectomy (11.9%). Mastectomy was most common in patients with stage II cancer ($P < .001$).

Conclusion.—Breast-conserving surgery was recommended by surgeons and attempted in the majority of patients evaluated, with surgeon

TABLE 2.—Frequency and Outcomes of Second Opinions

Recommendation by Second Surgeon	No. of Patients (n = 378)[a]	Recommendation by First Surgeon, No. (Weighted %)		
		Breast-Conserving Surgery	Mastectomy	Neither[b]
Breast-conserving surgery	166	130 (73.9)	19 (20.2)	17 (28.0)
Mastectomy	102	24 (11.9)	69 (65.6)	9 (15.5)
No recommendation	82	27 (14.2)	14 (14.2)	41 (56.5)
Total	350	181 (100)	102 (100)	67 (100)

[a]There were 28 patients with missing information (7.4%).
[b]Indicates that the surgeon did not recommend one (breast-conserving surgery or mastectomy) procedure over another.

TABLE 3.—Percentage of Patients who Received Mastectomy as Initial Treatment by Surgeon Recommendation[a]

Recommendation by Second Surgeon	No. of Patients	Recommendation by First Surgeon, No. (Weighted %)[b]		
		Breast-Conserving Surgery	Mastectomy	Neither[c]
No second opinion	1544	1052 (2.1)	241 (88.8)	251 (34.8)
Breast-conserving surgery	167	131 (1.9)	19 (33.8)	17 (3.9)
Mastectomy	105	24 (26.6)	72 (77.6)	9 (92.9)
No recommendation	83	28 (36.5)	14 (32.3)	41 (45.9)

[a]There were 85 patients with missing information.
[b]Indicates the weighted percentage of those patients who received initial mastectomy. For instance, of the 1052 patients for whom their first surgeon recommended breast-conserving surgery and who did not obtain a recommendation from a second surgeon, 2.1% (weighted percentage) had a mastectomy as the initial treatment.
[c]Indicates that the surgeon did not recommend one (breast-conserving surgery or mastectomy) procedure over another.

TABLE 4.—Surgical Outcomes by Stage for Patients who Received Initial Breast-Conserving Surgery[a]

Surgical Outcomes	All (n = 1459)[b]	Ductal Carcinoma in Situ (n = 359)	Stage I (n = 652)	Stage II (n = 448)
No further surgery	934 (62.1)	218 (57.3)	444 (68.0)	273 (58.0)
Reexcision only	358 (26.0)	100 (30.7)	152 (23.7)	105 (24.0)
Reexcision and then mastectomy	63 (4.2)	22 (6.3)	22 (3.0)	19 (4.6)
Mastectomy only	104 (7.7)	19 (5.7)	34 (5.3)	51 (13.4)

[a]Values are expressed as number (weighted percentage). There were 9 patients with missing information.
[b]$P < .001$ for differences in patterns of surgery by stage.

recommendation, patient decision, and failure of BCS all contributing to the mastectomy rate.

▶ This is a survey of women with early-stage breast cancer using the National Cancer Institute's Surveillance, Epidemiology, and End Results registry for the metropolitan areas of Los Angeles, California, and Detroit, Michigan. It involves experts from Memorial Sloan-Kettering, University of Michigan, and the Keck School of Medicine at the University of Southern California.

Concordance between recommendations of the first opinion and that of a surgeon participating in a second opinion was very high. Only 20% of patients whose first surgeon recommended mastectomy received a second opinion for breast conservation (Table 2); 11.9% of patients who received an initial recommendation of breast conservation received a second opinion for mastectomy. As seen in Table 3, most patients received the recommended treatment when the first and second surgeon concurred on the recommendation. As seen in Table 4, 37.9% of the women who initially received breast conservation required a second surgical procedure. Reasons were multifactorial and lack of consensus as to what defines an adequate margin is still an important reason. Obviously, re-excision, even if successful, reduces cosmetic approval, delays therapy, and increases the cost. Overall, about one quarter of total mastectomy use is related to patient preferences. These seem to be influenced by concern for disease recurrence as well as fear of radiation therapy and the inconvenience of radiation therapy. Improved decision making will occur with better education of patients and providers.

T. J. Eberlein, MD

Decision Involvement and Receipt of Mastectomy Among Racially and Ethnically Diverse Breast Cancer Patients

Hawley ST, Griggs JJ, Hamilton AS, et al (Univ of Michigan, Ann Arbor; Univ of Southern California, Los Angeles; et al)

J Natl Cancer Inst 101:1337-1347, 2009

Background.—Few studies have evaluated the association between patient decision involvement and surgery received among racially and ethnically diverse patients or patients' attitudes about surgery and the role of family and friends in surgical treatment choices.

Methods.—Women diagnosed with nonmetastatic breast cancer from June 2005 through February 2007 and reported to the Los Angeles or Detroit Surveillance, Epidemiology, and End Results registries were mailed a survey after diagnosis (N = 3133). Latina and African American women were oversampled. The response rate was 72.4%. The analytic sample (N = 1651) excluded those with stage IIIA or higher disease, self-reported clinical contraindications to breast-conserving surgery with radiation, and unclear race or ethnicity. The dependent variable was receipt of mastectomy initially. The primary independent variables were patient involvement in decision making, race or ethnicity, attitudes about recurrence, the effects of radiation, the impact of surgery on body image, and the role of others in decision making. Latinas were categorized as low or high acculturated. The association between patient involvement in decision making and the receipt of mastectomy was evaluated using logistic regression while controlling for other independent variables. All statistical tests were two-sided.

Results.—The analytic sample was 23.9% Latina (12.0% low acculturated, 11.9% high acculturated), 27.1% African American, and 48.9% white, and 17.2% received a mastectomy initially. For each racial or ethnic

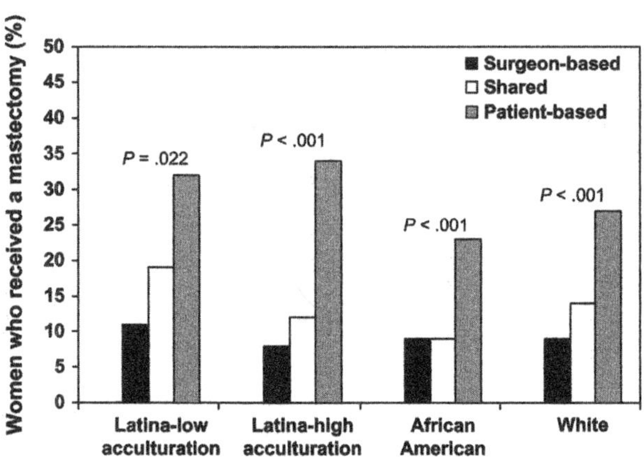

FIGURE 2.—Association between patient involvement in decision making and receipt of mastectomy, by race and ethnicity. Includes women with stage 0–II breast cancer and no clinical contraindications to breast-conserving surgery with radiation (N = 1651). *P* values are based on χ^2 tests (two-sided) for differences in decision involvement and receipt of mastectomy for each racial or ethnic group. (Reprinted from Hawley ST, Griggs JJ, Hamilton AS, et al. Decision involvement and receipt of mastectomy among racially and ethnically diverse breast cancer patients. *J Natl Cancer Inst.* 2009;101:1337-1347. Published by Oxford University Press.)

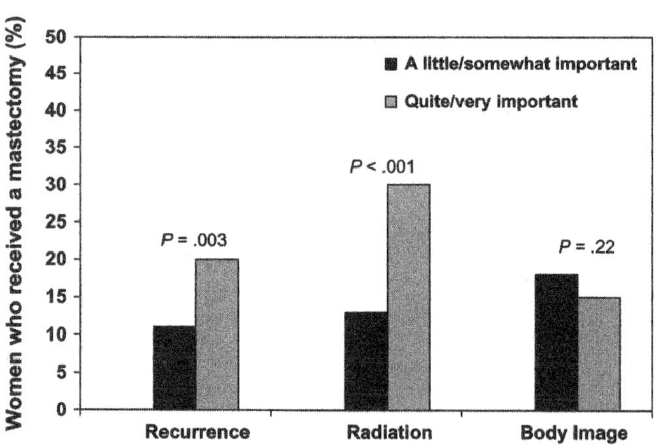

FIGURE 3.—Association between patient attitudes about surgery and receipt of mastectomy. Includes women with stage 0–II breast cancer and no clinical contraindications to breast-conserving surgery with radiation (N = 1651). *P* values are based on χ^2 tests (two-sided) for differences in degree of importance of each attitude (not/a little vs quite/very important) in surgical decision making and receipt of mastectomy. (Reprinted from Hawley ST, Griggs JJ, Hamilton AS, et al. Decision involvement and receipt of mastectomy among racially and ethnically diverse breast cancer patients. *J Natl Cancer Inst.* 2009;101:1337-1347. Published by Oxford University Press.)

group, more women who reported a patient-based decision received mastectomy than those who reported a shared or surgeon-based decision ($P = .022$ for low-acculturated Latinas, $P < .001$ for other groups). Women who reported that concerns about recurrence or radiation effects were very important in their surgery decision were more likely to receive mastectomy than those less concerned (for recurrence concerns, estimated relative risk [RR] = 1.66, 95% confidence interval [CI] = 1.28 to 2.10; for radiation concerns, estimated RR = 2.35, 95% CI = 1.88 to 2.85). Women who reported that body image concerns and their spouse's opinion were very important in their surgery decision less often received mastectomy than those less concerned about body image or who placed less weight on their spouse's opinion (for body image concerns, estimated RR = 0.47, 95% CI = 0.30 to 0.74; for spouse's opinion, estimated RR = 0.53, 95% CI = 0.36 to 0.78).

Conclusion.—Greater patient involvement in decision making was associated with receipt of mastectomy for all racial and ethnic groups. Patient attitudes about surgery and the opinions of family and friends contribute to surgical choices made by women with breast cancer.

▶ This study looking at the Los Angeles and Detroit Surveillance, Epidemiology, and End Results registries surveyed Latina and African American women. Greater patient involvement in decision making was associated with greater receipt of mastectomy in all racial and ethnic groups. This is seen in Fig 2. As seen in Fig 3, women who had concerns about recurrence and radiation received mastectomy more than in woman who had less concern about these issues. These feelings by patients were frequently influenced by the patients' family and friends.

The study does have some limitations. First, the survey is patient self-reported and therefore may suffer from bias. While the study was conducted in 2 geographic locations (Los Angeles and Detroit), this survey was administered to women who could speak English or Spanish and therefore, the generalizability to other patient populations may not be as valid.

T. J. Eberlein, MD

Characteristics and Treatment Modalities for African American Women Diagnosed With Stage III Breast Cancer

Rizzo M, Lund MJ, Mosunjac M, et al (Emory Univ, Atlanta, GA; Winship Cancer Inst, Atlanta, GA; et al)

Cancer 115:3009-3015, 2009

Background.—Stage III breast cancers account for about 6% to 7% of all invasive breast cancers diagnosed annually in the United States. In African American (AA) women, the incidence of stage III breast cancers is almost double that in Caucasian women. The aim of this study was to correlate age, receptor status, nuclear grade, and differences in treatment modalities for stage III breast cancer in an inner-city hospital serving a large AA population.

Methods.—A retrospective review was performed for all stage III primary breast cancers diagnosed and or treated from 2000 to 2006.

TABLE 3.—Population, Tumor, and Treatment Characteristics by Race

Variable	AA, n = 93, 86.9% No.	%	Non-AA, n = 14, 13.1% No.	%	*P**
Stage					
IIIA	39	41.9	4	28.5	.39
IIIB	31	33.3	4	28.5	
T4d	15	16.1	3	21.5	
IIIC	8	8.7	3	21.5	
Age at diagnosis, y					
Mean	55	NA	53.1	NA	.63†
Median	51.5	NA	51	NA	
Range	32-80	NA	27-93	NA	
<50	40	43.1	6	42.8	.99
≥50	53	56.9	8	57.2	
ER status					
Positive	45	48.3	10	71.4	.25‡
Negative	43	46.2	4	28.6	
Unknown	5	5.6	0	0.0	
PR status					
Positive	39	41.9	10	71.4	.04‡
Negative	47	50.5	3	21.5	
Unknown	7	7.6	1	7.1	
HER2 status					
Positive	11	11.8	1	7.1	.99‡
Negative	71	76.4	11	78.5	
Unknown	11	11.8	2	14.4	
Triple negative§					
Yes	28	30.1	3	21.4	.54‡
No	57	61.3	11	78.6	
Unknown	8	8.6	0		
Grade					
Low	9	9.6	2	14.2	.04‡
Intermediate	22	23.6	7	50.2	
High	41	44.3	2	14.2	
Unknown	21	22.5	3	21.4	
Chemotherapy					
Neoadjuvant	36	38.7	9	64.2	.26‡
Adjuvant	29	31.3	2	14.4	
Refused	19	20.4	3	21.4	
Unknown	9	9.6	0	0.0	
Radiation therapy					
Yes	49	52.6	11	78.5	.42‡
Not eligible	15	16.1	1	7.3	
Refused	22	23.6	2	14.2	
Unknown	7	7.7	0	0.0	

AA indicates African American; NA, not applicable; ER, estrogen receptor; PR, progesterone receptor; HER2, HER-2/*neu*.

*Fisher exact *P* values.

†*t*-test *P* value.

‡Unknowns deleted.

§ER, PR, and HER2 negative.

Results.—Of 840 primary invasive breast cancers, the authors identified 107 as stage III, 40.2% IIIA, 32.7% IIIB, 16.8% T4D, and 10.3% IIIC. The majority of the patients were AA (n = 93, 86.9%). Stage IIIC patients were younger ($P < .05$). Triple negative tumors (TNT) accounted for 29.0%. TNT were more likely among the inflammatory breast cancers (50.0%) compared with the other 3 groups ($P < .05$). Twenty-two patients (20.5%) refused chemotherapy, and 24 of the 91 patients (26.3%) who should have received chest wall radiation refused. There was no difference in race, marital status, religion, or age in the patients that refused chemotherapy or radiation therapy versus the majority of patients in this series who received standard care.

Conclusions.—Stage III breast cancers in AA women have distinct clinical characteristics. A high number of these patients refused chemotherapy and radiation therapy. Reasons for refusal need to be better defined so strategies can be implemented to improve compliance for these advanced stage patients.

▶ This is an article from the Winship Cancer Institute and Emory University. It is a retrospective review of stage III breast cancer. While the conclusion of this article is that African American women refused chemotherapy and radiation therapy in larger numbers, there are other issues involved. As seen in Table 3, approximately 78% of non-African American women received neoadjuvant or adjuvant chemotherapy. This number was only slightly less for African American women. However, there was a substantial reduction in neoadjuvant African American treatments. As shown in Table 3 for radiation therapy, there was a substantially higher number of "not eligible" African America patients and an almost double rate of "refusal" patients.

In future studies, identifying the reasons for this higher rate of refusal, and intervening with education, outreach, and communications programs should help to alleviate this disparity of known effective treatments.

T. J. Eberlein, MD

Patterns of Treatment for Early Stage Breast Cancers at the M. D. Anderson Cancer Center From 1997 to 2004

Shen Y, Dong W, Feig BW, et al (The Univ of Texas M. D. Anderson Cancer Ctr, Houston)

Cancer 115:2041-2051, 2009

Background.—The objectives of this study were to examine the patterns of use for adjuvant therapy and the changes in surgical practice for patients with early stage breast cancer and to describe how recent large clinical trial results impacted the patterns of care at The University of Texas M. D. Anderson Cancer Center (MDACC).

Methods.—The study included 5486 women who were diagnosed with stage I through IIIA breast cancer between 1997 and 2004 and received

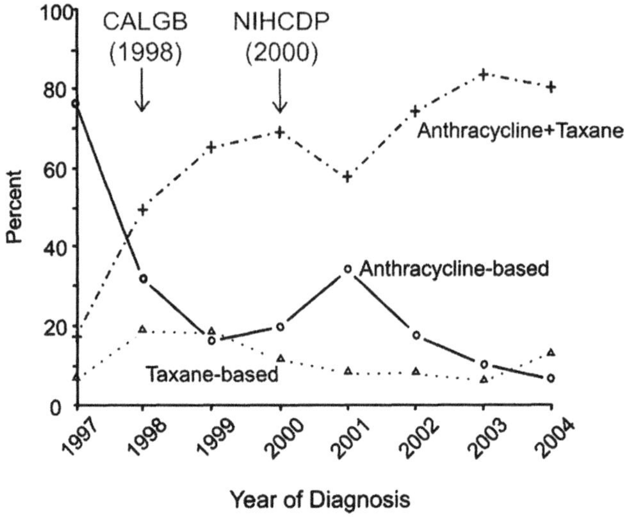

FIGURE 2.—Type of chemotherapy among lymph node-positive women. CALGB indicates Cancer and Leukemia Group B; NIHCDP, National Institutes of Health Consensus Development Conference. (Reprinted from Shen Y, Dong W, Feig BW, et al. Patterns of treatment for early stage breast cancers at the M. D. Anderson Cancer Center from 1997 to 2004. *Cancer.* 2009;115:2041-2051. Copyright 2009 American Cancer Society. This material is reproduced with permission of Wiley-Liss, Inc, a subsidiary of John Wiley & Sons, Inc.)

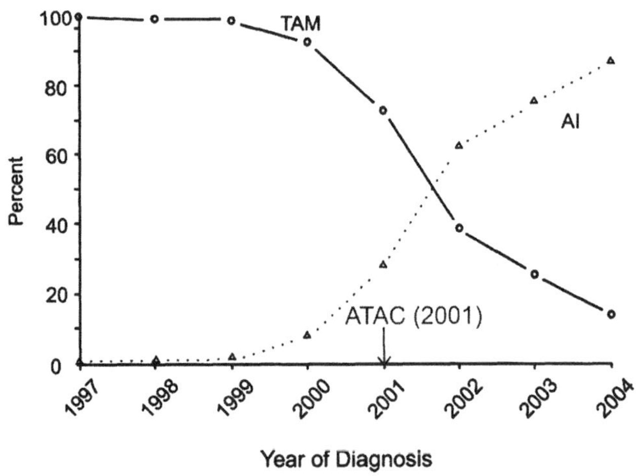

FIGURE 3.—Type of endocrine therapy among postmenopausal women. TAM indicates tamoxifen; AI, aromatase inhibitor; ATAC, the Arimidex, Tamoxifen, Alone or in Combination study. (Reprinted from Shen Y, Dong W, Feig BW, et al. Patterns of treatment for early stage breast cancers at the M. D. Anderson Cancer Center from 1997 to 2004. *Cancer.* 2009;115:2041-2051. Copyright 2009 American Cancer Society. This material is reproduced with permission of Wiley-Liss, Inc, a subsidiary of John Wiley & Sons, Inc.)

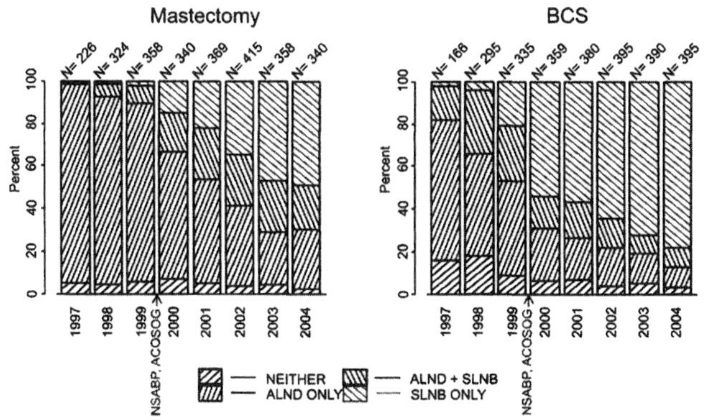

FIGURE 4.—Percentage of patients who underwent sentinel lymph node biopsy (SLNB) and/or axillary lymph node dissection (ALND) by year of diagnosis, according to type of surgery. BCS indicates breast-conserving surgery; NSABP, National Surgical Adjuvant Breast and Bowel Project; ASOSOG, American College of Surgeons Oncology Group. (Reprinted from Shen Y, Dong W, Feig BW, et al. Patterns of treatment for early stage breast cancers at the M. D. Anderson Cancer Center from 1997 to 2004. *Cancer.* 2009;115:2041-2051. Copyright 2009 American Cancer Society. This material is reproduced with permission of Wiley-Liss, Inc, a subsidiary of John Wiley & Sons, Inc.)

their treatment at MDACC. A chi-square trend test and multivariate logistic regression model were used to assess changes in treatment patterns over time.

Results.—Among lymph node-positive patients, the use of anthracycline plus taxane chemotherapy increased from 17% in 1997 to 81% in 2004 ($P < .001$). Meanwhile, the use of anthracyclines without taxanes dropped from 76% to 20% ($P < .001$) between 1997 and 2000. For postmenopausal patients who received endocrine therapy, the use of tamoxifen was replaced increasingly by the use of aromatase inhibitors (from 100% on tamoxifen in 1997 to 14% in 2004; $P < .001$). The percentage of women who underwent initial sentinel lymph node biopsy increased significantly during the period from 1997 to 2004 (from 1.8% to 69.7%, respectively, among patients who underwent mastectomy; and from 18.1% to 87.1%, respectively, among patients who underwent breast-conserving surgery; $P < .001$).

Conclusions.—The results from this study suggested that key findings from adjuvant therapy and surgical procedures from large clinical trials often prompt immediate changes in the patient care practices of research hospitals like MDACC.

▶ This article from M.D. Anderson Cancer Center documents the changes in that institution for breast cancer patients over a period of time from 1997-2004. As can be seen in Figs 2 and 3, the impact of clinical trials that documented the synergy between anthracycline, taxane, and the use of aromatase inhibitors alone, or in combinations with antiestrogen therapy, had a tremendous impact on treatment for patients with breast cancer in that institution. The same can be said for Fig 4, showing the impact of the National Surgical Adjuvant Breast and Bowel Project (NSABP) and American College of Surgeons Oncology Group (ACOSOG) clinical trials with respect to sentinel lymph node technologies.

This article is highlighted because these nationally recognized clinical trials changed the paradigm of treatment in this tertiary cancer center. However, these clinical trials should have the same impact on treatment paradigms for surgeons in clinical oncologic practice.

T. J. Eberlein, MD

Pancreatic

Relationship Between Hospital Volume, System Clinical Resources, and Mortality in Pancreatic Resection

Joseph B, Morton JM, Hernandez-Boussard T, et al (Henry Ford Hosp, Detroit, MI; Stanford Univ, Palo Alto, CA
J Am Coll Surg 208:520-527, 2009

Background.—The relationship between hospital volume and perioperative mortality in pancreaticoduodenectomy has been well established. We studied whether associations exist between hospital volume and hospital clinical resources and between both of these factors to mortality to help explain this relationship.

Study Design.—This two-part study reviewed publicly available hospital information from the Leapfrog Group, HealthGrades, and hospital Web sites. Hospitals were evaluated for Leapfrog ICU staffing criteria and Safe Practice Score; HealthGrades five-star rating for complex gastrointestinal procedures and operations; and presence of a general surgery residency, gastroenterology fellowship, and interventional radiology. Evaluation used trend analysis and multiple logistic regression analysis. The second part determined the mortality rate for pancreaticoduodenectomy using inpatient mortality data from the National Inpatient Sample and Leapfrog. Hospitals were categorized by low volume ($\leq$ 10/year), high volume ($\geq$ 11/year), strong clinical support (presence of all support factors), and weak clinical support (absence of any factor). Data were correlated by number of pancreatic resections per hospital, hospital system clinical resources, and operative mortality.

Results.—As hospital volume increased, statistically significant increases occurred in the frequency of hospitals meeting Leapfrog ICU staffing criteria ($p < 0.0001$), Leapfrog Safe Practice Score ($p = 0.0004$), HealthGrades 5-star rating ($p < 0.00001$), general surgery residency ($p < 0.00001$), gastroenterology fellowship ($p < 0.00001$), and interventional radiology services ($p < 0.00001$). No significant relationships were found between resection volume and any one of the clinical support factors and perioperative death. Presence of strong clinical support was associated with lower mortality (odds ratio $= 0.32$; $p = 0.001$).

Conclusions.—System clinical resources were more influential in operative mortality for pancreatic resection. This might help explain why high-volume hospitals, low-volume surgeons in high-volume institutions, and

TABLE 1.—Relationship of Pancreatic Resection Volumes to System Clinical Resources

Variable	Pancreatic resections (%) 0–5 (n = 256)	6–10 (n = 70)	11–30 (n = 70)	> 30 (n = 38)	p Value
ICU staffing	21	46	47	74	< 0.00001
Safe practice score	37	46	60	55	0.0004
HealthGrades five-star rating	11	17	23	39	< 0.00001
General surgery residency	11	17	50	79	< 0.00001
Gastroenterology fellowship	4	10	34	79	< 0.00001
Interventional radiology	58	81	87	97	0.00001

some lower-volume hospitals with excellent clinical resources have lower perioperative mortality rates for pancreatic resection.

▶ There appears to be an important relationship between hospital volume and perioperative mortality, especially for complex surgical procedures such as pancreaticoduodenectomy. This is a study resulting from collaboration between the Henry Ford Hospital and Stanford University, where the authors looked at the relationship between hospital volume, hospital clinical resources, and mortality. As is seen in Table 1, as hospital volume for pancreatic resections increases, the likelihood of having system clinical resources also dramatically improves. Indeed, these authors have shown a very nice interdependence of hospital volume showing that higher volume predicts higher resources, and a higher resource count predicts higher health grade quality score (Fig 2 in the original article). Using multivaried analysis, these authors showed that strong system clinical support was significant in reducing mortality, and this was true if the clinical system support is a cumulative variable (Table 5 in the original article).

Therefore, while high-volume hospitals tend to have lower mortality of pancreatic resections, this may be somewhat less due to volume per se, but may be because high-volume institutions have associated system clinical support that successfully treats these complex patients.

T. J. Eberlein, MD

Variations in Referral Patterns to High-Volume Centers for Pancreatic Cancer

Chang DC, Zhang Y, Mukherjee D, et al (Johns Hopkins School of Medicine, Baltimore, MD; Johns Hopkins Bloomberg School of Public Health, Baltimore, MD)

J Am Coll Surg 209:720-726, 2009

Background.—Multiple reports have demonstrated pancreatic cancer patients undergoing surgery have superior outcomes at high-volume hospitals. This study noted trends in access to high-volume centers for pancreatic resection and identified gaps in improving access.

Study Design.—We performed a retrospective analysis of the Nationwide Inpatient Sample (NIS 2000 to 2005) linked to the Area Resource File (ARF). Inclusion criteria were patients with primary diagnosis of pancreatic cancer who received pancreatic resection. The primary outcomes variable was treatment at high-volume hospitals (average annual case volume greater than 20). Independent variables included age, gender, race, Charlson Comorbidity Index score, insurance status, calendar year, and region, obtained from the Nationwide Inpatient Sample; community poverty level and density of all physicians, gastroenterologists, surgeons, and radiation oncologists were data obtained from the Area Resource File.

Results.—A total of 8,370 patients were identified. A minority (38.51%) were referred to high-volume hospitals. A significant increase in overall referral and odds of referral to a high-volume center was observed over time (22.2% in 2000 to 44.4% in 2005). Patients referred to high-volume centers were younger (61.9 versus 63.2 years, $p < 0.001$) and more likely to be Caucasian (81.7% versus 73.6%, $p < 0.001$). Patients greater than 85 years old, African Americans, Hispanics, and Asians were less likely to be referred, relative to their younger, Caucasian counterparts ($p < 0.01$). The overall trend toward improved referral over time was driven by improved referral among Caucasians. In multivariate analysis, access to high-volume centers was associated with calendar year, patient age, and race. In addition, increase in density of gastroenterologists or radiation oncologists in the population was also associated with higher likelihood of referral.

Conclusions.—This study demonstrated that less than half of pancreatic cancer patients are being referred to high-volume centers. Unlike referral in Caucasians, improvement in referral for minorities has not occurred.

▶ This study from the Johns Hopkins University School of Medicine retrospectively analyzes the nationwide input sample linked to the area resource file. It is a large study of over 8000 patients. As seen in Fig 2 in the original article, multivariate analysis demonstrates a significant increase in the likelihood of patients being referred to a high-volume center, with time. However, as seen in Fig 4 in the original article, the same multivariate analysis shows that minority patients are less likely to be referred to high-volume centers.

This study confirms a racial disparity in access to care while improving the density of gastroenterologists and radiation oncologists in communities may improve access to high-volume centers. It's certainly not feasible in the immediate future, and may not be economically viable.

This study has some limitations. It is retrospective in its analysis. Missing data are also a possibility. There is no cancer staging data. This latter point is important because there could be an argument that minority patients present with later-stage disease, therefore making them unresectable.

Less than half the patients with pancreatic cancer are being referred to high-volume centers, and this is particularly true among minority patients. Identifying mechanisms toward improvement of surgical care of these patients will likely result in preference for high-volume centers and earlier diagnosis in minority populations.

T. J. Eberlein, MD

Clinical Significance of Frozen Section Analysis During Resection of Intraductal Papillary Mucinous Neoplasm: Should a Positive Pancreatic Margin for Adenoma or Borderline Lesion Be Resected Additionally?

Nara S, Shimada K, Sakamoto Y, et al (Natl Cancer Ctr Hosp, Tokyo, Japan; et al)

J Am Coll Surg 209:614-621, 2009

Background.—The clinical significance of a positive intraoperative frozen section analysis of the pancreatic margin, especially for adenoma or borderline lesion, is not well understood during operations for intraductal papillary mucinous neoplasm of the pancreas.

Study Design.—Data from 130 consecutive patients who underwent intraductal papillary mucinous neoplasm resection in a single institution were retrospectively analyzed.

Results.—In the first intraoperative frozen section analysis, 26 patients were positive for adenoma or borderline lesion, 10 for carcinoma in situ, 2 for cancer cells floating in the duct, and 6 for invasive cancer. Twenty-nine patients underwent additional resection, and 105 patients finally achieved a negative pancreatic margin. Among 18 patients with a positive pancreatic margin for adenoma or borderline lesion, only 1 had a recurrence. All 20 patients who suffered a recurrence harbored invasive intraductal papillary mucinous carcinoma in resected specimens. In multivariate analysis, predictive factors of recurrence after intraductal papillary mucinous carcinoma resection were the presence of lymph node metastasis, serosal invasion, and a high level of serum carbohydrate antigen 19-9.

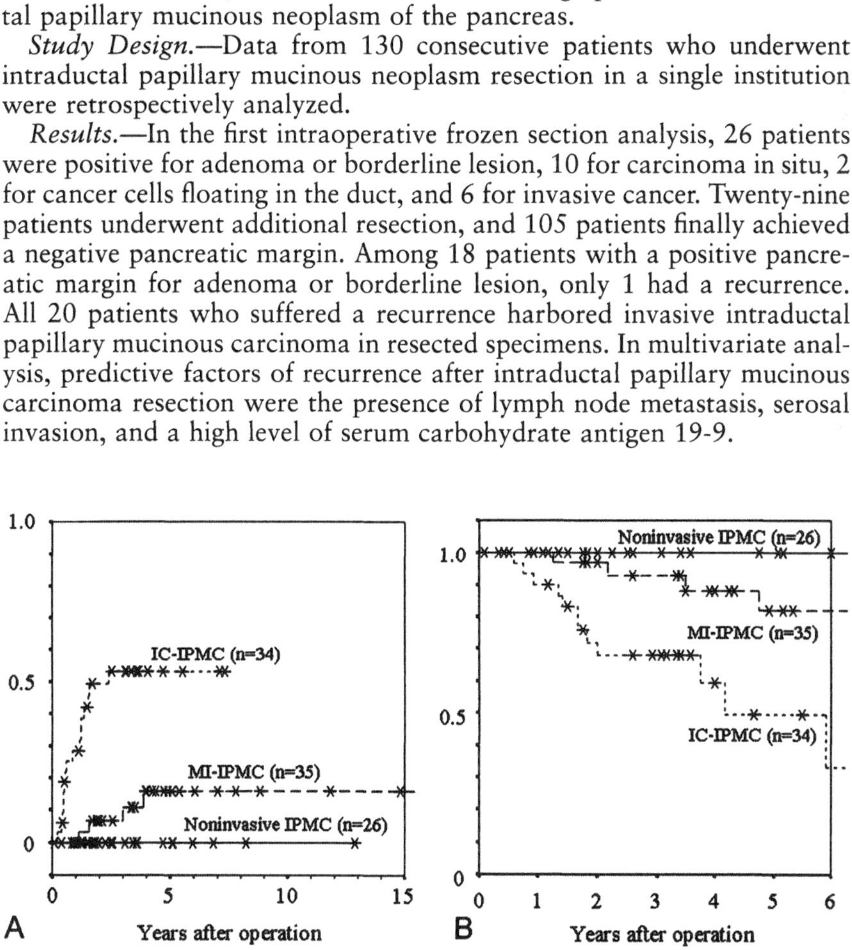

FIGURE 2.—Comparison of (A) recurrence and (B) overall survival rates among patients with noninvasive intraductal papillary mucinous carcinoma (IPMC), minimally invasive IPMC (MI-IPMC), and invasive cancer originating in IPMC (IC-IPMC). There was a significant difference in recurrence and overall survival rates by the log-rank test ($p < 0.001$). (Reprinted from Nara S, Shimada K, Sakamoto Y, et al. Clinical significance of frozen section analysis during resection of intraductal papillary mucinous neoplasm: should a positive pancreatic margin for adenoma or borderline lesion be resected additionally? *J Am Coll Surg.* 2009;209:614-621, with permission from the American College of Surgeons.)

TABLE 4.—Multivariate Analysis of Factors Associated with Recurrence in Patients with Noninvasive and Minimally Invasive Intraductal Papillary Mucinous Carcinoma and Patients with Invasive Cancer Originating in Intraductal Papillary Mucinous Carcinoma (n = 95)

Variable	p Value	Hazards Ratio	95% CI
Serosal invasion	<0.001	6.87	2.35–20.0
Lymph node metastasis	0.001	5.15	1.98–13.4
CA19-9 > 200 U/mL	0.023	3.00	1.17–7.73

CA19-9, carbohydrate antigen 19-9.

Conclusions.—The presence of adenoma or borderline lesion at the pancreatic margin does not always warrant further resection because of the low recurrence rate in the remnant pancreas. Recurrence after intraductal papillary mucinous neoplasm resection is influenced primarily by the presence and extent of invasive cancer rather than the status of the pancreatic margin (Fig 2, Table 4).

▶ Many surgeons advocate a drop in frozen section analysis of the pancreatic cut margin when performing surgery for intraductal papillary mucinous neoplasm (IPMN). As seen in Fig 2, comparison of recurrence (A) and overall survival (B) shows that degree of invasion significantly influences recurrence in overall survival. Looking at multivariate analysis, serosal invasion, lymph node metastases, and elevated carbohydrate antigen (CA) 19-9 were associated with recurrence of tumor (Table 4).

In this study, none of the patients who had noninvasive IPMN had recurrence, regardless of margin status. Yet, almost 30% of patients with invasive IPMC developed a recurrence. It is therefore very important that an experienced pathologist evaluate these tumors to determine whether a small area of microinvasion may be overlooked and would therefore be associated with a higher risk of recurrence.

T. J. Eberlein, MD

Margin Clearance and Outcome in Resected Pancreatic Cancer

Chang DK, Johns AL, Merrett ND, et al (Garvan Inst of Med Res, Sydney, Australia; Univ of New South Wales, Bankstown, Australia; Univ of Sydney, St Leonards, Australia; et al)

J Clin Oncol 27:2855-2862, 2009

Purpose.—Current adjuvant therapies for pancreatic cancer (PC) are inconsistently used and only modestly effective. Because a high proportion of patients who undergo resection for PC likely harbor occult metastatic disease, any adjuvant trials assessing therapies such as radiotherapy directed at locoregional disease are significantly underpowered. Stratification based on the probability (and volume) of residual locoregional disease could play an important role in the design of future clinical trials assessing adjuvant radiotherapy.

Patients and Methods.—We assessed the relationships between margin involvement, the proximity to operative resection margins and outcome in a cohort of 365 patients who underwent operative resection for PC.

Results.—Microscopic involvement of a resection margin by tumor was associated with a poor prognosis. Stratifying the minimum clearance of resection margins by 0.5-mm increments demonstrated that although median survival was no different to clear margins based on these definitions, it was not until the resection margin was clear by more than 1.5 mm that optimal long-term survival was achieved.

Conclusion.—These data demonstrate that a margin clearance of more than 1.5 mm is important for long-term survival in a subgroup of patients. More aggressive therapeutic approaches that target locoregional disease such as radiotherapy may be beneficial in patients with close surgical margins. Stratification of patients for entry onto future clinical trials based on this criterion may identify those patients who benefit from adjuvant radiotherapy.

▶ This study is conducted on 365 consecutive patients with pancreatic cancer from the New South Wales Pancreatic Cancer Network in Sydney, Australia. The authors assess the relationship between margin involvement and ultimate outcome. As expected, patients with negative margins did better than patients with positive margins. However, until the patient had a clear margin of 2 mm, the patients' outcome behaved more like a patient with positive margins (Fig 2 in the original article). Because many pancreatic surgeons consider body and tail cancers somewhat different from those arising in the pancreatic head, the authors identified 295 patients who underwent Whipple procedures (Fig 3 in the original article). The patients in the body/tail category with minimal negative margins were limited, which clearly implies that the major impact of this study was due to the cancers in the head of the pancreas, which underwent Whipple procedures.

Therefore, it appears that margin resection of greater that 1.5 mm is important for long-term survival. This is particularly true in tumors of the pancreatic head and patients who undergo Whipple procedures. Close margins may be a surrogate for the actual tumor biology. As genomic and other molecular data become available, a more accurate predictor for outcome may become available.

T. J. Eberlein, MD

Novel Pancreaticojejunostomy with a Low Rate of Anastomotic Failure-Related Complications

Grobmyer SR, Kooby D, Blumgart LH, et al (Univ of Florida, Gainesville, FL; Emory Univ, Atlanta, GA; Memorial Sloan-Kettering Cancer Inst, NY)

J Am Coll Surg 210:54-59, 2010

Background.—Pancreatic anastomotic failure has traditionally been a source of significant morbidity and potential mortality after pancreaticoduodenectomy. Both patient-derived and technical factors contribute to pancreatic anastomotic failure. From a technical standpoint, an "ideal" pancreaticojejunal anastomosis would meet the following criteria: applicable to all patients, easy to teach, and associated with a low rate of pancreatic anastomotic failure-related complications. The pancreaticojejunostomy described by one of the authors (LHB) meets the criteria for an "ideal" pancreaticojejunostomy.

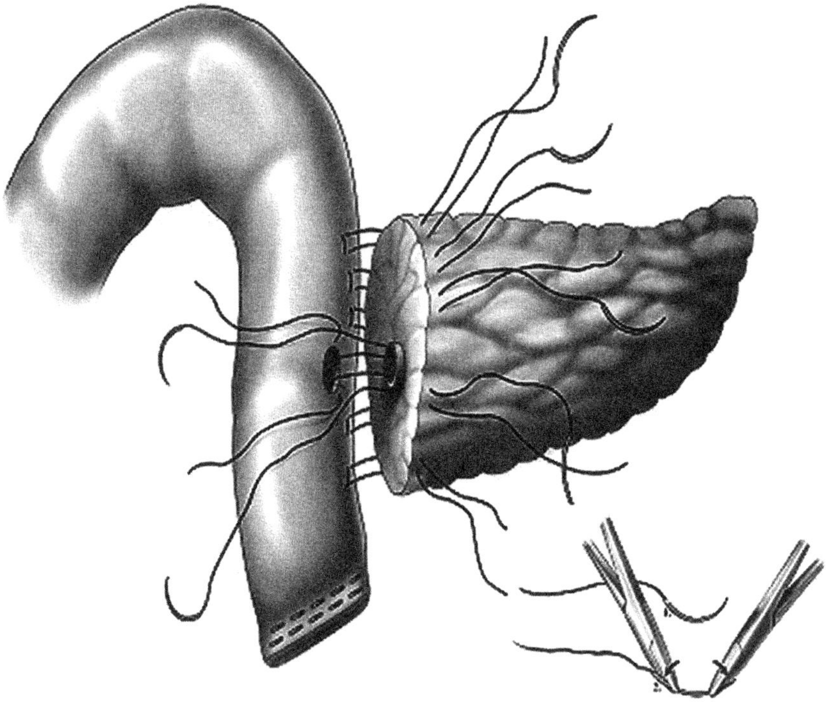

FIGURE 2.—Placement of full thickness pancreatic/jejunal seromuscular sutures and duct-to-mucosa sutures. Inset: Straightening the needle before placement through the pancreas facilitates full thickness suture placement. Note that the sutures are placed from anterior to posterior through the pancreatic gland, continuing with a seromuscular bite of jejunum and then back through the pancreas from posterior to anterior. Four to six sutures with 2-0 Vicryl are placed in this fashion. The needles are left on these sutures. Then the inner layer of full thickness bowel wall and pancreatic duct are done with 5-0 polydioxanone suture (PDS, Ethicon). (Reprinted from Grobmyer SR, Kooby D, Blumgart LH, et al. Novel pancreaticojejunostomy with a low rate of anastomotic failure-related complications. *J Am Coll Surg*. 2010;210:54-59, with permission from the American College of Surgeons.)

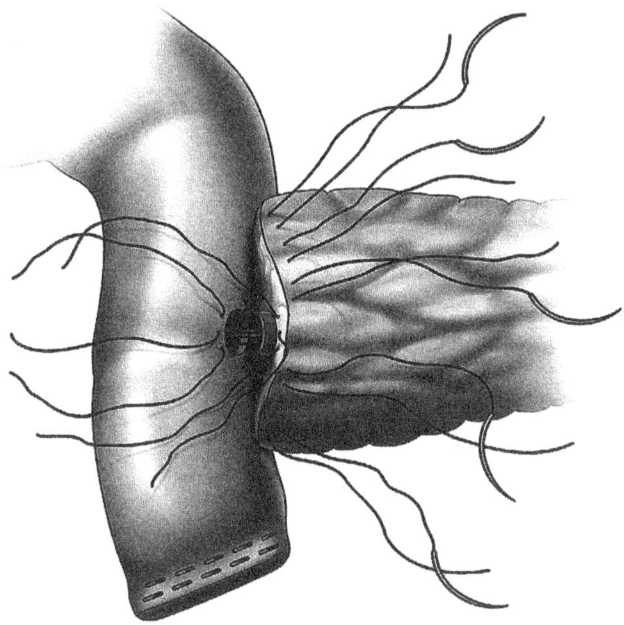

FIGURE 3.—The duct-to-mucosa sutures are tied initially, proceeding from the back row to front row. (Reprinted from Grobmyer SR, Kooby D, Blumgart LH, et al. Novel pancreaticojejunostomy with a low rate of anastomotic failure-related complications. *J Am Coll Surg*. 2010;210:54-59, with permission from the American College of Surgeons.)

Study Design.—We performed an audit of results of a consecutive series of patients at two institutions who underwent pancreaticojejunostomy using the described technique. Pancreaticojejunostomy after pancreaticoduodenectomy was performed in all cases using a novel two-layer technique consisting of an outer full thickness pancreas-to-seromuscular jejunal anastomosis and an inner duct-to-mucosal anastomosis. Incidences of pancreatic anastomotic failure (measured using the International Study Group of Pancreatic Fistula definition) and perioperative pancreatic anastomotic failure-related complications were analyzed.

Results.—One hundred eighty-seven patients underwent pancreaticojejunostomy after pancreaticoduodenectomy using the described technique. Overall mortality was 1.6%. The rate of clinically significant pancreatic anastomotic failure (International Study Group of Pancreatic Fistula grade B or C) was only 6.9%. There was no bleeding, reoperation, or mortality secondary to pancreatic anastomotic failure among patients in this series.

Conclusions.—The novel pancreaticojejunostomy is applicable to all patients in whom the pancreatic duct can be identified, and it is associated with very low rates of significant postoperative morbidity and mortality.

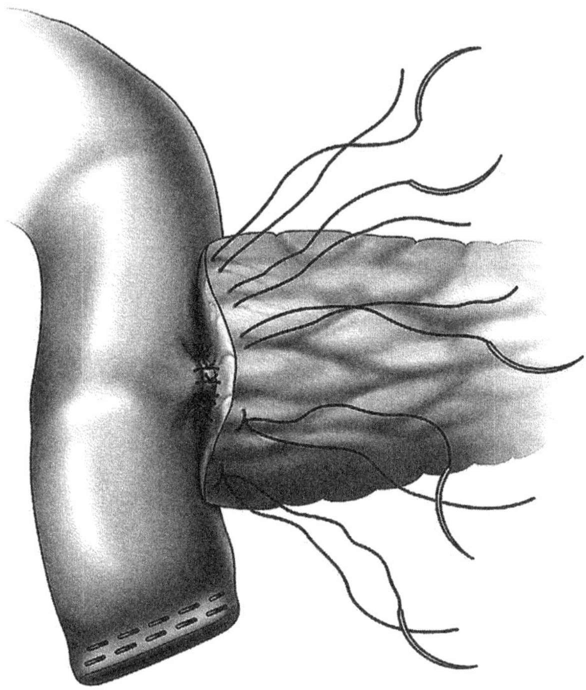

FIGURE 4.—The transpancreatic/jejunal seromuscular Vicryl sutures are tied to secure the approximation of pancreas and jejunum. Care is taken not to strangulate the pancreas when these sutures are tied. (Reprinted from Grobmyer SR, Kooby D, Blumgart LH, et al. Novel pancreaticojejunostomy with a low rate of anastomotic failure-related complications. *J Am Coll Surg*. 2010;210:54-59, with permission from the American College of Surgeons.)

TABLE 1.—Pancreatic Anastomotic Failure Rate[23] Among Patients in this Series

Grade	n	%	Length of Postoperative Hospital Stay, Median (d)
A	25	13.4	10.5
B	7	3.7	15.5
C	6	3.2	17.5

Editor's Note: Please refer to original journal article for full references.

These findings support its routine use for pancreaticojejunal reconstruction after pancreaticoduodenectomy (Figs 2–4, Table 1).

▶ One of the vexing issues in performing a Whipple procedure is the complication of postoperative pancreatic leaks. Dr Leslie Blumgart, from Memorial Sloan-Kettering, has been a proponent of a duct-to-mucosa technique that is 2-layered. This is a large series of patients prospectively gathered from 2 institutions. They are consecutive patients. The rate of clinically significant pancreatic anastomotic failure (Table 1) was only 6.9%. None of the patients required reoperations, and there was no mortality due to pancreatic anastomotic failure. Figs 2-4 show very explicit drawings of the technique involved. These authors describe a single, full-thickness, mattress-type suture as one of the layers. The authors hypothesize that this firmly anchors the gland to the jejunum, preventing full disruption of the gland from the pancreas. They also complete the duct-to-mucosa sutures before securing the posterior seromuscular jejunum.

The fact that 3 different pancreatic surgeons from 2 different institutions were able to replicate these outstanding results makes this a good technique to emulate for outstanding results.

T. J. Eberlein, MD

Rectal

Postoperative Morbidity with Diversion after Low Anterior Resection in the Era of Neoadjuvant Therapy: A Single Institution Experience

Tsikitis VL, Larson DW, Poola VP, et al (Mayo Clinic, Rochester, MN)

J Am Coll Surg 209:114-118, 2009

Background.—The use of defunctioning stomas has been advocated to mitigate the adverse sequela from anastomotic dehiscence after rectal cancer resection. The aim of this study was to report our experience with anastomotic dehiscence and overall morbidity of low anterior resections in the era of neoadjuvant therapy, where the use of fecal diversion is part of the standard operative strategy for low (< 5 cm) rectal anastomoses.

Study Design.—This retrospective case series included patients who were treated with neoadjuvant therapy and had rectal cancer resection with curative intent, from 1996 to 2007.

Results.—Two hundred thirty-seven patients (159 men, 78 women) with mean age of 59 years (SD ± 12.7 years), received 5-flurouracil–based infusional chemotherapy and external-beam radiation in the range of 45 to 54 Gy. Fifty-seven percent of patients underwent anterior resection and 43% had coloanal anastomosis. Anastomotic dehiscence occurred in 9 patients (3.8%). Seven of the anastomotic leaks were diagnosed as pelvic abscesses (2.1%) and 2 patients needed reexploration (0.8%). Early overall postoperative morbidity was 26%, and there was no postoperative mortality. One hundred ninety-one of 193 patients had their ileostomy reversed, with minimal morbidity (0.5% leak rate).

Conclusions.—Low postoperative morbidity after colorectal and coloanal anastomosis for adenocarcinoma is possible in patients who have received neoadjuvant therapy. Defunctioning stomas are safe and may

TABLE 3.—Factors Associated with Anastomotic Leakage

Variable	n	Univariate Analysis %	p Value
Gender			0.84
Male	160	67.3	
Female	78	32.7	
Age, y			0.003
< 65	153	64.3	
> 65	85	35.7	
Body mass index			0.71
Smoking	96	40.3	0.08
Cardiovascular disease	68	28.6	0.007
ASA class 3/4	81	34	0.01
Tumor height, cm from anal verge			0.23
< 5	171	72	
> 5	66	28	

ASA, American Society of Anesthesiologists.

TABLE 4.—Overall Postoperative Morbidity

Variable	n	%
Surgical		
Abdominal wound infection		
Treated with antibiotics	7/237	2.9
Anastomotic leak	9/237	3.7
Needed reexploration	3/237	1.2
CT-guided drainage	3/237	1.2
Pelvic abscess (not anastomotic leaks)	5/237	1.4
Prolonged ileus	18	7.5
Small bowel obstruction conservatively treated	10	4.2
Small bowel obstruction operated on	5	1.4
Blood transfusion	8	3.4
Urinary retention	20	9.0
Medical		
Deep vein thrombosis	1	0.4
Pulmonary embolism	2	0.8
Myocardial infarction	1	0.4
Acute renal insufficiency	2	0.8

mitigate the serious sequela of anastomotic dehiscence after low rectal anastomoses (Tables 3 and 4).

▶ This is very large series of patients from the Mayo Clinic. All of these patients had neoadjuvant treatment for rectal cancer and had defunctioning stomas at the time of their lower anterior resection or coloanal anastomosis.

As might be expected, overall morbidity was quite low. Anastomotic leakage was associated with high American Society of Anesthesiologists (ASA) class as well as cardiovascular disease and age (Table 3). As seen in Table 4, only

3 patients (1.2 %) required re-exploration. Obviously having a second procedure (ileostomy closure) can have potential for added morbidity. After stoma closure, these authors found a leak rate of 0.5%.

Common use of diverting ileostomy can certainly minimize the risk of morbidity in patients with rectal cancer who are treated with neoadjuvant therapy.

T. J. Eberlein, MD

Colon

Tumor Border Configuration Added to TNM Staging Better Stratifies Stage II Colorectal Cancer Patients Into Prognostic Subgroups

Zlobec I, Baker K, Minoo P, et al (Univ of Basel, Switzerland; McGill Univ, Quebec, Canada; Univ of California San Diego; et al)

Cancer 115:4021-4029, 2009

Background.—Reproducible and well characterized prognostic histomorphologic criteria added to current pathological staging could have an immediate effect on refining prognosis in colorectal cancer. The aim of this study was to determine the additive effect of tumor border configuration and peritumoral lymphocytic infiltration on the selection of patients for adjuvant therapy classified by TNM.

Methods.—A total of 1420 primary colorectal cancers with complete clinicopathological data from multiple treatment centers were analyzed. The prognostic effect of tumor border configuration (pushing or infiltrating) and peritumoral lymphocytic infiltration was assessed, validated by resampling of the data, and compared with TNM staging. All P values were 2-sided.

Results.—Multivariate analysis confirmed the adverse prognostic value of the tumor border configuration ($P < .001$), but not of peritumoral lymphocytic infiltration. The addition of tumor border configuration to T and N category identified 2 major prognostic subgroups (relative risk of death, 4.75; 95% confidence interval [CI], 2.53-8.94). Moreover, stage II patients with a pushing border had a 5-year survival rate of 82.1% (95% CI, 71.8%-90.3%), whereas an infiltrating border resulted in a significantly more adverse outcome (5-year survival rate, 62.7%; 95% CI, 48.0-76.2%), closely resembling that of stage III patients. Similar results were obtained after adjusting for adjuvant therapy ($P < .001$).

Conclusions.—The classification of patients into prognostic subgroups is improved with the addition of tumor border configuration to TNM stage. In particular, patients with stage II disease characterized by an infiltrating tumor border have poor clinical outcome and represent a subset of lymph node-negative patients who could be considered for adjuvant therapy (Fig 2).

▶ This article from Basel, Switzerland, attempts to better stratify patients with stage II colon cancer. A substantial number of patients with stage II colon

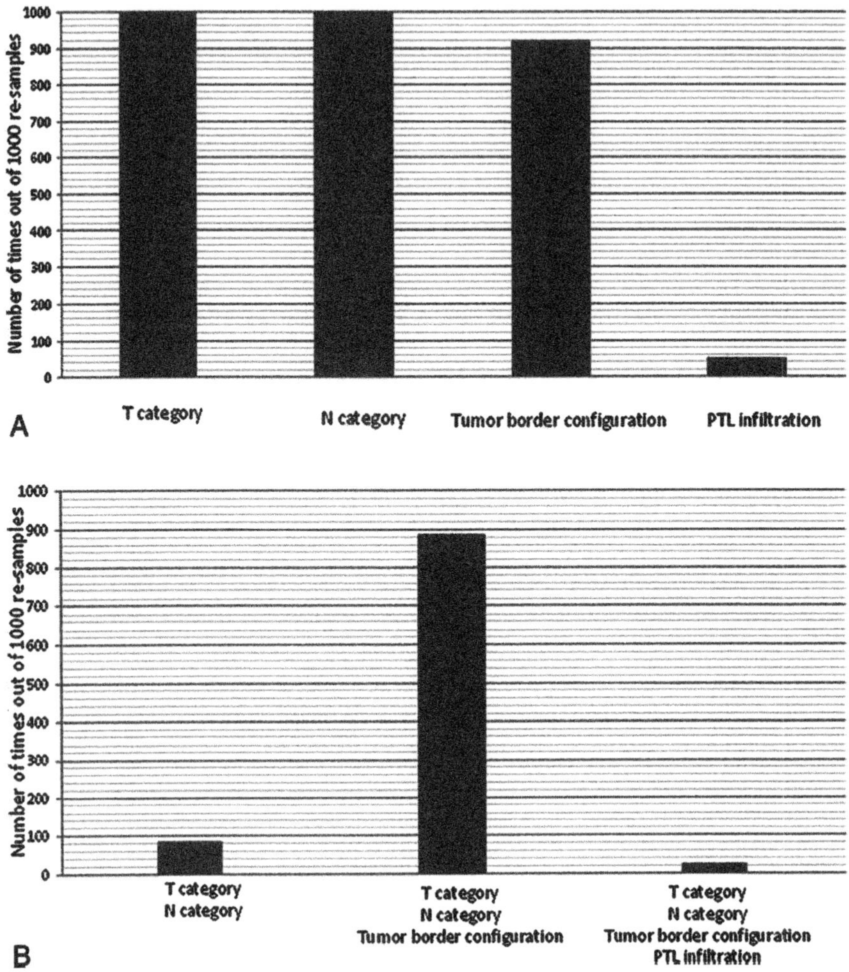

FIGURE 2.—After resampling of the data and multivariate Cox proportional hazards regression analysis, T category, N category, and tumor border configuration had the most reproducible prognostic effects, whereas peritumoral lymphocytic (PTL) infiltration was selected few times as an independent prognostic factor (*Top*). The model containing T, N, and tumor border configuration was identified as having the most reproducible prognostic effects (*Bottom*). (Reprinted from Zlobec I, Baker K, Minoo P, et al. Tumor border configuration added to TNM staging better stratifies stage II colorectal cancer patients into prognostic subgroups. *Cancer.* 2009;115:4021-4029, with permission from the American Cancer Society.)

cancer have recurrence of disease. Being able to identify the patients at highest risk would be beneficial. These authors showed that patients who had an infiltrating border associated with their stage II disease had a worse outcome. Therefore, the authors used multivariate Cox proportional hazard regression analysis and showed that combining tumor model and tumor border configuration had the most reproducible prognostic effects (Fig 2).

Evaluation of this tumor characteristic can be somewhat subjective, but in an experienced pathologist's hands this prognostic feature can be important in selecting patients for potential adjuvant treatment. Further confirmation in prospective trials will be necessary, particularly combining it with some of the newer genomic and gene-based panels that are being proposed for similar prognostic information in stage II colon patients.

T. J. Eberlein, MD

Quality of Life and Symptom Control after Stent Placement or Surgical Palliation of Malignant Colorectal Obstruction

Nagula S, Ishill N, Nash C, et al (Memorial Sloan-Kettering Cancer Ctr, NY; Univ of Calgary, Alberta, Canada)

J Am Coll Surg 210:45-53, 2010

Background.—Emergent surgical management of malignant large bowel obstruction (LBO) carries a high rate of morbidity and mortality. Self-expanding metal stents have emerged as an alternative for palliation of malignant LBO. However, there are few long-term studies documenting the effect of surgical palliation or colonic stents on symptoms or quality of life (QoL).

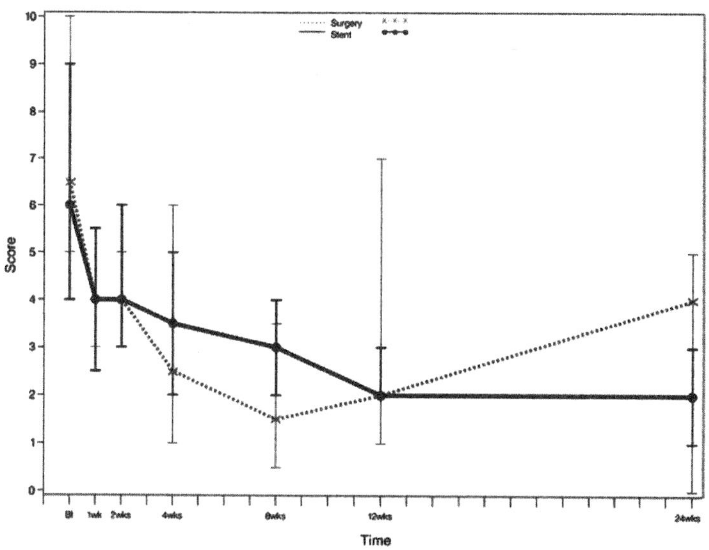

FIGURE 3.—Colon obstruction scores for stent and surgery groups (lower scores represent improved obstructive symptoms). Vertical bars represent interquartile range (IQR). (Reprinted from Nagula S, Ishill N, Nash C, et al. Quality of life and symptom control after stent placement or surgical palliation of malignant colorectal obstruction. *J Am Coll Surg*. 2010;210:45-53, with permission from the American College of Surgeons.)

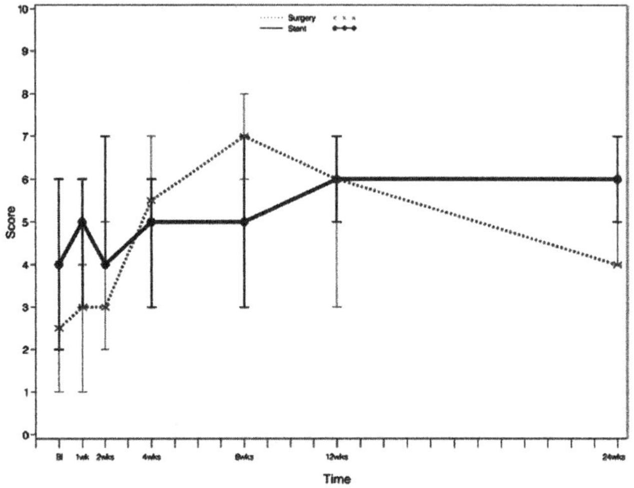

FIGURE 7.—Self-reported quality of life (QoL; higher scores represent improved QoL). Vertical bars represent interquartile range (IQR). (Reprinted from Nagula S, Ishill N, Nash C, et al. Quality of life and symptom control after stent placement or surgical palliation of malignant colorectal obstruction. *J Am Coll Surg*. 2010;210:45-53, with permission from the American College of Surgeons.)

Study Design.—Between 2003 and 2006, patients with unresectable-for-cure malignancies presenting with LBO were enrolled in this prospective study. Patients elected to undergo stent placement or surgical palliation. Patients completed a symptom questionnaire and a QoL instrument (Functional Assessment of Cancer Therapy-Colorectal [FACT-C]) at weeks 1, 2, 4, 8, 12, and 24 after palliation. Symptoms were assessed using the Colon Obstruction Score, a novel instrument comprising nausea, vomiting, pain, distension, and bowel movement frequency scores.

Results.—Thirty patients had successful stent placement; 14 underwent surgical diversion. Colon Obstruction Scores immediately improved after both stent placement and surgery ($p < 0.05$ for all time points). Composite FACT-C scores progressively improved after stent placement ($p = NS$), with the colon symptoms subscale improving after 1 month ($p < 0.05$). FACT-C scores declined initially after surgery and then returned to baseline, with modest improvements seen in the Colon Symptoms subscale ($p = NS$).

Conclusions.—Both stent placement and surgical diversion provide durable improvement in symptoms from LBO, as readily assessed by the Colon Obstruction Score. QoL is difficult to assess in terminal cancer patients, but colon stent placement is associated with improved overall QoL and QoL related to gastrointestinal symptoms.

▶ Patients with advanced abdominal cancers, particularly colorectal and gynecologic, may present with malignant large bowel obstructions. This is a single institution's study that compared surgery to self-expanding metal stents as palliation. Then patients were subsequently followed for symptom relief and quality-of-life assessments. The patients elected to undergo 1 procedure or the other rather than them being randomized to a prospective design. As seen in Fig 3, both stent and surgery significantly relieved obstructive symptoms, most notably pain, distention, and improved bowel movement frequency. With respect to quality of life, stent placement seemed to compare quite favorably to surgery. While at 4 and 8 weeks, it appeared that surgery was slightly better, statistically, after 8 weeks, the surgery group declined (Fig 7). This may be due to self-selection rather than the patients being randomized to intervention for relief of their obstruction.

There are a few caveats to this study. Stent placement is not 100% successful (usually greater than 90%, however). This study was unusual in that they also treated patients with extrinsic compression causing the colonic obstruction.

The choice of either of these procedures is usually a very individualized and personal decision for each particular patient. However, in general, sicker patients who may not withstand an operation may be better suited for colon stent placement. Similarly, younger patients may be better palliated by surgery. Up to 20% of patients with stent placement originally may ultimately require surgical palliation. However, colon stent placement is an excellent primary treatment, and should add to our possible interventions in patients with these difficult clinical situations.

T. J. Eberlein, MD

Gastric

Accuracy of Surgical Diagnosis in Detecting Early Gastric Cancer and Lymph Node Metastasis and Its Role in Determining Limited Surgery

Jeong O, Ryu SY, Park YK (Chonnam Natl Univ Hwasun Hosp, Jeollanam-do, Korea)

J Am Coll Surg 209:302-307, 2009

Background.—The aim of this study was to evaluate the accuracy of surgical diagnosis of early gastric cancer (EGC) and lymph node metastasis, and elucidate its role in determining limited surgery for EGC.

Study Design.—We reviewed 369 patients undergoing gastrectomy for primary gastric carcinoma. Surgical diagnosis was evaluated by determining its sensitivity, specificity, and accuracy, and was compared with preoperative examinations.

Results.—Sensitivity, specificity, and accuracy of intraoperative diagnosis for EGC were 74.5%, 95.7%, and 83.7%, respectively. The predictive value for EGC by intraoperative diagnosis was 95.7%. Surgical diagnosis of EGC showed higher specificity and predictive value than preoperative examinations did, which significantly reduced the risk of underestimating advanced gastric cancer (AGC) to EGC. The sensitivity, specificity, and accuracy for lymph node metastasis by surgical diagnosis were 73.2%, 78.1%, and 76.4%, respectively. In 70 patients with a discrepancy in the diagnosis of EGC between pre- and intraoperative

TABLE 2.—Comparisons of Pathologic Examinations with Preoperative Examinations and Surgical Diagnosis of the Depth of Invasion

Variable	Pathologic Diagnosis, n		Total, n
	pT1	pT2–4	
Intraoperative assessment			
sT1	155	7	162
sT2–4	53	154	207
Preoperative examinations			
cT1	105	13	118
cT2–4	103	148	151
Total	208	161	

TABLE 3.—Comparisons of Pathologic Examinations with Preoperative Examinations and Surgical Diagnosis of Lymph Node Metastasis

Variable	Pathologic Diagnosis, n		Total, n
	pN0	pN+	
Intraoperative assessment			
sN0	189	34	223
sN+	53	93	146
Preoperative examinations			
cN0	215	59	274
cN+	27	68	95
Total	242	127	

diagnoses, surgical diagnosis was correct in 63 (90%) patients, but preoperative examination was correct in only 7 (10%) patients.

Conclusions.—Surgical diagnosis shows better accuracy than preoperative examinations do in detecting EGC and lymph node metastasis. Our results suggest that the decision to perform limited surgery based on surgical diagnosis might reduce the risk of undertreatment of AGC to EGC better than preoperative examinations (Tables 2 and 3).

▶ This is a single-institution study from the Chonnam National University Hwasun Hospital, Korea. The goal of this study was to evaluate the accuracy of surgical diagnosis of early gastric cancer. As seen in Table 2, diagnostic accuracy of preoperative examination was helpful but not overwhelmingly accurate. Thirteen patients with advanced gastric cancer were underestimated as having early gastric cancer, and almost half of the early gastric cancer patients were overestimated as having advanced gastric cancer using preoperative examinations (Table 2). As seen in Table 3, accuracy was also improved with intraoperative evaluation compared with preoperative evaluation with respect to lymph node involvement.

Clearly, surgical evaluation can improve preoperative studies for evaluation of gastric cancer; however, the caveat is that the surgeons in this study were very experienced gastric surgeons performing well over 100 gastric cancer operations every year. While surgical evaluation may improve accuracy of staging, few surgeons in the United States have the expertise to completely use this evaluative process.

T. J. Eberlein, MD

Prognostic Significance of Intraoperatively Estimated Surgical Stage in Curatively Resected Gastric Cancer Patients

Lee SE, Ryu KW, Nam BH, et al (Natl Cancer Ctr, Goyang-si, Republic of Korea)

J Am Coll Surg 209:461-467, 2009

Background.—The aim of this study was to assess the prognostic significance of intraoperatively estimated surgical stage (sStage) as a complementary role for pathologic stage (pStage) in gastric cancer.

Study Design.—This was a retrospective study of 1,543 patients who underwent curative resection for gastric cancer. Clinicopathologic and therapeutic factors, including sStage, were analyzed for prognostic significance. Prognosis was stratified by sStage and pStage, and the prognoses of patients with an overestimated sStage were compared with those with a nonoverestimated sStage in the same pStage.

Results.—Overall accuracy of sStage versus pStage was 39% (T stage, 73.0%; N stage, 43.5%). Survival curves were obviously stratified by sStage and pStage: Ia (97.5% versus 97.9%), Ib (94.3% versus 92.4%), II (89.6% versus 84.2%), IIIa (74.2% versus 69.3%), IIIb (54.4% versus 50.4%), and IV (55.6% versus 36.7%), respectively ($p < 0.001$). In addition to pStage, age and sStage were found to be significantly associated with overall survival by univariate and multivariate analysis. In pStages II, IIIa, and IIIb, intraoperatively overestimated patients had significantly poorer survival than nonoverestimated patients.

Conclusions.—sStage should be considered as a complementary prognostic factor for pStage in gastric cancer after curative resection, especially in stages II and III patients (Fig 2, Table 7).

▶ This article from the National Cancer Center in Korea attempts to access the prognostic significance of intraoperative surgical staging in patients with gastric cancer.

This study showed a very favorable 5-year overall survival, possibly because the authors excluded patients with hepatic metastases, peritoneal seeding, and positive periaortic lymph node metastases. There were also a fair number of stage 1 gastric cancers in this series. Over 40% of the patients with greater than stage II disease underwent adjuvant chemotherapy in this series. Table 7 shows the survival of patients with surgically staged overestimation and non-overestimation with the same pathologic stage. This is also seen in Fig 2, which shows overall survival for patients with overestimation of a surgical stage, showing lower survivability for stage II, IIIa, and IIIb pathologic staged patients.

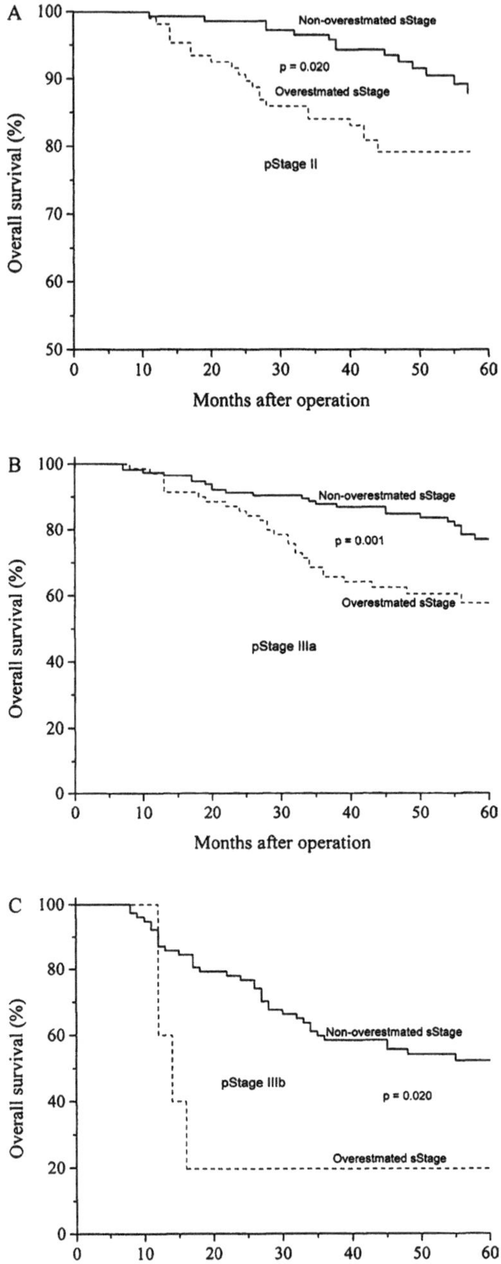

FIGURE 2.—Overall survival of patients with overestimated or nonoverestimated sStage in pStages (A) II, (B) IIIa, and (C) IIIb. (Reprinted from Lee SE, Ryu KW, Nam BH, et al. Prognostic significance of intraoperatively estimated surgical stage in curatively resected gastric cancer patients. *J Am Coll Surg.* 2009;209:461-467, with permission from the American College of Surgeons.)

TABLE 7.—Survivals of Patients with Overestimated and Nonoverestimated Surgical Stage in the Same Pathologic Stage

pStage	sStage	n	%	5-y Overall Survival, %	p Value
Ia	Ia	290	46.8	98.2	0.733
	> Ia	330	53.2	97.5	
Ib	≤ Ib	135	45.5	94.1	0.584
	> Ib	162	54.5	91.0	
II	≤ II	143	57.2	87.9	0.020
	> II	107	48.3	79.6	
IIIa	≤ IIIa	115	62.2	78.6	0.001
	> IIIa	70	37.8	57.8	
IIIb	≤ IIIb	77	93.9	52.3	0.020
	> IIIb	5	6.1	20.0	
IV	< IV	72	66.1	33.0	0.391
	IV	37	33.9	44.4	

pStage, pathologic stage; sStage, surgical stage.

While this study indicates that intraoperative surgical stage can predict prognosis, this requires an experienced and well-trained surgeon. Nonetheless, this can become complementary for prognosis in gastric cancer after curative resection.

T. J. Eberlein, MD

Association of Age and Survival in Patients With Gastroesophageal Cancer Undergoing Surgery With or Without Preoperative Therapy

Braiteh F, Correa AM, Hofstetter WL, et al (The Univ of Texas M. D. Anderson Cancer Ctr, Houston)

Cancer 115:4450-4458, 2009

Background.—Meticulous selection of patients for esophageal cancer surgery is critical, because major surgical intervention can cause considerable consequences. For this study, the authors explored their institution's large surgical experience to examine the impact of age on long-term patient survival and surgical complications.

Method.—Six hundred consecutive patients with esophageal cancer who underwent surgery (409 patients received preoperative therapy, and 191 patients underwent surgery first) were analyzed. All demographic information (including American Society of Anesthesiology risk scores) and therapy-related information was collected retrospectively. Multiple statistical methods were used to assess survival rates and surgical complications and their correlation with patient age. Twenty-one patients (30-day mortality) first were excluded ($n = 600$) and then were included ($n = 621$) in the analysis.

Results.—By using the median age (≤60 years) as the cutoff point and creating 2 subgroups (ages 61 years to 70 years and aged >70 years) in

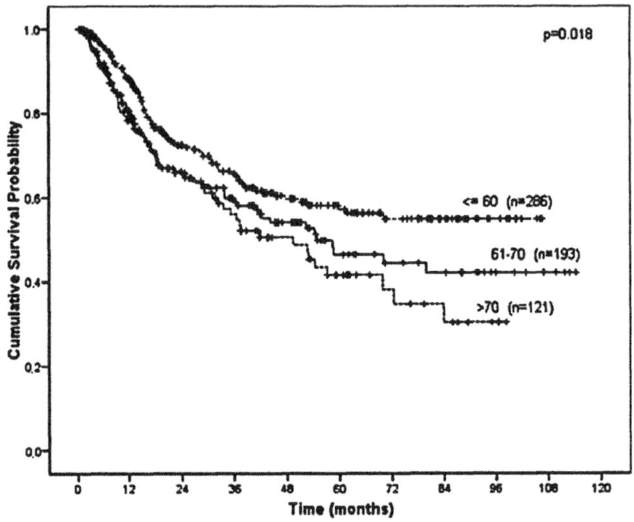

FIGURE 1.—This Kaplan-Meier plot illustrates overall survival according to 3 age groups, patients who were the median age (≤60 years) and patients who were older than the median age (subgrouped as ages 61-70 years and aged >70 years), for the entire population (n = 600). (Reprinted from Braiteh F, Correa AM, Hofstetter WL, et al. Association of age and survival in patients with gastroesophageal cancer undergoing surgery with or without preoperative therapy. *Cancer.* 2009;115:4450-4458, with permission from the American Cancer Society.)

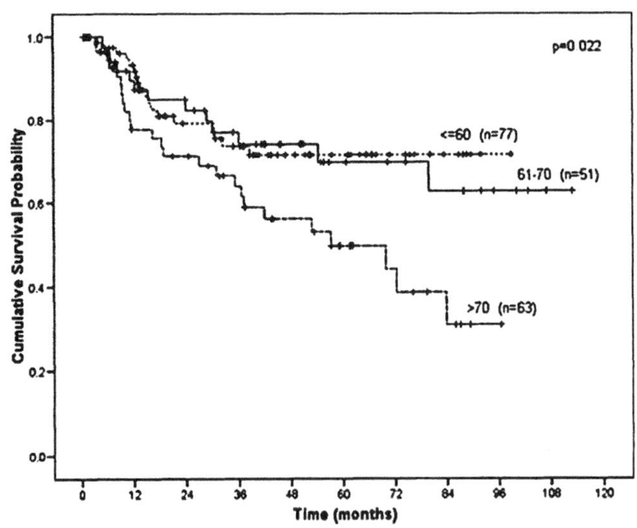

FIGURE 2.—This Kaplan-Meier plot illustrates overall survival according to 3 age groups, patients who were the median age (≤60 years) and patients who were older than the median age (subgrouped as ages 61-70 years and aged >70 years), in those who underwent surgery as primary therapy (n = 191). (Reprinted from Braiteh F, Correa AM, Hofstetter WL, et al. Association of age and survival in patients with gastroesophageal cancer undergoing surgery with or without preoperative therapy. *Cancer.* 2009;115:4450-4458, with permission from the American Cancer Society.)

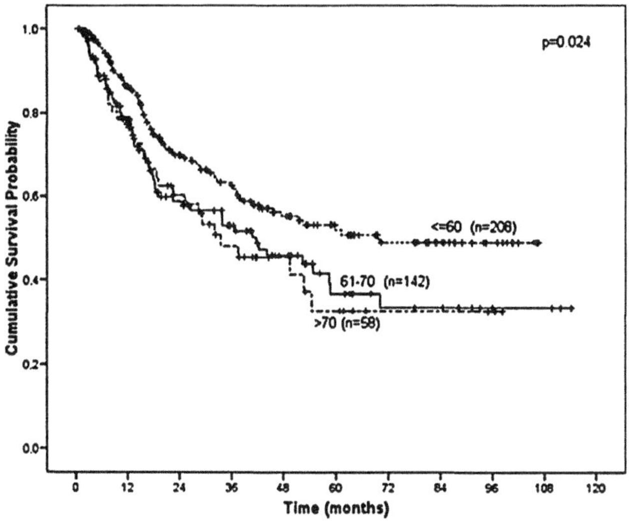

FIGURE 3.—This Kaplan-Meier plot illustrates overall survival according to 3 age groups, patients who were the median age (≤60 years) and patients who were older than the median age (subgrouped as ages 61-70 years and aged >70 years), in those who received preoperative therapy (n = 409). (Reprinted from Braiteh F, Correa AM, Hofstetter WL, et al. Association of age and survival in patients with gastroesophageal cancer undergoing surgery with or without preoperative therapy. *Cancer.* 2009;115:4450-4458, with permission from the American Cancer Society.)

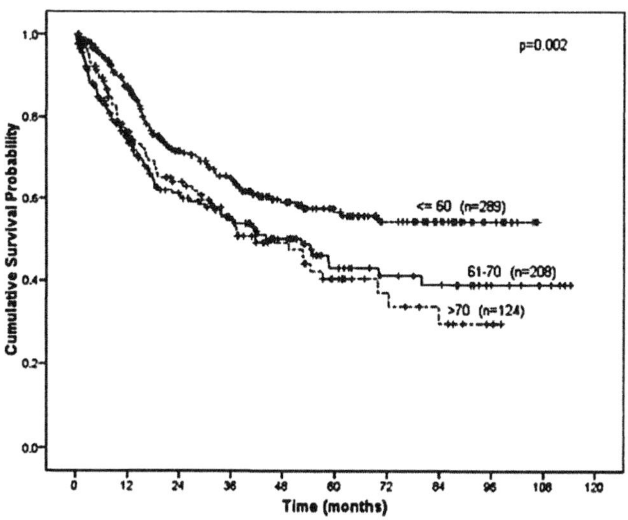

FIGURE 4.—This Kaplan-Meier plot illustrates overall survival according to 3 age groups, patients who were the median age (≤60 years) and patients who were older than the median age (subgrouped as ages 61-70 years and aged >70 years), for the population that included 21 patients with surgical mortality (n = 621). (Reprinted from Braiteh F, Correa AM, Hofstetter WL, et al. Association of age and survival in patients with gastroesophageal cancer undergoing surgery with or without preoperative therapy. *Cancer.* 2009;115:4450-4458, with permission from the American Cancer Society.)

patients older than the median age, univariate analysis demonstrated a higher risk of death with increasing age ($P = .019$). In multivariate analysis, increasing age was an independent prognosticator of poor overall survival ($P = .041$). The inclusion of 30-day mortality did not alter the results. Surgical complications were statistically significantly higher in older patients compared with younger patients in the following categories: aspiration pneumonia, adult respiratory distress syndrome, cardiovascular, neurologic, and miscellaneous complications.

Conclusions.—The data in this study demonstrated that patients aged ≤60 years who underwent surgery for esophageal cancer achieved the best overall survival and experienced fewer surgical complications than patients aged >70 years. Age was identified as an important variable in the selection of patients for esophageal cancer surgery (Figs 1-4).

▶ This is a single-institution series from the MD Anderson Cancer Center that studies 600 consecutive patients. Over 400 received preoperative therapy and 191 patients underwent surgery first. They compare outcome of patients younger than 60 years of age and over 70 years of age with a third group in between. As seen in Fig 1, the overall survival for all patients shows a reduction in survival for older-aged patients. This was true in patients who had primary therapy (Fig 2), preoperative therapy (Fig 3), and when analyzing the patients who died (Fig 4).

There are some caveats with this study; it is retrospective in nature and has a somewhat heterogeneous patient population. In addition, the authors did not have disease-specific survival data available.

Obviously, the more elderly the patient the more likely comorbidity becomes, which might exclude such a large surgical intervention as esophagectomy. Future studies should include age as a variable.

T. J. Eberlein, MD

Miscellaneous

Regulation of *RUNX3* Tumor Suppressor Gene Expression in Cutaneous Melanoma

Kitago M, Martinez SR, Nakamura T, et al (John Wayne Cancer Inst at Saint John's Health Ctr, Santa Monica, CA)
Clin Cancer Res 15:2988-2994, 2009

Purpose.—*RUNX3* is a known tumor suppressor gene in several carcinomas. Aberration in RUNX3 expression has not been described for cutaneous melanoma. Therefore, we assessed the expression of RUNX3 in cutaneous melanoma and its regulatory mechanisms relative to tumor progression.

Experimental Design.—The expression of RUNX3 mRNA and miR-532-5p (microRNA) was assessed in melanoma lines and in primary and metastatic melanoma tumors.

Results.—RUNX3 mRNA expression was down-regulated in 11 of 11 (100%) metastatic melanoma lines relative to normal melanocytes ($P < 0.001$). Among 123 primary and metastatic melanoma tumors and 12 normal skin samples, RUNX3 expression was significantly down-regulated in primary melanomas ($n = 82$; $P = 0.02$) and in melanoma metastasis ($n = 41$; $P < 0.0001$) versus normal skin ($n = 12$). This suggested that RUNX3 down-regulation may play a role in the development and progression of melanoma. RUNX3 promoter region hypermethylation was assessed as a possible regulator of RUNX3 expression using methylation-specific PCR. Assessment of RUNX3 promoter region methylation showed that only 5 of 17 (29%) melanoma lines, 2 of 52 (4%) primary melanomas, and 5 of 30 (17%) metastatic melanomas had hypermethylation of the promoter region. A microRNA (miR-532-5p) was identified as a target of RUNX3 mRNA sequences. miR-532-5p expression was shown to be significantly up-regulated in melanoma lines and metastatic melanoma tumors relative to normal melanocytes and primary melanomas, respectively. To investigate the relation between RUNX3 and miR-532-5p, anti–miR-532-5p was transfected into melanoma lines. Inhibition of miR-532-5p up-regulated both RUNX3 mRNA and protein expression.

Conclusions.—RUNX3 is down-regulated during melanoma progression and miR-532-5p is a regulatory factor of RUNX3 expression.

▶ This is a study from the John Wayne Cancer institute looking at a tumor suppressor gene, *RUNX3*, and its impact in the development of a melanoma. A microRNA (miR-532-5p) was identified as a target of RUNX3 mRNA sequences. The miR-532-5p expression was significantly upregulated in metastatic tumor. In further molecular studies, in this article, miR-532-5p, appears to be a regulatory factor of RUNX3 expression. Because these molecular changes are associated with metastatic disease, targeting these mechanisms specifically may result in more effective treatments for our patients.

T. J. Eberlein, MD

Autologous Melanoma Vaccine Induces Antitumor and Self-Reactive Immune Responses That Affect Patient Survival and Depend on MHC Class II Expression on Vaccine Cells

Lotem M, Machlenkin A, Hamburger T, et al (Hadassah Hebrew Univ Hosp, Jerusalem, Israel; et al)

Clin Cancer Res 15:4968-4977, 2009

Purpose.—Autologous melanoma cells display a broad variety of tumor antigens and were used for treatment of American Joint Committee on Cancer stages III and IV melanoma as an adjuvant or active therapy. Survival data and immune response were evaluated in vaccinated patients.

Experimental Design.—Forty-seven patients received 2,4-dinitrophenyl–conjugated autologous melanoma vaccine as an adjuvant (23 patients) or therapy (24 patients). CD4 and CD8 T-cell response in blood sampled before vaccination and after five or eight vaccine doses was evaluated against melanoma cells and autologous peripheral blood mononuclear cells using IFNγ enzyme–linked immunospot. Serum levels of antilivin, an inhibitor of apoptosis, and anti-gp100 IgG were determined.

Results.—The immunologic effect of the vaccine differed between the two groups of patients. In the adjuvant group, there was a significant increase in CD8 melanoma-reactive T cells ($P = 0.035$) after vaccination and an increase in antimelanoma CD4 T cells correlating with improved overall survival ($P = 0.04$). In the therapeutic group, there was no objective tumor regression; antimelanoma T-cell reactivity increased by a small amount, stayed the same, or in some cases decreased. In all patients, a significant increase was noted in CD4 T-cell reactivity against autologous peripheral blood mononuclear cells ($P = 0.02$), which did not affect survival. Increased antilivin IgG was associated with improved survival. Expression of MHC class II on melanoma cells was vital for the immunogenicity of the vaccine.

Conclusion.—Autologous melanoma cell vaccine is capable of inducing effective antimelanoma CD4 T-cell activity associated with improved survival. Patients with active metastatic disease generally displayed reduced immune response and gained little from active immunization.

▶ This study from Hebrew University Hospital in Jerusalem, supported by the Israel Cancer Association, looks at an autologous melanoma vaccine as an adjuvant in a substantial number of patients as either an adjuvant or therapy for metastatic disease. As seen in Fig 1 in the original article, in the patients who received adjuvant vaccine treatment, there was a statically significant disease-free overall survival in the patients who had a significant delayed-type hypersensitivity (DTH) reaction. It is interesting that this appeared to be due an increase in CD8 T-cells and CD4 T-cells (Fig 2 in the original article), and although this was not statically significant (possibly because of the number of patients) it is interesting to note that in the metastatic cancer patients in Fig 2 in the original article, there was little immune reactivity of CD8 T-cells and, if anything, a nonstatistically significant decrease in CD4 T-cells. This was relatively common in patients with metastatic disease as it is more difficult to mount an immune response to vaccine therapy.

While this vaccine will need further investigation, it may provide a viable alternative in an adjuvant setting. It does not appear that in patients with metastatic disease this vaccine therapy would be effective.

T. J. Eberlein, MD

Erlotinib and Bevacizumab Have Synergistic Activity against Melanoma

Schicher N, Paulitschke V, Swoboda A, et al (Med Univ Vienna, Austria; et al)

Clin Cancer Res 15:3495-3502, 2009

Purpose.—Melanoma is one of the most aggressive types of cancer with currently no chance of cure once the disease has spread to distant sites. Therapeutic options for advanced stage III and IV are very limited, mainly palliative, and show response in only ~20% of all cases. The presented preclinical study was done to investigate the influence of a combined treatment of the epidermal growth factor receptor inhibitor erlotinib and the vascular endothelial growth factor monoclonal antibody bevacizumab in melanoma.

Experimental Design and Results.—The epidermal growth factor receptor was expressed in all cell lines tested, and treatment with erlotinib did inhibit the activation of the MEK/extracellular signal-regulated kinase and AKT signaling pathways. Whereas *in vitro* no influence on tumor cell proliferation was seen with erlotinib or bevacizumab monotherapy, a decreased invasive potential on erlotinib treatment in a three-dimensional Matrigel assay was observed. Furthermore, both drugs inhibited proliferation and sprouting of endothelial cells. *In vivo*, in a severe combined immunodeficient mouse xenotransplantation model, reduction in tumor volume under combined treatment with erlotinib and bevacizumab was superior to the additive effect of both single agents. This was associated with reduced cell proliferation, increased apoptosis, and a reduction in tumor angiogenesis compared with control or single treatment groups. Likewise, the reduction in the extent of lymph node and lung metastasis was most pronounced in animals treated with both drugs.

Conclusion.—The presented data strongly support the use of a combination of erlotinib and bevacizumab as a novel treatment regimen for metastatic melanoma.

► This article from Austria is actually a preclinical article looking at the epidermal growth factor receptor inhibitor erlotinib and the vascular endothelial growth factor monoclonal antibody bevacizumab. They are using a mirroring model. I have included this article simply because melanoma is one of the most difficult tumors to treat in advanced stage disease. As seen in Fig 3 in the original article, the combination of these treatments reduces the tumor volume significantly, and also significantly reduces the number of lymph node metastases and lung metastases (Fig 3 in the original article).

Several other comments are warranted about this article. As single treatments these drugs did not show a statistically significant influence on reduction in tumor burden. However, the combination of these treatments was not only effective in reducing the primary tumor burden but also local regional lymph nodes, which is a significant advancement if verified in clinical trials. Clinical trials with this combination are currently under way.

T. J. Eberlein, MD

Combined Blunt-Clamp Dissection and LigaSure Ligation for Hepatic Parenchyma Dissection: Postcoagulation Technique

Patrlj L, Tuorto S, Fong Y (Univ Hosp Dubrava Zagreb, Croatia; Memorial Sloan-Kettering Cancer Ctr, NY)
J Am Coll Surg 210:39-44, 2010

Background.—Blunt-clamp dissection allows for visualization of intrahepatic vessels and individual ligation of major blood or bile vessels. Recently, many instruments have been developed for "precoagulation" of liver parenchyma before sharp transection, but suffer from the possibility of injuring major blood and biliary vessels that are not well-visualized, along with high cost. In this article, we describe a "postcoagulation" technique combining clamp dissection and sealing of vessels under direct vision using a tissue-sealing device.

Study Design.—Clinical evaluation of 400 patients from 2 centers subjected to liver resection using this technique.

Results.—There were no cases complicated by hemorrhage. There was an incidence of 1.8% for bile leaks. This low incidence of biloma formation was seen even with the high incidence (49%) of abnormal parenchyma encountered in this cohort.

Conclusions.—Combining the clamp-crushing method with use of the LigaSure device (Valleylab) allows identification of intraparenchymal vessels followed by sealing. This method of parenchymal transaction optimizes ease of use with confidence in vessel ligation.

▶ This is a prospective evaluation of 400 patients from 2 centers evaluating proper technique for liver resection. This article provides excellent insights into the technical aspect of liver resection. The caveat, however, is that the authors of this study, particularly those from Memorial Sloan-Kettering, are experts with enormous experience. The figures in the article are outstanding and should be helpful to less experienced surgeons.

T. J. Eberlein, MD

Natural History of Patients with Subcentimeter Pulmonary Nodules Undergoing Hepatic Resection for Metastatic Colorectal Cancer

Maithel SK, Ginsberg MS, D'Amico F, et al (Emory Univ, Atlanta, GA; Memorial Sloan-Kettering Cancer Ctr, NY)
J Am Coll Surg 210:31-38, 2010

Background.—CT imaging frequently detects subcentimeter pulmonary nodules (SPN) in patients undergoing resection of colorectal cancer liver metastases. Their clinical significance is unknown.

Study Design.—Patients were identified who underwent hepatic resection for colorectal cancer liver metastases between October 2004 and March 2006. The presence and imaging features of preoperative SPN were analyzed for their association with progression-free survival (PFS), disease-specific survival (DSS), and SPN progression.

Results.—One hundred sixty patients underwent liver resection and 68 (43%) had SPN identified preoperatively. Median number of nodules was 1 (75th percentile: ≤2 nodules) and median size of the largest was 3 mm (25th to 75th percentile: 2 to 5 mm). SPN were unilateral in 77%, calcified in 19%, solid in 92%, and smooth in contour in 95% of patients. At median follow-up of 31 months for survivors, SPN were proven to be metastatic disease in 35% of patients (24 of 68), either by radiographic increase in size or number (n = 12) or histologic confirmation after resection (n = 12). Median PFS for the 160 patients was 16 months and 3-year DSS was 78%. There was a trend toward shorter median PFS in patients with preoperative SPN compared with patients with no SPN (12 versus 20 months; $p = 0.242$). There was no difference in 3-year DSS (70% versus 83%; $p = 0.46$). SPN progression after hepatic resection did not substantially affect 3-year DSS. Calcified nodules were less likely to progress compared with noncalcified nodules (8% versus 42%; $p = 0.03$).

Conclusion.—SPN are common among patients undergoing resection of colorectal cancer liver metastases and approximately one-third of these will prove to be metastatic disease. Presence of limited preoperative SPN might be associated with shorter PFS after hepatectomy, but does not

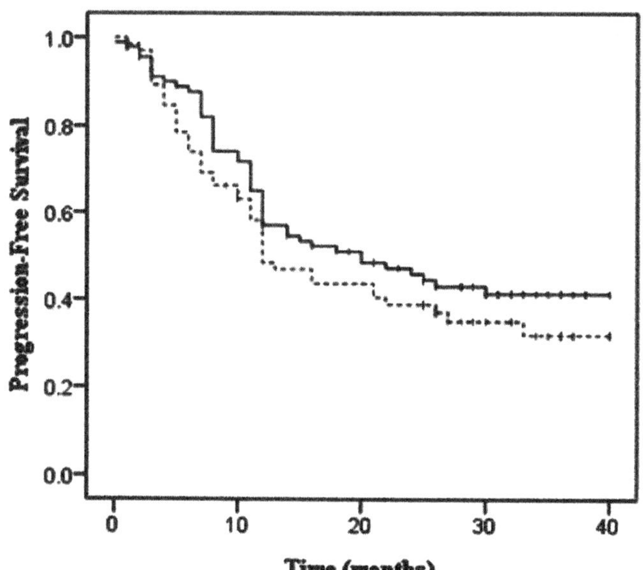

FIGURE 1.—Progression-free survival of patients with subcentimeter pulmonary nodules present at the time of hepatic resection. Black line, no preoperative subcentimeter pulmonary nodules, n = 92; dotted line, preoperative subcentimeter pulmonary nodules, n = 68 ($p = 0.24$). (Reprinted from Maithel SK, Ginsberg MS, D'Amico F, et al. Natural history of patients with subcentimeter pulmonary nodules undergoing hepatic resection for metastatic colorectal cancer. *J Am Coll Surg*. 2010;210:31-38, with permission from the American College of Surgeons.)

TABLE 3.—Regression Analysis for Predicting Subcentimeter Pulmonary Nodules Progression from Radiologic and Clinical Characteristics (n = 68)

Variable	Univariate Logistic Regression HR (95% CI)	p Value
No. of nodules*	0.80 (0.53–1.20)	0.29
Size of largest nodule*	1.01 (0.77–1.32)	0.94
Bilateral*	0.86 (0.25–2.92)	0.81
Calcified*	0.12 (0.01–1.03)	0.05
Solid/partly solid/ground glass*	0.83 (0.13–5.36)	0.84
Spiculated/smooth/lobular	—	—
Rectal versus colon primary	0.38 (0.12–1.22)	0.10
Positive smoking history	0.38 (0.14–1.05)	0.63
No. of hepatic tumors	0.99 (0.71–1.38)	0.96
Elevated clinical risk score	1.04 (0.37–2.97)	0.94

HR, hazard ratio.
*Analysis includes 64 patients for whom adequate chest CT images were available for review.

substantially impact 3-year DSS, and should not necessarily preclude resection of hepatic metastases (Fig 1, Table 3).

▶ One of the vexing issues in oncology care is a patient who has colorectal cancer and then subsequently presents with liver metastases. These patients routinely have staging work-up, and not infrequently will have some subcentimeter pulmonary nodules. This article from Memorial Sloan-Kettering addresses the management and follow-up of these subcentimeter pulmonary nodules.

This large series was unable to identify specific characteristics of the pulmonary nodule that would predict for true metastatic disease (Table 3). Although patients with a higher clinical risk score had a significantly lower disease-specific survival at 3 years, the patients with preoperative subcentimeter pulmonary nodules tended toward shorter median progression-free survival, but this was not statistically significant (Fig 1).

The vast majority of these small pulmonary nodules are likely not metastatic disease. Positron emission tomography (PET) imaging has been somewhat disappointing, and fine needle aspiration and video-assisted thoracoscopic surgery are frequently difficult or not feasible.

The conclusion of this very large series was that the presence of subcentimeter pulmonary nodules was not associated with earlier progression or decreased survival. However, approximately one-third of the subcentimeter pulmonary nodules will ultimately prove to be metastatic disease. This has less impact on overall survival because most of the patients who present with small pulmonary nodules present with only 1 or 2 nodules (78% of patients in this study).

T. J. Eberlein, MD

Complete Cytoreduction Offers Longterm Survival in Patients with Peritoneal Carcinomatosis from Appendiceal Tumors of Unfavorable Histology

Omohwo C, Nieroda CA, Studeman KD, et al (Mercy Med Ctr, Baltimore, MD; et al)

J Am Coll Surg 209:308-312, 2009

Background.—Cytoreductive surgery (CRS) combined with hyperthermic intraperitoneal chemotherapy (HIPEC) is a rapidly evolving treatment for metastatic appendiceal neoplasms. The aim of this study was to show the effect of complete cytoreduction (CC) on survival in patients undergoing CRS and HIPEC for high-grade appendiceal neoplasm.

Study Design.—A retrospective study of a prospective database of 56 patients (from 1999 to 2007) with appendiceal neoplasms treated with CRS and HIPEC was carried out. Histology of the disease, CC score, and peritoneal cancer index (PCI) score were assessed independently and collectively for each group of patients. Survival analysis was performed using the Cox proportional hazard model.

Results.—Three-year overall survival was 60%. The median peritoneal cancer index score was 25 or higher. Survival analysis by tumor histology was 80% for patients with low-grade tumors and 52% for patients with high-grade tumors ($p = 0.024$). Survival by completeness of cytoreduction was 78% for patients with a low CC score (0 to 1) and 28% in patients with a high CC score (2 to 3; $p = 0.01$). There was no statistically significant difference in survival between the low-grade and high-grade tumors when a complete cytoreduction was performed in both groups of patients: 80% versus 68% ($p = 0.69$).

Conclusions.—CRS and HIPEC is an effective treatment for patients with disseminated appendiceal tumors. High-grade tumors also benefit from this approach and should not be excluded from CRS and HIPEC. Every effort should be made to achieve a complete cytoreduction regardless of the tumor histology (Figs 1 and 2, Table 3).

► Appendiceal neoplasms are frequently difficult to diagnose because they are relatively rare. In addition, it is not uncommon to have rupture of the appendix with peritoneal dissemination. This study looked at a relatively large group of patients with appendiceal tumors, specifically studying the role of cytoreductive surgery combined with hypothermic intraperitoneal chemotherapy. As seen in Fig 1, the author showed that low-grade tumors have a better prognosis as well as patients who undergo complete cytoreduction. In combining the prognostic indicators, patients who had low-grade tumors and cytoreductive surgery had the best prognosis. High-grade tumors, particularly those incompletely resected, had the poorest prognosis (Fig 2).

Of note, this study had a higher-than-usual percentage of high-grade tumors compared with other studies. However, their 3-year follow-up time is relatively short, compared with similar studies (Table 3). While this short follow-up may be adequate for high-grade tumors, it may not be adequate for the low-grade

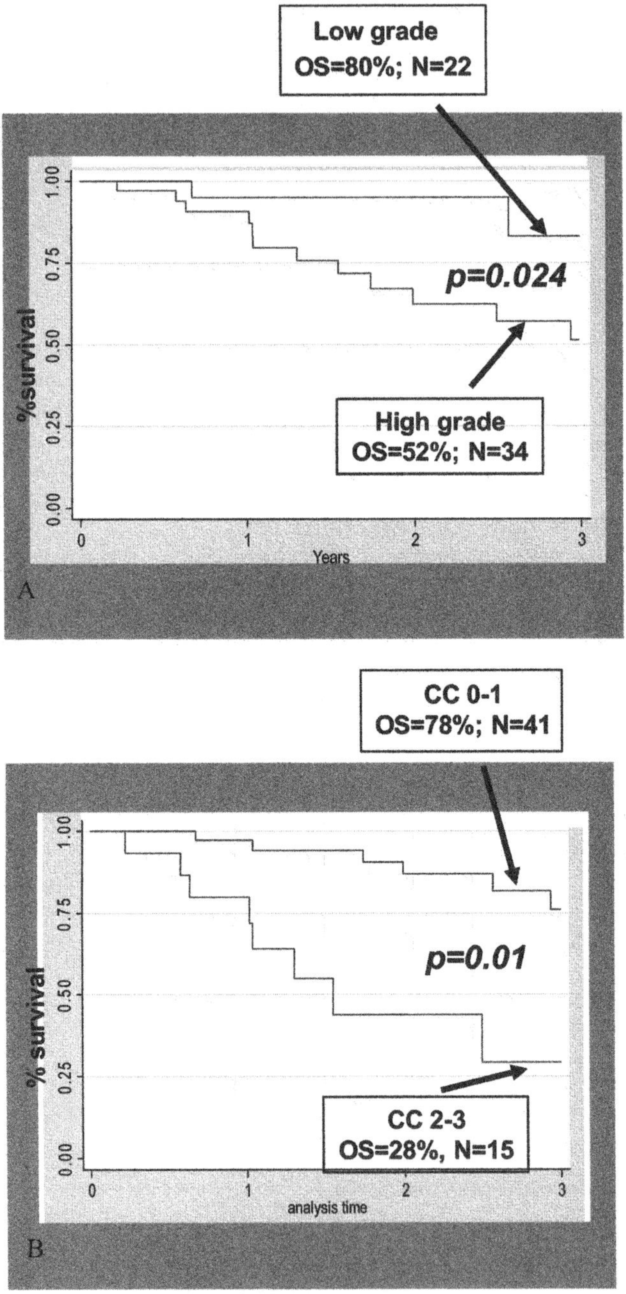

FIGURE 1.—Kaplan-Meier curves each showing 3-year survival of patients by (A) tumor histology and (B) completeness of cytoreduction. HR, 5.6 (95% CI, 1.8 to 17.20). CC, completeness of cytoreduction; OS, overall survival. (Reprinted from Omohwo C, Nieroda CA, Studeman KD, et al. Complete cytoreduction offers longterm survival in patients with peritoneal carcinomatosis from appendiceal tumors of unfavorable histology. *J Am Coll Surg*. 2009;209:308-312, with permission from the American College of Surgeons.)

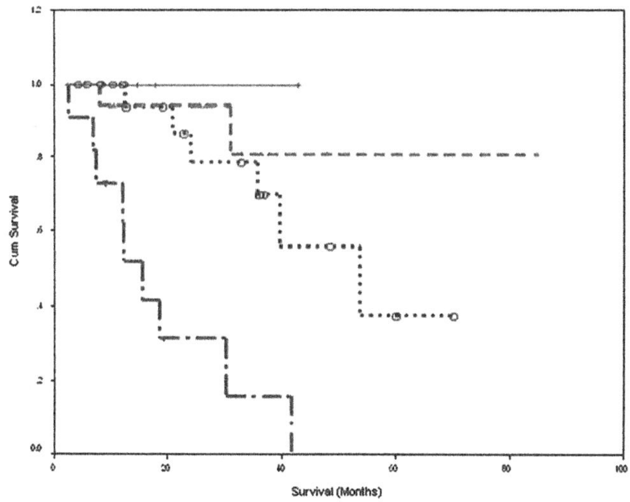

FIGURE 2.—Kaplan-Meier curves showing survival (OS) of patients according to a combination of tumor histology and the completeness of cytoreduction (CC). Blue dashed line, high-grade (CC, 2–3; OS, 9%; n, 3/11); red dotted line, high-grade (CC, 0–1, OS, 68%, n, 19/23); green dashed line, low-grade (CC, 0–1, OS, 80%, n, 16/18); purple line, low-grade (CC, 2–3, OS, 100%, n, 4/4). (Reprinted from Omohwo C, Nieroda CA, Studeman KD, et al. Complete cytoreduction offers longterm survival in patients with peritoneal carcinomatosis from appendiceal tumors of unfavorable histology. *J Am Coll Surg*. 2009;209:308-312, with permission from the American College of Surgeons.)

TABLE 3.—Comparison of Multicenter Survival Statistics of Patients with Peritoneal Carcinomatosis

First Author, Year	n	Histology, % of Total Patient Population: DPAM n	DPAM %	PMCA n	PMCA %	Overall Survival, % 3y	5y	Mean PCI Score
Stewart IV[9] 2005	110	55	50	55*	50	59	53	—
Smeenk[3] 2007	103	66	64†	36*	35†	71	60	—
Baratti[10] 2008	95	78	74	26	26	n/a	72	21
Elias[11] 2003	36	22	61	14*	39	n/a	66	21
This study	56	22	39	34	61	60		25

DPAM, disseminated peritoneal; PCI, peritoneal cancer index; PMCA, peritoneal mucinous.
Editor's note: Please check the original article for full references.
*Including patients with PMCA and PMCA-1 as a group.
†Data missing in one patient.

tumors, particularly those with complete cytoreduction surgeries. Nonetheless, achieving the goal of complete cytoreduction in this patient population should be the goal of surgeons treating these types of tumors.

T. J. Eberlein, MD

Effect of High Perioperative Oxygen Fraction on Surgical Site Infection and Pulmonary Complications After Abdominal Surgery: The PROXI Randomized Clinical Trial

Meyhoff CS, for the PROXI Trial Group (Copenhagen Univ Hosp, Rigshospitalet; et al)

JAMA 302:1543-1550, 2009

Context.—Use of 80% oxygen during surgery has been suggested to reduce the risk of surgical wound infections, but this effect has not been consistently identified. The effect of 80% oxygen on pulmonary complications has not been well defined.

Objective.—To assess whether use of 80% oxygen reduces the frequency of surgical site infection without increasing the frequency of pulmonary complications in patients undergoing abdominal surgery.

Design, Setting, and Patients.—The PROXI trial, a patient- and observer-blinded randomized clinical trial conducted in 14 Danish hospitals between October 2006 and October 2008 among 1400 patients undergoing acute or elective laparotomy.

Interventions.—Patients were randomly assigned to receive either 80% or 30% oxygen during and for 2 hours after surgery.

Main Outcome Measures.—Surgical site infection within 14 days, defined according to the Centers for Disease Control and Prevention. Secondary outcomes included atelectasis, pneumonia, respiratory failure, and mortality.

Results.—Surgical site infection occurred in 131 of 685 patients (19.1%) assigned to receive 80% oxygen vs 141 of 701 (20.1%) assigned to receive 30% oxygen (odds ratio [OR], 0.94; 95% confidence interval [CI], 0.72-1.22; $P = .64$). Atelectasis occurred in 54 of 685 patients (7.9%) assigned to receive 80% oxygen vs 50 of 701 (7.1%) assigned to receive 30% oxygen (OR, 1.11; 95% CI, 0.75-1.66; $P = .60$), pneumonia in 41 (6.0%) vs 44 (6.3%) (OR, 0.95; 95% CI, 0.61-1.48; $P = .82$), respiratory failure in 38 (5.5%) vs 31 (4.4%) (OR, 1.27; 95% CI, 0.78-2.07; $P = .34$), and mortality within 30 days in 30 (4.4%) vs 20 (2.9%) (OR, 1.56; 95% CI, 0.88-2.77; $P = .13$).

Conclusion.—Administration of 80% oxygen compared with 30% oxygen did not result in a difference in risk of surgical site infection after abdominal surgery.

Trial Registration.—clinicaltrials.gov Identifier: NCT00364741 (Tables 3 and 4).

▶ This is a randomized clinical trial conducted in 14 Danish hospitals undergoing acute and elective laparotomy. As can be seen in Table 3 and Table 4, administration of 80% oxygen compared with 30% did not result in a difference in surgical site infection following these surgical procedures. Additionally, there was no difference with respect to atelectasis, pneumonia, or admission to the ICU (Table 3).

TABLE 3.—Clinical Outcomes for Patients Scheduled for Laparotomy (N = 1386)

Outcome	No. (%) 80% Oxygen (n = 685)	30% Oxygen (n = 701)	Univariate OR (95% CI)	*P* Value	Adjusted OR (95% CI)[a]	*P* Value
Surgical site infection	131 (19.1)	141 (20.1)	0.94 (0.72 to 1.22)	.64	0.91 (0.69 to 1.20)	.51
Infection location						
Superficial	75 (57.3)	76 (53.9)				
Deep	20 (15.3)	26 (18.4)				
Organ/space	36 (27.5)	39 (27.7)				
ASEPSIS score >20[b]	32 (4.7)	36 (5.1)				
Atelectasis	54 (7.9)	50 (7.1)	1.11 (0.75 to 1.66)	.60	1.13 (0.75 to 1.72)	.56
Pneumonia	41 (6.0)	44 (6.3)	0.95 (0.61 to 1.48)	.82	0.95 (0.60 to 1.49)	.81
Health care–associated	30 (73.2)	30 (68.2)				
Ventilator-associated	7 (17.1)	9 (20.5)				
Aspiration	2 (4.9)	1 (2.3)				
Community-acquired	2 (4.9)	2 (4.5)				
Immunocompromised	0	2 (4.5)				
Respiratory failure	38 (5.5)	31 (4.4)	1.27 (0.78 to 2.07)	.34	1.22 (0.74 to 2.03)	.44
Reoperation	104 (15.2)	104 (14.8)	1.03 (0.77 to 1.38)	.86	1.01 (0.75 to 1.37)	.93
Admission to ICU[c]	50 (7.3)	44 (6.3)	1.18 (0.77 to 1.79)	.45	1.21 (0.78 to 1.89)	.40
30-d mortality	30 (4.4)	20 (2.9)	1.56 (0.88 to 2.77)	.13	1.55 (0.86 to 2.85)	.15
Postoperative hospitalization, d	6 (1-34)	7 (2-36)	−0.69 (−2.3 to 0.93)	.09[d]		

Abbreviations: ASEPSIS, additional treatment, serous discharge, erythema, purulent exudate, separation of deep tissues, isolation of bacteria, and duration of postoperative stay; CI, confidence interval; ICU, intensive care unit; OR, odds ratio.

[a]Adjusted for study center, body mass index (<30 or ≥30, calculated as weight in kilograms divided by height in meters squared), diabetes mellitus, acute or elective surgery, chronic obstructive pulmonary disease, current smoker, incision extending above the umbilicus, duration of surgery, and age (≥ 40 years or <40 years).

[b]Range of possible scores, 0-70. Combines wound appearance the first 5 postoperative days with additional surgical treatment; a score higher than 20 indicates wound infection.[27] Editor's note: Please check the original article for full references.

[c]Admissions to ICU excluded if part of routine postoperative care and lasting less than 24 hours (13 vs 9 patients in the 80% oxygen and 30% oxygen groups, respectively).

[d]Calculated with Wilcoxon unpaired rank sum test.

TABLE 4.—Adverse Events Other Than Primary and Secondary Outcomes for Patients Scheduled for Laparotomy (N = 1386)

Adverse Event	No. (%) 80% Oxygen (n = 685)	30% Oxygen (n = 701)
Any	361 (52.7)	369 (52.6)
Wound-related	61 (8.9)	77 (11.0)
Infection		
Urinary tract	23 (3.4)	34 (4.9)
Other	79 (11.5)	83 (11.8)
Postoperative nausea or vomiting	136 (19.9)	135 (19.3)
Respiratory	63 (9.2)	57 (8.1)
Circulatory	57 (8.3)	67 (9.6)
Gastrointestinal tract	61 (8.9)	62 (8.8)
Other	150 (21.9)	152 (21.7)
Any serious adverse event	165 (24.1)	154 (22.0)
Sepsis	21 (3.1)	15 (2.1)
Other infection	29 (4.2)	34 (4.9)
Respiratory	27 (3.9)	25 (3.6)
Circulatory	24 (3.5)	20 (2.9)
Gastrointestinal tract	53 (7.7)	46 (6.5)
Other	47 (6.9)	44 (6.3)

So, while this is a negative study, it answers important questions regarding administration of oxygen and surgical site infection and secondary pulmonary complications.

T. J. Eberlein, MD

12 Vascular Surgery

Introduction

During the past year, there were 3 landmark studies published that should help define the practice of vascular surgery. These studies were included among the abstracts, but should be read in their entirety. In the much anticipated OVER trial, open and endovascular aneurysm repair (EVAR) were compared at Veterans Affairs hospitals. Similar to the European trials, there were no differences in mortality or the other major outcome measures at 2 years. The ASTRAL trial clearly demonstrated that endovascular revascularization did not improve blood pressure control or salvage renal function in patients with atherosclerotic renovascular occlusive disease. Lastly, the INSTEAD trial examined the role of thoracic endovascular aortic repair (TEVAR) in patients with stable type B aortic dissections and demonstrated that were no differences in survival at 2 years, the primary study end point, or the secondary end points of aortic-related death and freedom from progressive aortic disease.

The treatment of aortic diseases was marked by a series of studies "pushing the envelope" in terms of new therapies for juxtarenal and thoracoabdominal aneurysms. These approaches have involved using endografts modified with fenestrations or "scallops" to facilitate revascularization of the visceral vessels or some combination of open visceral or arch "debranching" with more standard EVAR or TEVAR techniques. The role of these fenestrated grafts and hybrid procedures remains to be determined, but they may safely extend the indications for operative repair to older, sicker patients. A publication from the Swedish Twin Registry further confirmed the role of genetics in the development of abdominal aortic aneurysms and reported that the odds ratio (ie, the relative risk of an AAA for individuals whose twin had an AAA compared with persons whose twin did not have an AAA) was 71 for monozygotic twins and 7.6 for dizygotic twins. Lastly, a report from the Vascular Study Group of Northern New England (VSGNNE) examined mortality at 1 year after aneurysm repair and reported that predicted values after open repair ranged 1–67% and was associated with advanced age ($\geq$ 70 yrs), renal insufficiency (creatinine $\geq$ 1.8), COPD, and suprarenal aortic clamp.

The treatment of cerebrovascular occlusive disease continues to be focused on defining the role of carotid artery stenting (CAS). Not surprisingly, CAS for recurrent carotid artery stenoses appears to be at least as safe as CAS for primary lesions and, indeed, this appears to be one of its more compelling indications. Comparison of carotid revascularization before and after the widespread implementation of CAS using the Medicare database suggests that the outcomes may be worse after implementation, particularly in geographic areas where CAS was widely adopted. A publication analyzing compliance with the clinical practice guidelines for the timing of carotid endarterectomy (CEA) at stroke centers in Canada found that it was performed outside of the period of maximal effectiveness in the majority of patients, thereby suggesting that there is room for improvement in the clinical care delivery system.

The outcome after lower extremity revascularization was the focus of 2 papers included this year. Using the California statewide database, "long-term" outcome after aortoiliac or femoropopliteal bypass was associated with a remedial bypass/revision rate of 29%, and a 5-year amputation-free survival rate of 52%. In a separate, single institutional series, outcome after lower extremity revascularization for ischemic tissue loss was defined from a "patient" standpoint using the measures of patent revascularization until wound healing, limb salvage for 1 year, independent ambulation for 1 year, and survival to 6 months. Unfortunately, only 41% of the patients had a successful outcome or met all of the criteria. The role of arterial duplex as an adjunct to preoperative planning was demonstrated in a separate publication.

The papers dealing with venous disease included in this year's edition of the *Year Book* make several practical contributions. First, wearing compression stockings (eg, support hose) does not appear to be necessary after open surgical varicose vein stripping. Second, foam sclerotherapy appears to be comparable to open surgical varicose vein stripping; however, almost 40% of patients undergoing foam sclerotherapy in a separate study had evidence of a right to left shunt as detected by transcranial Doppler with almost 15% having evidence of severe shunting. Third, the infrarenal inferior vena cava is very responsive to the circulating volume status and the conformation changes are anisotropic with little change along the major axis and significant change along the minor axis. Clearly, this has major implications for the appropriate sizing of caval filters. Finally, the natural history of catheter-based upper extremity deep venous thromboses has been partially clarified and appears to be fairly benign.

The role of endovascular treatment for failing and thrombosed hemodialysis accesses has been clarified during the past year. In contrast to an earlier meta-analysis, endovascular treatment appears to be comparable to open surgical thrombectomy for patients with thrombosed prosthetic accesses. Surveillance and remediation appear to be beneficial for "failing" autogenous accesses although many of these lesions can be safely monitored. Interestingly, the treatment of venous outflow lesions in patients with failing prosthetic access using covered stents were superior to noncovered stents and suggest that the biological response to these covered stents may be different.

The final group of the included unrelated or "miscellaneous" articles addresses iatrogenic trauma and visceral artery dissections. The evolution of the endovascular approaches has truly revolutionized the treatment of traumatic injury to the arch and great vessels, and a series of articles is included documenting several creative solutions to arterial injuries associated with attempted central venous line placement. Lastly, the advances in imaging have led to an increased diagnosis or identification of spontaneous visceral artery dissections. Although the natural history remains to be defined, these lesions appear to be benign in terms of need for emergent intervention, but they do merit long-term follow-up because of their potential for aneurysmal degeneration.

During the past year, the vascular surgery community lost one of its quiet leaders in James M. Seeger, MD. He served as the Associate Editor for the *Year Book of Surgery* since 1993, and we have all benefited from his keen insight. He will be sorely missed by his friends and colleagues.

Thomas S. Huber, MD, PhD

Access

Maintenance of Hemodialysis Arteriovenous Fistulas by an Interventional Strategy: Clinical and Duplex Ultrasonographic Surveillance Followed by Transluminal Angioplasty

Scaffaro LA, Bettio JA, Cavazzola SA, et al (Hosp Mãe de Deus, Porto Alegre, Brazil; et al)

J Ultrasound Med 28:1159-1165, 2009

Objective.—A native arteriovenous fistula (NAF) is a widely used access location for hemodialysis (HD). Monitoring of the NAF followed by percutaneous transluminal angioplasty (PTA) as needed may reduce the incidence of NAF failure according to nonrandomized studies. The aim of this randomized study was to determine whether an interventional strategy consisting of clinical and duplex ultrasonographic (DUS) surveillance of NAFs followed by PTA reduces the rate of the need of central venous dialysis catheters (CVCs) and NAF thrombosis in patients undergoing HD.

Methods.—A total of 108 patients with 111 functioning NAFs in an HD program were randomized to control and interventional strategy groups. The control group received standard care: clinical and hemodynamic NAF assessment followed by vascular surgeon consultation in cases of dysfunction. In the interventional group, the patients underwent clinical monitoring and systematic DUS surveillance every 3 months. Cases with access dysfunction underwent angiography followed by PTA for stenosis of 50% or greater. Primary outcomes were the need of temporary CVCs and fistula thrombosis.

Results.—Fifty-eight NAFs were randomized to the control group, and 53 were randomized to the interventional group. Groups had similar baseline characteristics. The interventional strategy showed a significant reduction in the CVC need (25.9% versus 7.5% for control and interventional groups, respectively; $P = .021$). No significant difference was observed for thrombosis rates (24.1% versus 17.0%; $P = .487$). The composite end point of NAF thrombosis or CVC need was reduced by the interventional strategy (44.8% versus 20.8%; $P = .033$).

Conclusions.—This randomized study indicates the benefit of a surveillance program for maintenance of NAFs based on clinical and DUS surveillance followed by PTA of major stenosis.

▶ This study and a study by Tuka et al[1] examine the role of surveillance and intervention for patients with prosthetic and autogenous hemodialysis accesses. As noted in both articles, some type of surveillance is mandatory for all hemodialysis accesses, but the role of intervention for failing accesses and the appropriate threshold are somewhat controversial. Scaffaro et al demonstrated that an ultrasound-based surveillance protocol for autogenous accesses (ie, native fistulas) with remedial intervention for significant stenoses (ie, percutaneous transluminal angioplasty for stenoses > 50% and a flow rate < 500 mL/min) resulted in a decrease in the incidence of central venous catheters for patients with autogenous accesses (ie, native fistulas). Notably, there was no decrease in the incidence of access thromboses. Tuka et al[1] reported that borderline stenoses (ie, > 50% stenoses without additional ultrasound-based criteria) in prosthetic grafts could be safely monitored with serial ultrasounds without adverse consequences. Although only 1 of 102 grafts with borderline stenoses thrombosed, > 60% of the lesions progressed, many requiring remedial intervention. Collectively, these studies suggest that surveillance and remedial treatment are indicated for failing hemodialysis accesses (both autogenous and prosthetic) with > 50% stenoses and evidence of hemodynamic significance. Not surprisingly, this suggestion is almost identical to the National Kidney Foundation Kidney Disease Outcome Quality Initiative Guidelines (KDOQI).[2] They do not justify remedial treatment for every stenosis > 50%, despite the widespread practice across the country that has proliferated with the dissemination of endovascular skills across specialties.

T. S. Huber, MD, PhD

References

1. Tuka V, Slavikova M, Krupickova Z, et al. Short-term outcomes of borderline stenoses in vascular accesses with PTFE grafts. *Nephrol Dial Transplant.* 2009; 24:3193-3197.
2. III. NKF-K/DOQI Clinical Practice Guidelines for Vascular Access: update 2000. *Am J Kidney Dis.* 2001;37:S137-S181.

Short-term outcomes of borderline stenoses in vascular accesses with PTFE grafts

Tuka V, Slavikova M, Krupickova Z, et al (Charles Univ in Prague, Czech Republic)

Nephrol Dial Transplant 24:3193-3197, 2009

Background.—There are controversial data about vascular access stenosis surveillance by ultrasonography. The definition of stenosis significance varies among centres. We performed a retrospective study to describe short-term outcomes of borderline asymptomatic stenoses defined by precise criteria and to determine possible risk factors of stenosis progression.

Methods.—We studied the outcome of borderline stenoses in accesses with PTFE grafts. Stenosis was considered significant if there was a combination of >50% lumen reduction and peak systolic ratio >2, together with at least one of the following additional criteria: (1) residual diameter <2.0 mm and (2) flow reduction of >25% or actual flow volume <600 ml/min. Stenosis was considered borderline in the absence of the additional criteria.

Results.—Of the 102 borderline stenoses, after 11 ± 6 weeks, 55 remained non-progressive, in 38 the degree of the stenosis progressed, in 8 a percutaneous transluminal angioplasty (PTA) was performed due to clinical indication and only 1 thrombosed. A significant relative risk of developing significant stenosis was found in grafts with prior PTA [RR = 1.91 (95% CI: 1.27, 2.88), $P = 0.002$] and in female gender [RR = 2.29, (95% CI: 1.29, 4.06), $P = 0.025$].

Conclusions.—Delaying PTA of borderline stenoses is safe using this watch-and-wait strategy and stenoses remain stable over at least short time, but with higher risk of progression especially after prior PTA. We believe that the definition of precise criteria of stenosis significance is necessary for the benefit of ultrasound surveillance.

▶ This study and a study by Scaffaro et al[1] examine the role of surveillance and intervention for patients with prosthetic and autogenous hemodialysis accesses. As noted in both articles, some type of surveillance is mandatory for all hemodialysis accesses, but the role of intervention for failing accesses and the appropriate threshold are somewhat controversial. Scaffaro et al[1] demonstrated that an ultrasound-based surveillance protocol for autogenous accesses (ie, native fistulas) with remedial intervention for significant stenoses (ie, percutaneous transluminal angioplasty for stenoses >50% and a flow rate <500 mL/min) resulted in a decrease in the incidence of central venous catheters for patients with autogenous accesses (ie, native fistulas). Notably, there was no decrease in the incidence of access thromboses. Tuka et al reported that borderline stenoses (ie, >50% stenoses without additional ultrasound-based criteria) in prosthetic grafts could be safely monitored with serial ultrasounds without adverse consequences. Although only 1 of 102 grafts with borderline stenoses thrombosed, >60% of the lesions progressed, many requiring remedial intervention. Collectively, these studies suggest that surveillance and remedial treatment are indicated for failing hemodialysis accesses (both autogenous and prosthetic) with > 50% stenoses and evidence of hemodynamic significance. Not surprisingly, this suggestion is almost identical to the National Kidney Foundation Kidney Disease Outcome Quality Initiative Guidelines (KDOQI).[2] They do not justify remedial treatment for every stenosis > 50%, despite the widespread practice across the country that has proliferated with the dissemination of endovascular skills across specialties.

T. S. Huber, MD, PhD

References

1. Scaffaro LA, Bettio JA, Cavazzola SA, et al. Maintenance of hemodialysis arteriovenous fistulas by an interventional strategy: clinical and duplex ultrasonographic surveillance followed by transluminal angioplasty. *J Ultrasound Med.* 2009;28: 1159-1165.
2. III. NKF-K/DOQI Clinical Practice Guidelines for Vascular Access: update 2000. *Am J Kidney Dis.* 2001;37:S137-S181.

Stent Graft versus Balloon Angioplasty for Failing Dialysis-Access Grafts

Haskal ZJ, Trerotola S, Dolmatch B, et al (Univ of Maryland Med Ctr, Baltimore; Hosp of the Univ of Pennsylvania, Philadelphia; Univ of Texas–Southwestern Med Ctr, Dallas; et al)
N Engl J Med 362:494-503, 2010

Background.—The leading cause of failure of a prosthetic arteriovenous hemodialysis-access graft is venous anastomotic stenosis. Balloon angioplasty, the first-line therapy, has a tendency to lead to subsequent recoil and restenosis; however, no other therapies have yet proved to be more effective. This study was designed to compare conventional balloon angioplasty with an expanded polytetrafluoroethylene endovascular stent graft for revision of venous anastomotic stenosis in failing hemodialysis grafts.

Methods.—We conducted a prospective, multicenter trial, randomly assigning 190 patients who were undergoing hemodialysis and who had a venous anastomotic stenosis to undergo either balloon angioplasty alone or balloon angioplasty plus placement of the stent graft. Primary end points included patency of the treatment area and patency of the entire vascular access circuit.

Results.—At 6 months, the incidence of patency of the treatment area was significantly greater in the stent-graft group than in the balloon-angioplasty group (51% vs. 23%, $P<0.001$), as was the incidence of patency of the access circuit (38% vs. 20%, $P = 0.008$). In addition, the incidence of freedom from subsequent interventions at 6 months was significantly greater in the stent-graft group than in the balloon-angioplasty group (32% vs. 16%, $P = 0.03$ by the log-rank test and $P = 0.04$ by the Wilcoxon rank-sum test). The incidence of binary restenosis at 6 months was greater in the balloon-angioplasty group than in the stent-graft group (78% vs. 28%, P<0.001). The incidences of adverse events at 6 months were equivalent in the two treatment groups, with the exception of restenosis, which occurred more frequently in the balloon-angioplasty group (P<0.001).

Conclusions.—In this study, percutaneous revision of venous anastomotic stenosis in patients with a prosthetic hemodialysis graft was improved with the use of a stent graft, which appears to provide longer-term and superior patency and freedom from repeat interventions than standard balloon angioplasty. (ClinicalTrials.gov number, NCT00678249.)

▶ The authors have demonstrated that stent grafts covered with expanded polytetrafluoroethylene (ePTFE) were superior to balloon angioplasty alone for failing hemodialysis access grafts. Notably, both the 6-month primary patency rate (51% vs 23%, $P < .001$) at the treatment area (ie, venous anastomosis) and the primary patency of the access circuit (38% vs 20%, $P = .008$) were superior. The failing grafts were patent grafts (ie, nonthrombosed) with a stenotic lesion > 50%, an evidence that the lesion was hemodynamically significant, consistent with the National Kidney Foundation Kidney Disease Outcome Quality Initiative (KDOQI) guidelines.[1] Inclusion criteria attesting to the significance of the lesion included elevated venous pressures and decreased access blood flow. Notably, the randomization process was performed after the initial angioplasty and quantitative arteriograms were performed at 2- and 6-month intervals after the index procedure. The beneficial effect of the stent grafts appeared to be related to a decrease in the hyperplastic response (or recurrent hyperplastic response) at the treatment area as reflected by the significantly greater luminal diameter, lower percent stenosis, shorter length of stenosis, and lower incidence of stenotic lesions (ie, > 50% diameter). Collectively, the results from this well-performed study are very compelling and demonstrate that covered stents are superior in this clinical setting and suggest that they somehow modulate the inflammatory response or intimal hyperplasia. This ability to modulate the biological response is very intriguing and suggests multiple other potential applications on both the arterial and venous sides of the circulation. Despite the results, it remains to be determined which failing or thrombosed (ie, failed) accesses should be treated with covered stents, given the modest improvement in patency and their associated costs. Interestingly, the 6-month primary access patency rates (or access circuit patency rates) reported in this study (stent graft—38% and balloon angioplasty—20%) are significantly lower than 50% primary patency rate target defined by the 2006 KDOQI guidelines (guideline 6.5.1.2).

T. S. Huber, MD, PhD

Reference

1. III. NKF-K/DOQI Clinical Practice Guidelines for Vascular Access: update 2000. *Am J Kidney Dis.* 2001;37:S137-S181.

Surgical or endovascular repair of thrombosed dialysis vascular access: Is there any evidence?

Tordoir JHM, Bode AS, Peppelenbosch N, et al (Maastricht Univ Med Ctr, The Netherlands)

J Vasc Surg 50:953-956, 2009

Introduction.—Endovascular and surgical strategies have been used to manage patients with thrombosed vascular access for hemodialysis. We analyzed the evidence to see whether endovascular or surgical treatment has the best outcome in terms of primary success rate and long-term patency.

Methods.—We performed a systematic literature search of endovascular and surgical repair of thrombosed hemodialysis vascular access. The analysis included meta-analysis, randomized, and population-based studies of thrombosed arteriovenous fistulae and grafts.

Results.—One meta-analysis and eight randomized studies on the treatment of arteriovenous graft thrombosis were identified. Studies conducted before 2002 demonstrated a significantly better primary success rate and primary and secondary patencies of surgical thrombectomy vs endovascular intervention. After 2002, similar results of both techniques have been reported. Only population-based studies on the treatment of thrombosed autogenous arteriovenous fistulae have been published, showing similar outcome of surgical and endovascular intervention in terms of primary success. The long-term primary and secondary patencies are slightly better for surgical treatment, but this concerns only forearm fistulae.

Conclusions.—The outcome of endovascular and surgical intervention for thrombosed vascular access is comparable, in particular for thrombosed prosthetic grafts. Surgical treatment of autogenous arteriovenous fistulae is likely to have benefit compared with endovascular means. Definitive randomized trials are needed to provide the level 1 evidence to resolve this latter issue.

▶ This systematic review examining the optimal treatment of thrombosed hemodialysis accesses concluded that endovascular treatment of prosthetic accesses (ie, grafts) was comparable to the open approach. Notably, these findings are different than an earlier review meta-analysis by Green et al[1] that demonstrated that the open surgical treatment was clearly superior. Furthermore, they are not consistent with the clinical outcome goals (guideline 8.4.1) defined by the Kidney Disease Outcome Quality Initiative (KDOQI)[2] for thrombosed access that include a 50% unassisted patency rate at 6 months after endovascular treatment and a 50% rate at 1 year after open surgical repair. Interestingly, the KDOQI guidelines concede that the open approach is held to a higher standard because of the use of venous capital (ie, outflow vein). The current findings suggest that the endovascular treatment of thrombosed grafts has improved over the past several years, although it is worth emphasizing that despite the excellent initial technical results (>90%) the long-term results are only moderate with a primary patency rate of 34% to 44% at 6 months (well below the KDOQI targets). The mechanisms responsible for these improved results are not clear but potentially include better mechanical thrombectomy devices, improved thrombolytic agents, and an appreciation for the importance of clearing the whole access circuit from the arterial anastomosis to the central venous outflow. Although comparable, the fairly dismal results for both the endovascular and open approaches suggest that the life expectancy for a thrombosed graft is fairly short and consideration should be given to creating a new access rather than repeatedly attempting to salvage the problematic one. In our own practice, we thrombectomized a graft only once before creating a new access, preferably an autogenous one. The systematic review was unable to identify any randomized trial comparing endovascular and surgical treatment for thrombosed autogenous accesses (ie, fistulas). The case series suggested that the initial results were comparable between the 2 approaches, but the long-term results may be better with open surgery. The mere fact that there are even case series examining the role of thrombectomy for autogenous accesses reflects a change in practice patterns. Notably, an earlier version of the KDOQI had suggested that the success rates for clearing thrombosed autogenous accesses were so poor that it should not be attempted.

T. S. Huber, MD, PhD

References

1. Green LD, Lee DS, Kucey DS. A metaanalysis comparing surgical thrombectomy, mechanical thrombectomy, and pharmacomechanical thrombolysis for thrombosed dialysis grafts. *J Vasc Surg*. 2002;36:939-945.
2. III. NKF-K/DOQI Clinical Practice Guidelines for Vascular Access: update 2000. *Am J Kidney Dis*. 2001;37:S137-S181.

Aneurysm

Contemporary results of standard open repair of acute traumatic rupture of the thoracic aorta

Verdant A (Université de Montréal, Quebec, Canada)

J Vasc Surg 51:294-298, 2010

Background.—Open repair of acute traumatic rupture of the thoracic aorta has been the standard of care for the past half century. Traditional criteria of operative success have been patient survival and prevention of spinal cord ischemia. Historical series have reported a variability of surgical results with relation to the variety of operative approaches. This study aims to update the results obtained with a uniform surgical technique based on a systematic utilization of distal perfusion during aortic cross-clamping.

Methods.—During a 35-year period (1974-2009), 138 consecutive patients with an acute traumatic rupture of the thoracic aorta were repaired with a Dacron graft interposition through a standard left thoracotomy. All patients received a method of circulatory support. A passive 9-mm Gott shunt inserted between the ascending and the descending aorta and delivering a median flow of 3 L/min was used in the first 40 cases. A partial left heart bypass realized from the left atrium to the descending aorta and driven with a centrifugal pump was used in the last 98 consecutive cases. A median flow of 4 L/min was recorded. Mean age of the patients was 27 years and 90.6% of them had associated injuries for a calculated mean ISS of 44.

Results.—Two outcome variables were analyzed: hospital mortality and postoperative spinal cord ischemic injury. Overall hospital mortality is 5% (7/138 patients). This was improved from 7.5% (3/40) in patients perfused with the Gott shunt to 4% (4/98) in patients protected with the left heart bypass and lowered to 1.5% (1/68) in the last 68 patients. Among 134 cases with an intact preoperative spinal cord, one patient (0.7%) developed a new paraplegia due to a nonfunctional Gott shunt. Among 98 patients perfused with a centrifugal pump-driven left heart bypass, none of the 97 patients (0%) with a preoperative intact spinal cord developed a spinal cord ischemic deficit.

Conclusion.—Conventional open surgical repair of acute traumatic rupture of the thoracic aorta performed with an orderly monitored circulatory support can be accomplished with a very low rate of mortality and spinal cord injury. Compared with the Gott shunt, a left heart bypass propelled with a centrifugal pump is technically a more versatile method of perfusion, and it provides higher hemodynamic performance.

▶ This study and a study by Demetriades et al[1] detail different management strategies for the traumatic thoracic aortic injury. Open operative repair has been the traditional approach but has been largely replaced by the endovascular approach over the past several years at most major trauma centers. The study by Verdant documents spectacular outcomes (5% mortality and <1% paraplegia) for the open approach in a series of 138 patients spanning 35 years (average <4 repairs/year). Although it is unlikely that this single-surgeon experience can be duplicated at other centers, the results clearly establish a benchmark for comparison and likely define the best-case scenario. The results after endovascular repair reported by Neschis et al are not quite as good (12% mortality and 0% paraplegia), but, notably, none of the deaths were related to the aortic injury. Despite the series by Verdant, the introduction of the endovascular approach for traumatic thoracic aortic injuries appears to have had a significant impact nationwide in terms of the associated mortality and paraplegia rates. Indeed, Demetriades et al[1] reported from the American Association of Trauma in 2008 that mortality has decreased from 22% to 13%, and paraplegia had decreased from 8.7% to 1.6% in parallel with the widespread application of the endovascular approach. The results from Neschis et al suggest that the mid-term outcomes after endovascular repair are reasonable, but long-term follow-up and intense surveillance are mandatory. It is important to remember that a large percentage of the thoracic aortic trauma occurs in younger individuals with small, angulated aortas and that none of the commercially available thoracic or infrarenal aortic endovascular grafts are specifically designed for this purpose. In this endovascular study, the authors detailed that early device failure was associated with a sharp angulation of the aorta in conjunction with a short distance from the left subclavian and aortic injury. The failures involved collapse of the device, necessitating open conversion. Importantly, this has been seen during the follow-up and merits consideration during serial review of the imaging studies. Hopefully, these issues about the appropriate-sized device will be resolved in the near future because there are several industry-sponsored trials for this specific application in either development or progress.

T. S. Huber, MD, PhD

Reference

1. Demetriades D, Velmahos GC, Salea TM, et al. Diagnosis and treatment of blunt thoracic aortic injuries: changing perspectives. *J Trauma.* 2008;64:1415-1418.

Endograft Repair of Traumatic Aortic Injury—A Technique in Evolution: A Single Institution's Experience

Neschis DG, Moainie S, Flinn WR, et al (Univ of Maryland School of Medicine, Baltimore; et al)

Ann Surg 250:377-382, 2009

Objective.—We evaluated a large single center experience of endograft repair of blunt traumatic injury of the thoracic aorta.

Summary Background Data.—Traumatic aortic transection is a devastating injury with high morbidity and mortality. Endograft repair of these injuries has reduced the rates of death and paraplegia seen with open surgical treatment in the past. However, endograft repair has been associated with a higher incidence of device related failure.

Methods.—The records of 43 consecutive cases of endograft treatment of traumatic aortic injury from December 2004 to November 2008 were reviewed. Patient demographics, procedure details, and outcomes were recorded. Aortic morphology was analyzed for predictors of device failure.

Results.—Forty-three patients (32 men) with a mean age of 44 years (range: 17–88) were treated. Primary technical success was 86%. Six proximal endoleaks (14.3%) occurred. Two were repaired with a more proximal cuff, but 3 required explantation and open repair (7%). Mortality in this series was 11.6%, but no death was aorta related. No patient having endograft treatment suffered postoperative paraplegia. Early device failure is associated with sharp angulation of the aorta and shortened distance between the left subclavian artery and the site of injury. Follow-up ranged from 1 to 38 months (mean: 7.4 months). There were no late device failures or complications.

Conclusions.—Endovascular repair of blunt traumatic aortic injury can be performed with a low morbidity and mortality. Anatomic patterns in the aortic arch appear to be predictive of early device failure. Midterm

durability is excellent, but reliable follow-up remains challenging in this group of patients.

▶ This study and a study by Verdant[1] detail different management strategies for the traumatic thoracic aortic injury. Open operative repair has been the traditional approach but has been largely replaced by the endovascular approach over the past several years at most major trauma centers. The study by Verdant[1] documents spectacular outcomes (5% mortality and <1% paraplegia) for the open approach in a series of 138 patients spanning 35 years (average <4 repairs/year). Although it is unlikely that this single-surgeon experience can be duplicated at other centers, the results clearly establish a benchmark for comparison and likely define the best-case scenario. The results after endovascular repair reported by Neschis et al are not quite as good (12% mortality and 0% paraplegia), but, notably, none of the deaths were related to the aortic injury. Despite the series by Verdant,[1] the introduction of the endovascular approach for traumatic thoracic aortic injuries appears to have had a significant impact nationwide in terms of the associated mortality and paraplegia rates. Indeed, Demetriades et al[2] reported from the American Association of Trauma in 2008 that mortality has decreased from 22% to 13% and paraplegia had decreased from 8.7% to 1.6% in parallel with the widespread application of the endovascular approach. The results from Neschis et al suggest that the mid-term outcomes after endovascular repair are reasonable, but long-term follow-up and intense surveillance are mandatory. It is important to remember that a large percentage of the thoracic aortic trauma occurs in younger individuals with small, angulated aortas and that none of the commercially available thoracic or infrarenal aortic endovascular grafts are specifically designed for this purpose. In this endovascular study, the authors detailed that early device failure was associated with a sharp angulation of the aorta in conjunction with a short distance from the left subclavian and aortic injury. The failures involved collapse of the device, necessitating open conversion. Importantly, this has been seen during the follow-up and merits consideration during serial review of the imaging studies. Hopefully, these issues about the appropriate-sized device will be resolved in the near future because there are several industry-sponsored trials for this specific application in either development or progress.

T. S. Huber, MD, PhD

References

1. Verdant A. Contemporary results of standard open repair of acute traumatic rupture of the thoracic aorta. *J Vasc Surg.* 2010;51:294-298.
2. Demetriades D, Velmahos GC, Salea TM, et al. Diagnosis and treatment of blunt thoracic aortic injuries: changing perspectives. *J Trauma.* 2008;64:1415-1418.

Endovascular Repair of Thoracoabdominal Aortic Aneurysms

Haulon S, D'Elia P, O'Brien N, et al (Université Lille 2, France)

Eur J Vasc Endovasc Surg 39:171-178, 2010

Objectives.—To evaluate the early outcomes following thoracoabdominal aortic aneurysm (TAAA) repair utilising fenestrated and branched endografts.

Design and Materials and Methods.—A prospective analysis of all patients undergoing endovascular repair of TAAA in a single academic centre. All patients were deemed unfit for open surgical repair. Customised endografts were designed using CT data reconstructed on 3D workstations. Post-operatively all patients were evaluated radiologically at hospital discharge, at 6, 12, 18 and 24 months, and annually thereafter.

Results.—Thirty-three consecutive patients (30 males) were treated over 33 months (August 2006 to April 2009). Median age and aneurysm size were 70 years (range 50–83 years) and 64 mm (range 55–100 mm) respectively. 114/116 (98%) of the targeted visceral vessels were successfully catheterised and perfused. The in-hospital mortality rate was 9% (3/33). Transient spinal cord ischaemia was diagnosed in 4/33 (12%) patients, and permanent paraplegia in one (3%). The median follow-up period was 11 months (range 1–33 months). Endoleaks were identified in 5/33 (15%) patients: type II in four patients and a type III endoleak in one patient which required the only secondary intervention. During follow-up, two patients died: one from stroke and the other from myocardial infarction 9 and 29 months respectively after the procedure.

Conclusion.—This preliminary study, which includes our learning curve, confirms the feasibility and safety of the endovascular repair of TAAA in high-risk patients. Meticulous follow-up to assess sac behaviour and visceral perfusion is critical in order to ensure optimal results of these complex endovascular repairs requiring numerous mating components.

▶ This study and a study by Greenberg et al[1] document the exciting application of endovascular treatment for juxtarenal and thoracoabdominal aortic aneurysms. Although the patients were very highly selected, the favorable outcomes suggest that the approach has evolved from proof of concept to clinical applicability. The perioperative mortality rates were 0% and 12% for juxtarenal and thoracoabdominal aortic aneurysms, respectively, and compare favorably with open repair. Indeed, the potential benefit of the endovascular approach for these complex aneurysms far exceeds that for infrarenal aneurysms, given that the mortality rates for open repair have exceeded 20% for thoracoabdominal aortic aneurysms in most nationwide series. The underlying concept of the endovascular approach for juxtarenal aneurysms is that the landing zone is extended by anchoring the device in the perirenal/perivisceral aorta while maintaining perfusion through the renal and visceral vessels with some combination of scallops (ie, semicircular defect in the most proximal aspect of the graft), large fenestrations, or small fenestrations through which stents are placed as needed. The endovascular approach for thoracoabdominal aortic aneurysms is based upon using a branched or fenestrated graft for the perirenal/perivisceral aorta with standard aortic grafts extended both proximally and distally. Collectively, this study and Greenberg et al's[1] study have demonstrated that technical success rates are excellent despite the inherent challenges as reflected by the operative time of almost 4 hours. The various strategies implemented to maintain renal and visceral perfusion (ie, stent, bypass, and fenestration) appear to be effective within the mid-term range. Furthermore, the excluded aneurysm appears to behave during mid-term follow-up like the more familiar infrarenal aneurysm after a standard endovascular repair. It will be interesting to see how this exciting technology evolves. However, given the complexity of the case planning, the need for custom-ordered devices, and the technical challenges of implantation, it is likely that the approach will be concentrated in centers of excellence.

T. S. Huber, MD, PhD

Reference

1. Greenberg RK, Sternbergh WC III, Makaroun M, et al. Intermediate results of a United States multicenter trial of fenestrated endograft repair for juxtarenal abdominal aortic aneurysms. *J Vasc Surg*. 2009;50:730-737.

Intermediate results of a United States multicenter trial of fenestrated endograft repair for juxtarenal abdominal aortic aneurysms

Greenberg RK, Sternbergh WC III, Makaroun M, et al (Cleveland Clinic Foundation, OH; Oschner Clinic, New Orleans, LA; Univ of Pittsburgh Med Ctr, PA; et al)

J Vasc Surg 50:730-737, 2009

Objective.—This article reports the intermediate-term (24-month) outcomes of a prospective multicenter trial designed to evaluate the Zenith Fenestrated AAA Endovascular Graft (Cook Medical, Bloomington, Ind) for treating juxtarenal abdominal aortic aneurysms with short proximal necks. The study goals were to evaluate the safety and preliminary effectiveness of the device and refine patient selection criteria.

Methods.—Five centers in the United States enrolled 30 patients with juxtarenal aortic aneurysms with ≥50-mm diameter and short proximal necks. Devices were custom-designed for each patient based on measurements from reconstructed computed tomography (CT) data. Follow-up studies included physical examinations, laboratory studies, CT imaging, mesenteric-renal duplex ultrasound imaging, and abdominal flat plate radiographs at hospital discharge, at 1, 6, and 12 months, and yearly thereafter up to 5 years.

Results.—During a 1-year period, 30 patients (80% men; mean age, 75 years) with a mean aneurysm size of 61.4 mm were enrolled. In these 30 patients, 77 visceral vessels were accommodated by fenestrations located within the sealing segment of the grafts. The most common design accommodated two renal arteries and the superior mesenteric artery (66.7%). All prostheses were implanted successfully. No visceral arteries were lost. Of the 30 patients treated, 27 were available for 12-month follow-up and 23 were available for 24-month follow-up. No aneurysm-related deaths, aneurysm ruptures, or conversions were observed through 24 months of follow-up. No type I or type III endoleaks were observed. Type II endoleaks were noted in six (26.1%) at 12 months and four (20.0%) at 24 months. No patients had aneurysm growth >5 mm. Aneurysm size decreased in 16 of 23 (69.6%) and was stable in the remaining patients at 24 months. Eight patients experienced a renal event (4 renal artery stenoses, 2 renal artery occlusions, and 2 renal infarcts). Five underwent secondary interventions. No renal failure developed requiring dialysis.

Conclusions.—The intermediate-term (24-month) results of the 30 patients in this multicenter study are concordant with previous single-center studies and support the concept that placement of fenestrated endovascular grafts is safe and effective at centers with experience in endovascular repair and renal/mesenteric stent placement.

▶ This study and a study by Haulon et al[1] document the exciting application of endovascular treatment for juxtarenal and thoracoabdominal aortic aneurysms. Although the patients were very highly selected, the favorable outcomes suggest that the approach has evolved from proof of concept to clinical applicability. The perioperative mortality rates were 0% and 12% for juxtarenal and thoracoabdominal aortic aneurysms, respectively, and compare favorably with open repair. Indeed, the potential benefit of the endovascular approach for these complex aneurysms far exceeds that for infrarenal aneurysms, given that mortality rates for open repair have exceeded 20% for thoracoabdominal aortic aneurysms in most nationwide series. The underlying concept of the endovascular approach for juxtarenal aneurysms is that the landing zone is extended by anchoring the device in the perirenal/perivisceral aorta while maintaining perfusion through the renal and visceral vessels with some combination of scallops (ie, semicircular defect in the most proximal aspect of the graft), large fenestrations, or small fenestrations through which stents are placed as needed. The endovascular approach for thoracoabdominal aortic aneurysms is based upon using a branched or fenestrated graft for the perirenal/perivisceral aorta with standard aortic grafts extended both proximally and distally. Collectively, this study and Haulon et al's[1] study have demonstrated that technical success rates are excellent despite the inherent challenges as reflected by the operative time of almost 4 hours. The various strategies implemented to maintain renal and visceral perfusion (ie, stent, bypass, and fenestration) appear to be effective within the mid-term range. Furthermore, the excluded aneurysm appears to behave during mid-term follow-up like the more familiar infrarenal aneurysm after a standard endovascular repair. It will be interesting to see how this exciting technology evolves. However, given the complexity of the case planning, the need for custom-ordered devices, and the technical challenges of implantation, it is likely that the approach will be concentrated in centers of excellence.

T. S. Huber, MD, PhD

Reference

1. Haulon S, D'Elia P, O'Brien N, et al. Endovascular repair of thoracoabdominal aortic aneurysms. *Eur J Vasc Endovasc Surg*. 2010;39:171-178.

Genetic and environmental contributions to abdominal aortic aneurysm development in a twin population

Wahlgren CM, Larsson E, Magnusson PKE, et al (Karolinska Univ Hosp, Stockholm, Sweden; Karolinska Inst, Stockholm, Sweden)
J Vasc Surg 51:3-8, 2010

Background.—The contribution of hereditary and environmental factors to the development of abdominal aortic aneurysms (AAAs) is still partly unknown. The aim of this study was to analyze the role of these factors in a large population-based sample of twins.

Methods.—The Swedish Twin Registry, containing data on twins born in the country since 1886, was cross-linked with the Inpatient Registry, providing national coverage of discharge diagnoses coded according to the International Classification of Diseases (ICD). All twins with an infrarenal AAA were identified. Concordance rates and tetrachoric correlations were calculated for monozygotic (MZ) and dizygotic (DZ) twins. Tetrachoric correlations were calculated assuming an underlying normal distribution of liability, with multiple factors contributing additively and a threshold value that discriminates between AAA and no AAA. Higher concordance rates and correlations of liability in MZ twins than in DZ twins suggest that genetic factors influence disease development. Structural equation modeling techniques, Mx-analyses, were used to estimate the contributions of genetic effects as well as shared and nonshared environmental factors for development of AAA.

Results.—There were 172,890 twins registered at the time of the study including 265 twins (81% men; mean age 72 years; range, 48-94) with AAA. There were 7 MZ and 5 DZ concordant pairs as well as 44 MZ and 197 DZ discordant pairs with AAA. The probandwise concordance rates for MZ and DZ pairs were 24% and 4.8%, respectively. The tetrachoric correlations were 0.71 in MZ pairs and 0.31 in DZ pairs. The odds ratio (OR) was 71 (95% confidence interval [CI] 27-183) for MZ twins and 7.6 (95% CI 3.0-19) for DZ twins. In the structural equation models, genetic effects accounted for 70% (95% CI 0.33-0.83), shared environmental effects for 0% (95% CI 0-0.27), and nonshared environmental effects for 30% (95% CI 0.17-0.46) of the phenotypic variance among twins.

Conclusion.—These data provide robust epidemiologic evidence that heritability contributes to aneurysm formation. Concordances and correlations were higher in MZ compared with DZ twins, indicating genetic effects. There was a 24% probability that an MZ twin of a person with AAA will have the disease. The twin of an MZ twin with AAA had a risk of AAA that was 71 times that of the MZ twin of a person without AAA. A heritability of 70% of the total trait variance was estimated. The remaining variance was explained by nonshared environmental factors with no support for a role of shared environmental influences.

▶ This study helps define the role of genetic and environmental factors on the development of abdominal aortic aneurysms (AAA) using the Swedish Twin Registry. The authors found that the probability of an individual developing an AAA if his/her twin had an AAA (ie, probandwise concordance) was 24% for monozygotic twins (ie, identical) and 4.8% for dizygotic twins (ie, fraternal). Additionally, the odds ratio (ie, the relative risk of an AAA for individuals whose twin had an AAA compared with persons whose twin did not have an AAA) was 71 for monozygotic twins and 7.6 for dizygotic twins. Based on their statistical models, the authors reported that genetic factors accounted for 70% of the phenotypic variation between the twins with the balance due to nonshared environmental influences. Notably, shared environmental influences were not contributory. Given the single pair of female twins with an AAA, the authors were unable to reach any conclusion about the potential role of gender and the inheritability of an AAA. The overall findings, albeit based on somewhat sophisticated statistical analyses, provide fairly definitive evidence incriminating genetics in the pathophysiology of AAA. They are consistent with several other single-center and population studies that have estimated the prevalence of AAA among first-degree relatives to be as high as 15% to 20%. Furthermore, they provide strong support for screening family members of patients with an AAA. Indeed, this recommendation is usually part of the good news/bad news that I share with families in the recovery room after repairing an AAA: the good news is that your family member is doing well; the bad news is that there is a 15% to 20% chance that you could have the same problem.

T. S. Huber, MD, PhD

Hybrid Repair of Aortic Aneurysms Involving the Visceral and Renal Vessels

Kabbani LS, Criado E, Upchurch GR Jr, et al (Univ of Michigan School of Medicine, Ann Arbor)

Ann Vasc Surg 24:219-224, 2010

Background.—We sought to analyze our experience with hybrid treatment of aortic aneurysms involving the renal and visceral arteries.

Methods.—We conducted a retrospective review of 36 consecutive patients who underwent renal/visceral bypasses followed by aortic endografting. Patient demographics, medical history, operations, complications, graft patency, and patient survival were recorded. Observational and comparative analyses were performed.

Results.—Mean patient age was 71 years. Mean aneurysm diameter was 6.3 cm (range 4.1-9.4 cm). Crawford aneurysm types included 1 type I, 10 type II, 12 type III, 10 type IV, and 3 pararenal aneurysms. Four patients were symptomatic. One hundred twenty-three bypasses were performed (median of three per patient), including 62 renal, 32 superior mesenteric, and 29 celiac arteries. Retrograde inflow (using the iliac arteries, aorta, or a limb of an aortobifemoral graft) was obtained in 30 patients and antegrade inflow was performed in six (three from the supraceliac aorta and three celiac branch to renal bypasses). In-hospital mortality occurred in 3 patients (8.3%). Patient survival was 80% at a mean follow-up of 6 months. Major morbidity occurred in 17 patients (47%) and included need for dialysis (5), ischemic colitis (3), failure to thrive (5), temporary paraparesis (1), and need for reoperation (7). No patient sustained permanent paraplegia. Mean length of stay was 26 days (range 8-100 days). Primary renovisceral bypass graft patency rate at 8 months was 93%. During follow-up, 14 patients developed at least one endoleak, 2 patients required percutaneous intervention, and the rest remained under observation. At last follow-up, four type 2 endoleaks and one type 3 endoleak with stable or decreasing aneurysm size.

Conclusion.—Hybrid repair of aortic aneurysms involving the renal and visceral arteries is feasible with a reasonable mortality and satisfactory short-term visceral graft patency rate. However, the morbidity of the debranching procedures is high. More stringent patient selection may improve these results.

▶ This study and a study by Younes et al[1] document the potential role of hybrid or combined endovascular and open surgical procedures to extend the indications and/or patient population amenable to thoracic (thoracic endovascular aortic repair [TEVAR]) and abdominal aortic aneurysm (endovascular aortic repair [EVAR]) repair. Both studies report favorable outcomes and conclude that the approach is encouraging, albeit associated with an increased incidence of complications. Further review of the data illustrates that these are significant procedures from a technical standpoint and that the complications are major, far from the minimally invasive description usually ascribed to the endovascular approach. Notably, the stroke and spinal cord ischemia rates were 19% and 5%, respectively in the report by Younes et al,[1] while 29% of the patients were discharged to a rehabilitation facility and 11% to a skilled care facility. Similarly, Kabbani et al reported a median operative time for the debranching of 7 hours, a 47% major morbidity rate, a combined median length of stay of 19 days, and a 6-month survival rate of 80%. Although the studies seem to extend the indications for TEVAR and EVAR, the magnitude of the procedure and associated adverse outcomes mandate ongoing reappraisal of the indications for the procedure. It is important to remember that the indications for operative repair for both thoracic and abdominal aortic aneurysms are contingent upon the rupture risk of the aneurysm, the operative mortality, patient life expectancy, and patient preference. It is not completely clear whether a 20% mortality rate at 6 months justifies the hybrid approach. Furthermore, it is also worth emphasizing that the current results reflect relatively short- to mid-term results, and it is not clear how the off-label uses of the endovascular devices will behave over time and whether the patency rates for the visceral and arch revascularizations will be acceptable. Based upon our own experience, we have assumed a more conservative approach for the hybrid repair of abdominal and/or thoracoabdominal aortic aneurysms but have maintained an aggressive approach to the thoracic aorta as highlighted here, reflecting our impression that the arch debranching procedures are tolerated far better than the visceral ones. It is unclear what role these hybrid procedures will play if and when the fenestrated and branched-chain endografts evolve, although it is likely that they will continue to fill a niche for appropriately selected patients.

T. S. Huber, MD, PhD

Reference

1. Younes HK, Davies MG, Bismuth J, et al. Hybrid thoracic endovascular aortic repair: pushing the envelope. *J Vasc Surg*. 2010;51:259-266.

Hybrid thoracic endovascular aortic repair: Pushing the envelope

Younes HK, Davies MG, Bismuth J, et al (The Methodist Hosp, Houston, TX)

J Vasc Surg 51:259-266, 2010

Objective.—Thoracic endovascular aortic repair (TEVAR) can be limited by inadequate proximal and distal landing zones. Debranching or hybrid TEVAR has emerged as an important modality to expand landing zones and facilitate TEVAR. We report a single-center experience with hybrid TEVAR.

Methods.—We retrospectively reviewed all patients with thoracic aortic disease who received a TEVAR between February 2005 and October 2008.

Results.—Forty-two patients underwent a hybrid procedure (mean age 68 ± 13 years; 55% men). All patients were denied open surgery due to preoperative comorbidities or low physiologic reserve; 62% had a history of coronary artery disease, 67% had chronic obstructive pulmonary disease, 61% had undergone prior aortic surgery, and 90% had an American Society of Anesthesiology score of 4 and above. The average Society for Vascular Surgery comorbidity score was 12 ± 2 with a range of 9 to 14. Fifty-five percent of cases were symptomatic on presentation and 83% were done emergently. Seventy-six percent underwent debranching of the aortic arch, 17% of the visceral vessels, and 7% required both. Primary technical success was achieved in all cases and of these, 43% were staged. The 30-day mortality was 5%. Myocardial infarction developed in 5%, respiratory failure in 31%, cerebrovascular accident (stroke or transient ischemic attack) in 19%, and spinal cord ischemia with ensuant paraplegia occurred in 5% of patients. Fifty-eight percent of patients were discharged home, 11% required rehabilitation, and 29% were transferred to a skilled nursing facility. There was a significant association between visceral vessel debranching and both spinal cord ischemia ($P = .004$) and gastrointestinal complications ($P = .005$). On the other hand, there was no difference between staged and non-staged hybrid procedures.

Conclusions.—Hybrid procedures can successfully extend the range of patients suitable for a subsequent TEVAR. These procedures are associated with higher complication rates than isolated infrarenal or thoracic endovascular repair, but given the medical and anatomical complexity of these patients, the current results are quite encouraging.

▶ This study and a study by Kabbani et al[1] document the potential role of hybrid or combined endovascular and open surgical procedures to extend the indications and/or patient population amenable to thoracic (thoracic endovascular aortic repair [TEVAR]) and abdominal aortic aneurysm (endovascular aortic repair [EVAR]) repair. Both studies report favorable outcomes and conclude that the approach is encouraging, albeit associated with an increased incidence of complications. Further review of the data illustrates that these are significant procedures from a technical standpoint and that the complications are major, far from the minimally invasive description usually ascribed to the endovascular approach. Notably, the stroke and spinal cord ischemia rates were 19% and 5%, respectively in the report by Younes et al, while 29% of the patients were discharged to a rehabilitation facility and 11% to a skilled care facility. Similarly, Kabbani et al[1] reported a median operative time for the debranching of 7 hours, a 47% major morbidity rate, a combined median length of stay of 19 days, and a 6-month survival rate of 80%. Although the studies seem to extend the indications for TEVAR and EVAR, the magnitude of the procedure and associated adverse outcomes mandate ongoing reappraisal of the indications for the procedure. It is important to remember that the indications for operative repair for both thoracic and abdominal aortic aneurysms are contingent upon the rupture risk of the aneurysm, the operative mortality, patient life expectancy, and patient preference. It is not completely clear whether a 20% mortality rate at 6 months justifies the hybrid approach. Furthermore, it is also worth emphasizing that the current results reflect relatively short- to mid-term results, and it is not clear how the off-label uses of the endovascular devices will behave over time and whether the patency rates for the visceral and arch revascularizations will be acceptable. Based upon our own experience, we have assumed a more conservative approach for the hybrid repair of abdominal and/or thoracoabdominal aortic aneurysms but have maintained an aggressive approach to the thoracic aorta as highlighted here, reflecting our impression that the arch debranching procedures are tolerated far better than the visceral ones. It is unclear what role these hybrid procedures will play if and when the fenestrated and branched-chain endografts evolve, although it is likely that they will continue to fill a niche for appropriately selected patients.

T. S. Huber, MD, PhD

Reference

1. Kabbani LS, Criado E, Upchurch GR Jr, et al. Hybrid repair of aortic aneurysms involving the visceral and renal vessels. *Ann Vasc Surg*. 2010;24:219-224.

Outcomes Following Endovascular vs Open Repair of Abdominal Aortic Aneurysm: A Randomized Trial

Lederle FA, Freischlag JA, Kyriakides TC, et al (Veterans Affairs Med Ctr, Minneapolis, MN; Veterans Affairs Med Ctr, Baltimore, MD; Veterans Affairs Med Ctr, West Haven, CT; et al)

JAMA 302:1535-1542, 2009

Context.—Limited data are available to assess whether endovascular repair of abdominal aortic aneurysm (AAA) improves short-term outcomes compared with traditional open repair.

Objective.—To compare postoperative outcomes up to 2 years after endovascular or open repair of AAA in a planned interim report of a 9-year trial.

Design, Setting, and Patients.—A randomized, multicenter clinical trial of 881 veterans (aged ≥49 years) from 42 Veterans Affairs Medical Centers with eligible AAA who were candidates for both elective endovascular repair and open repair of AAA. The trial is ongoing and this report describes the period between October 15, 2002, and October 15, 2008.

Intervention.—Elective endovascular (n = 444) or open (n = 437) repair of AAA.

Main Outcome Measures.—Procedure failure, secondary therapeutic procedures, length of stay, quality of life, erectile dysfunction, major morbidity, and mortality.

Results.—Mean follow-up was 1.8 years. Perioperative mortality (30 days or inpatient) was lower for endovascular repair (0.5% vs 3.0%; $P = .004$), but there was no significant difference in mortality at 2 years (7.0% vs 9.8%, $P = .13$). Patients in the endovascular repair group had reduced median procedure time (2.9 vs 3.7 hours), blood loss (200 vs 1000 mL), transfusion requirement (0 vs 1.0 units), duration of mechanical ventilation (3.6 vs 5.0 hours), hospital stay (3 vs 7 days), and intensive care unit stay (1 vs 4 days), but required substantial exposure to fluoroscopy and contrast. There were no differences between the 2 groups in major morbidity, procedure failure, secondary therapeutic procedures, aneurysm-related hospitalizations, health-related quality of life, or erectile function.

Conclusions.—In this report of short-term outcomes after elective AAA repair, perioperative mortality was low for both procedures and lower for endovascular than open repair. The early advantage of endovascular repair was not offset by increased morbidity or mortality in the first 2 years after repair. Longer-term outcome data are needed to fully assess the relative merits of the 2 procedures.

Trial Registration.—clinicaltrials.gov Identifier: NCT00094575.

▶ The Open Versus Endovascular Aneurysm Repair (OVER) trial represents one of the seminal surgical studies published during the past year and should be read in its entirety. It further clarifies the role of endovascular aneurysm repair (EVAR) and corroborates the earlier findings of both the EVAR-1[1,2] and DREAM[3,4] trials. The eagerly awaited OVER trial demonstrated that the perioperative mortality was lower for EVAR (0.5% vs 3.0%, $P = .004$), but there was no difference in mortality at 2 years (7.0% vs 9.8%, $P = .13$). Notably, the perioperative mortality rates were even lower than reported from the other comparable randomized trials (DREAM—1.2% vs 4.6%; EVAR Trial—1.7% vs 4.7%) and negate any criticism for our side of the Atlantic that the findings of the earlier trials were confounded by excess morbidity and mortality. Predictably, the soft perioperative outcome measures (ie, procedure time, estimated blood loss, length of stay, and intensive care length of stay) favored EVAR. However, there were no differences in the major outcome measures, including major morbidity, procedure failure, secondary interventions, quality of life, and erective dysfunction in contrast to some of the findings in the earlier trials. Approximately 13% of the patients in both the open and endovascular groups required remedial procedures during the early time course of the study, although the types of secondary procedures were dramatically different. Most remedial procedures were secondary endovascular procedures in the EVAR group, while the bulk of those in the open group were hernia repairs. Importantly, 2% of the patients in the open group required additional aortic procedures, further emphasizing the important point that it is not only EVAR patients that require remedial aortic interventions. Although the study population was almost an exclusively male veteran population, the findings are likely applicable to the larger cohort of patients with intact abdominal aortic aneurysms and suggest that EVAR is at least comparable, if not superior, to open repair. I would echo the authors' conclusions that "the early advantage of endovascular repair was not offset by increased morbidity and mortality in the first 2 years after repair." It is reassuring that we now have level 1 data to support the widespread application of EVAR, a technology that has eclipsed open repair, largely driven by patient, provider, and industry preference. It remains to be seen whether the apparent benefit of EVAR is sustained and cost-effective. I look forward to further additional reports from the OVER study group.

T. S. Huber, MD, PhD

References

1. Greenhalgh RM, Brown LC, Kwong GP, Powell JT, Thompson SG. Comparison of endovascular aneurysm repair with open repair in patients with abdominal aortic aneurysm (EVAR trial 1), 30-day operative mortality results: randomised controlled trial. *Lancet.* 2004;364:843-848.
2. EVAR trial participants. Endovascular aneurysm repair versus open repair in patients with abdominal aortic aneurysm (EVAR trial 1): randomised controlled trial. *Lancet.* 2005;365:2179-2186.
3. Prinssen M, Verhoeven EL, Buth J, et al. A randomized trial comparing conventional and endovascular repair of abdominal aortic aneurysms. *N Engl J Med.* 2004;351:1607-1618.

4. Blankensteijn JD, de Jong SE, Prinssen M, et al. Two-year outcomes after conventional or endovascular repair of abdominal aortic aneurysms. *N Engl J Med.* 2005; 352:2398-2405.

Randomized Comparison of Strategies for Type B Aortic Dissection: The INvestigation of STEnt Grafts in Aortic Dissection (INSTEAD) Trial

Nienaber CA, for the INSTEAD Trial (Univ of Rostock, Germany; et al)

Circulation 120:2519-2528, 2009

Background.—Thoracic endovascular aortic repair (TEVAR) represents a novel concept for type B aortic dissection. Although life-saving in acute emergencies, outcomes and survival of TEVAR in stable dissection are unknown.

Methods and Results.—One hundred forty patients in stable clinical condition at least 2 weeks after index dissection were randomly subjected to elective stent-graft placement in addition to optimal medical therapy (n=72) or to optimal medical therapy alone (n=68) with surveillance (arterial pressure according to World Health Organization guidelines ≤120/80 mm Hg). The primary end point was all-cause death at 2 years, whereas aorta-related death, progression (with need for conversion or additional endovascular or open surgery), and aortic remodeling were secondary end points. There was no difference in all-cause deaths, with a 2-year cumulative survival rate of 95.6 ± 2.5% with optimal medical therapy versus 88.9 ± 3.7% with TEVAR (P=0.15); the trial, however, turned out to be underpowered. Moreover, the aorta-related death rate was not different (P=0.44), and the risk for the combined end point of aorta-related death (rupture) and progression (including conversion or additional endovascular or open surgery) was similar (P=0.65). Three neurological adverse events occurred in the TEVAR group (1 paraplegia, 1 stroke, and 1 transient paraparesis), versus 1 case of paraparesis with medical treatment. Finally, aortic remodeling (with true-lumen recovery and thoracic false-lumen thrombosis) occurred in 91.3% of patients with TEVAR versus 19.4% of those who received medical treatment (P<0.001), which suggests ongoing aortic remodeling.

Conclusions.—In the first randomized study on elective stent-graft placement in survivors of uncomplicated type B aortic dissection, TEVAR failed to improve 2-year survival and adverse event rates despite favorable aortic remodeling.

▶ The INvestigation of STent Grafts in Aortic Dissection (INSTEAD) trial has helped define the role of thoracic endovascular aortic repair (TEVAR) in patients with stable type B dissections and, thereby, illustrated several key management points. Patients with stable dissections (diameter < 6 cm, no acute complications, duration > 2 weeks, and TEVAR eligible by anatomic criteria) were randomly assigned to medical therapy or medical therapy in conjunction with TEVAR. There were no differences in survival at 2 years, the primary study end point, or in the secondary end points of aortic-related death and freedom from progressive aortic disease. Notably, aortic expansion >60 mm did occur more frequently in the medical group, necessitating remedial TEVAR in 16% of the patients and open repair in 4%. TEVAR was associated with a significant increase in the thoracic true-lumen diameter and the regression of the false-lumen diameter, with false-lumen thrombosis occurring in 91% of the cases. Unfortunately, the study was underpowered, largely due to the better-than-predicted survival in the medical group that underscored the effectiveness of these therapies. Although the results failed to identify an early benefit for TEVAR in the setting of stable type B dissections, they suggest that a complication-specific approach may be effective and that patients can safely cross over to TEVAR or open repair during the follow-up period. The observed crossovers emphasize the importance of long-term surveillance given the significant potential for aneurysmal degeneration. Lastly, the TEVAR-associated aortic remodeling and thrombosis of the false lumen were impressive and may actually lead to a significant benefit during long-term follow-up, given the association between perfusion of the false lumen and adverse outcome.

T. S. Huber, MD, PhD

Carotid

Predicting 1-year mortality after elective abdominal aortic aneurysm repair

Beck AW, for the Vascular Study Group of Northern New England (Dartmouth-Hitchcock Med Ctr Dept of Surgery, Lebanon, NH; et al)

J Vasc Surg 49:838-844, 2009

Objective.—Benefit of prophylactic abdominal aortic aneurysm (AAA) repair requires sufficient survival to overcome operative risk. Since death within 1 year of elective open or endovascular (EVAR) infrarenal AAA repair likely indicates ineffective treatment, we developed a prediction model for 1-year mortality to aid clinical decision-making.

Methods.—We used a prospective registry of 1387 consecutive patients who had undergone elective AAA repair from 2003 to 2007 by 50 surgeons from 11 hospitals in Northern New England. Cox proportional hazards were used to analyze potential risk factors for 1-year mortality, including medical comorbidities, aortic clamp site, preoperative risk factor modification (eg, beta-blockade), and aneurysm diameter.

Results.—Thirty-day and 1 year mortality after open repair (n = 748) was 2.3% and 5.8%, and after EVAR (n = 639) was 0.5% and 5.7%, respectively. Factors associated with death within 1 year after open repair were: age ≥ 70 (P =.007; hazard ratio [HR] 2.9, 95% confidence interval [CI] 1.3-6.3), history of chronic obstructive pulmonary disease (COPD) (P < .0001; HR 3.6, 95% CI 1.9-7.0), chronic renal insufficiency (creatinine ≥ 1.8) (P =.008; HR 2.8, 95% CI 1.3-6.2) and suprarenal aortic clamp site (P < .0001; HR 3.8, 95% CI 1.9-7.5). Depending on the number of risk factors present, predicted 1-year mortality after open repair varied from 1% in patients with no risk factors to 67% in patients with four risk factors. Our model demonstrated excellent correlation between observed and expected deaths ($r = 0.97$). For EVAR, identified risk factors for death within 1 year included a history of congestive heart failure (CHF) ($P = .002$; HR 3.2, 95% CI 1.6-6.5), and aneurysm diameter ≥6.5 cm ($P = .04$ 95% CI 1.0-4.8). Depending on the number of risk factors present, predicted mortality ranged from 3.6% to 23%. A model using CHF and aneurysm diameter correlated well with actual mortality rates, with an observed to expected ratio of 0.96.

Conclusion.—Predictors of 1-year mortality can identify patients less likely to benefit from elective AAA repair. These factors differ for open repair vs EVAR and should be considered in individual patient decision-making. Our EVAR model had less impact on 1-year survival, even if CHF and large AAA diameter were present. However, a combination of age, COPD, renal insufficiency, and need for suprarenal clamping have significant impact on 1-year mortality after open AAA repair. Consideration of these variables should assist decision-making for elective AAA repair, especially in borderline cases.

▶ The authors have used data from the Vascular Study Group of Northern New England (VSGNNE) to develop a predictive model for 1-year mortality after both open and endovascular aneurysm repair (endovascular aortic repair [EVAR]). In essence, they have attempted to combine patient comorbidities to refine clinical or operative decision making. They appropriately contend that a successful outcome after aneurysm repair requires surviving for at least a year, given the costs associated with repair from a social, financial, morbidity, and rehabilitation standpoint. In our own practice, we have traditionally balanced the risk of operative repair and the annual rupture risk of the aneurysm, but this simple decision algorithm is too narrow. We readily concede that it is more appropriate to factor in life expectancy (ie, 1-year survival) as the authors have suggested, and an increased emphasis should be placed upon patient preference. The predicted mortalities after open repair are somewhat sobering (range 1%-67%) and suggest that we should perhaps be more aggressive for patients without any of the 4 risk factors (age >70, renal insufficiency—creatinine >1.8, chronic obstructive pulmonary disease [COPD], and suprarenal aortic clamp) and progressively less aggressive as the number of risk factors increase for a specific patient. As illustrated in Table 5 in the original article, the appropriate threshold for open aneurysm repair in patients with more than 2 risk factors may be >9 cm. These observations are even more enlightening considering the evolution and widespread application of EVAR. In our own practice, the small subset of patients that require open repair (ie, not EVAR candidates) usually have juxtarenal aneurysms and advanced comorbidities, the same risk factors outlined above. Unfortunately, the authors' predictive model was not very helpful for EVAR with the only predictors of 1-year mortality being congestive heart failure and aneurysm diameter (>6.5 cm). Paradoxically, the presence of a large aneurysm in the EVAR model was associated with both increased rupture risk and 1-year mortality after repair. It is noteworthy that the 1-year mortality rates were comparable for both open repair and EVAR, a trend similar to the randomized controlled trials.

T. S. Huber, MD, PhD

Comparative effectiveness of carotid arterial stenting versus endarterectomy

Groeneveld PW, Yang L, Greenhut A, et al (Philadelphia Veterans Affairs Med Ctr, PA; Univ of Pennsylvania School of Medicine, Philadelphia)
J Vasc Surg 50:1040-1048, 2009

Background.—Carotid arterial stent (CAS) systems are an alterative to carotid endarterectomy for the treatment of moderate to severe carotid stenosis, but the effectiveness of CAS compared to endarterectomy in preventing stroke and death is uncertain. This study's objective was to compare the clinical outcomes among Medicare beneficiaries undergoing carotid revascularization before and after CAS became widely available.

Objectives.—This observational, retrospective cohort study compared 46,784 patients undergoing carotid revascularization from August 2005-March 2006 (the coverage era) to propensity-score-matched patients undergoing carotid revascularization between October 2002-September 2004 (the pre-coverage era), before widespread Medicare coverage of CAS.

Methods.—Mortality was compared at 90 and 270 days after revascularization, as were the combined outcomes of periprocedural acute myocardial infarction and any stroke or death within 90 and 270 days after revascularization, between the two eras. Comparisons were also made between localities with high (23% of carotid procedures being CAS) and lower (9% of carotid procedures being CAS) adoption rates of carotid stents during the coverage era.

Results.—There were no significant differences in 90-day mortality (2.2% vs 2.2%; $P = .79$), 90-day combined outcomes (4.5% vs 4.3%; $P = .13$), or 270-day mortality (4.8% vs 4.6%; $P = .17$) between the coverage and pre-coverage eras, but there were more 270-day combined outcomes in the coverage era (7.7% vs 7.3%; $P = .03$). In localities with higher adoption of carotid stents, there was higher 90-day mortality (adjusted odds ratio [OR] 1.15; $P = .16$), 90-day combined outcomes (OR = 1.17; $P = .03$), 270-day mortality (OR = 1.13; $P = .07$), and 270-day combined outcomes (OR = 1.10; $P = .09$) in the coverage era. There were no differences in event rates between eras in areas with lower carotid stent adoption.

Conclusion.—The adoption of carotid stents for treatment of carotid stenosis was associated with increased rates of adverse clinical outcomes after carotid revascularization.

▶ The study has attempted to determine the clinical impact of carotid arterial stenting (CAS) among Medicare beneficiaries by comparing outcome for carotid revascularization before and after the technique became widely available. The goal of the study was to compare carotid endarterectomy (CEA) and CAS in the real-world setting, outside the context of clinical trials. Using some fairly sophisticated statistical techniques, the authors found that there were no differences in 90-day mortality, 90-day combined outcome measures, or 270-day mortality, but there was a difference in 270-day combined outcomes (7.7% vs 7.3%, $P = .03$), albeit a small difference, likely not clinically relevant. Analysis of the geographic areas in which the technique was widely adopted demonstrated worse outcomes for all of the measures detailed above after introduction of CAS. Furthermore, comparison of CEA and CAS during the time period when CAS was available revealed that CAS was also associated with worse outcomes for all of the measures (ie, relative to CEA). It is conceivable that these adverse outcomes were associated with the use of CAS in patients who would not have undergone CEA in the precoverage era, but this explanation does not seem to be supported by the statistical modeling. These findings must be interpreted with some caution, given the limitations of the Medicare claims databases that include the lack of an indication for the procedure, limitations in assessing the comorbidities, inability to document medical treatment, and inaccuracies in assessing postoperative complications, particularly stroke. However, they are consistent with the Endarterectomy vs Angioplasty in patients with Severe Symptomatic Carotid Stenosis (EVA-3S) trial that suggested CAS was associated with a higher incidence of stroke or death at 30 days.[1] These real-world data suggest that CEA is the optimal treatment for carotid artery stenosis regardless of the clinical trials. It will be interesting to see the response from both Medicare and practitioners across the country to the Carotid Revascularization Endarterectomy vs Stenting Trial (CREST), whose preliminary results have suggested equivocal results for CEA and CAS.[2]

T. S. Huber, MD, PhD

References

1. Mas JL, Chatellier G, Beyssen B, et al. Endarterectomy versus stenting in patients with symptomatic severe carotid stenosis. *N Engl J Med.* 2006;355:1660-1671.
2. Hobson RW, Howard VJ, Brott TG, Howard G, Roubin GS, Ferguson RD, For the CREST Executive Committee. Organizing the Carotid Revascularization Endarterectomy versus Stenting Trial (CREST). *Curr Control Trials Cardiovasc Med.* 2001; 2:160-164.

Primary carotid artery stenting versus carotid artery stenting for postcarotid endarterectomy stenosis

AbuRahma AF, Abu-Halimah S, Bensenhaver J, et al (West Virginia Univ, Charleston; et al)

J Vasc Surg 50:1031-1039, 2009

Background.—Carotid artery stenting (CAS) has been advocated as an alternative to carotid endarterectomy (CEA) in high-risk surgical patients, including stenosis after CEA. This study compared early and midterm clinical outcomes for primary CAS vs CAS for post-CEA stenosis.

Methods.—This study analyzed 180 high-risk surgical patients: 68 had primary CAS (group A), and 112 had CAS for post-CEA stenosis (group B). Patients were followed-up prospectively and had duplex ultrasound imaging at 1 month and every 6 months thereafter. All patients had cerebral protection devices. Kaplan-Meier life-table analysis was used to estimate rates of freedom from stroke, stroke-free survival, ≥50% in-stent stenosis, ≥80% in-stent stenosis, and target vessel reintervention (TVR).

Results.—Patients had comparable demographic and clinical characteristics. Carotid stent locations were similar. Indications for CAS were transient ischemic attacks (TIA) or stroke in 50% for group A and 45% for group B. The mean follow-up was comparable, at 21 (range, 1-73) vs 25 (range, 1-78) months, respectively. The technical success rate was 100%. The perioperative stroke rates and combined stroke/death/myocardial infarction (MI) rates were 7.4% for group A vs 0.9% for group B ($P = .0294$). No perioperative MIs occurred in either group. One death was secondary to stroke. The combined early and late stroke rates were 10.8% for group A and 1.8% for group B ($P = .0275$). The stroke-free rates at 1, 2, 3, and 4 years for groups A and B were 89%, 89%, 89%, and 89%; and 98%, 98%, 98%, and 98%, respectively ($P = .0105$). The rates of freedom from ≥50% carotid in-stent stenosis were 94%, 83%, 83%, and 66% for group A vs 96%, 91%, 83%, and 72% for group B ($P = .4705$). Two patients (3%) in group A and seven patients (6.3%) in group B had ≥80% in-stent stenosis (all were asymptomatic except one). The freedom from ≥80% in-stent stenosis at 1, 2, 3, and 4 years for groups A and B were 100%, 98%, 98%, and 78% vs 99%, 96%, 92%, and 87%, respectively ($P = .7005$). Freedom from TVR rates at 1, 2, 3, and 4 years for groups A and B were 100%, 100%, 100%, and 100% vs 99%, 97%, 97%, and 92%, respectively ($P = .261$).

Conclusions.—CAS for post-CEA stenosis carried a lower risk of early postprocedural neurologic events than primary CAS, with a trend toward a higher restenosis rate during follow-up.

▶ The study compared the results of carotid artery stenting (CAS) for primary lesions with those for recurrent lesions after carotid endarterectomy (CEA). Not surprisingly, the technical success rates were excellent (100%) for both groups, but the perioperative and long-term stroke rates were lower in the patients with recurrent lesions (perioperative stroke/death/myocardial infarction—7.4% vs 0.9%; early and late stroke rates—10.8% vs 1.8%). Notably, the patients with primary CAS were deemed high risk as defined by a variety of clinical trials, and half of the patients were symptomatic, although it has never been clear to me why high-risk patients with asymptomatic lesions merit treatment at all. The perioperative adverse event rates for the primary group were greater than those generally defined for CEA (ie, asymptomatic—< 3%, symptomatic—< 5%) but were within the range of the other CAS trials for high-risk patients. The low perioperative adverse event rates in the post-CEA group appear to justify the use of CAS in that setting, and, indeed, this appears to be one of its more compelling indications. It is worth noting that the proper control group for comparison is really patients undergoing open, surgical revascularization for post-CEA stenoses rather than those undergoing primary CAS. It is not surprising that the perioperative stroke rate was higher in the primary CAS group, given the usual differences in the composition of the stenotic lesion (ie, primary—atherosclerotic, recurrent—intimal hyperplasia), and it is worth noting that most of the perioperative strokes in the primary group were embolic in nature. A trend toward an increased incidence of recurrence was found in the post-CEA group, suggesting that this cohort of patients may be predisposed to developing recurrent stenoses regardless of the initial event (ie, CAS or CEA). Although the study is limited by its retrospective design, small sample size, and selection bias, the results provide further justification for CAS as the optimal treatment for recurrent stenoses after CEA.

T. S. Huber, MD, PhD

Urgency of Carotid Endarterectomy for Secondary Stroke Prevention: Results From the Registry of the Canadian Stroke Network

Gladstone DJ, Oh J, Fang J, et al (Inst for Clinical Evaluative Sciences, Toronto, Canada; Univ of Toronto, Canada; et al)

Stroke 40:2776-2782, 2009

Background and Purpose.—The benefit of carotid endarterectomy for preventing recurrent stroke is maximal when surgery is performed within 2 weeks after ischemic stroke or transient ischemic attack; the benefit is reduced when surgery is delayed >2 weeks and essentially lost if delayed >3 months. Guidelines recommend endarterectomy within 2 weeks post-stroke/transient ischemic attack for patients with symptomatic carotid stenosis. This study examined time to endarterectomy at designated stroke centers as a measure of evidence-based best practices for stroke prevention.

Methods.—From the Registry of the Canadian Stroke Network, we identified all consecutive patients presenting with acute ischemic stroke or transient ischemic attack at 12 provincial stroke centers (Ontario, Canada, 2003 to 2006) and selected those with unilateral symptomatic carotid stenosis of moderate (50% to 69%) or severe (70% to 99%) degree. Using linkages to administrative databases, we identified patients who underwent carotid endarterectomy within 6 months after the symptomatic event and calculated the time intervals between the index event and surgery. We compared the timing of surgery according to age, sex, degree of stenosis, index event, geographic region, and year. Logistic regression assessed variables associated with early surgery.

Results.—One hundred five patients underwent endarterectomy for unilateral symptomatic carotid stenosis (50% to 99%) within 6 months of the index event. The median time from index event to surgery was 30 days (interquartile range, 10 to 81). Only one third (38 of 105) received endarterectomy within the recommended 2-week target timeframe, and in one fourth (26 of 105), surgery was delayed >3 months. Surgery within 2 weeks was more likely if the index event was a transient ischemic attack rather than a stroke. Access to early endarterectomy varied markedly between hospitals across the province and improved over time from 2003 to 2006.

Conclusions.—In this hospital-based cohort, the majority of patients undergoing carotid endarterectomy after a transient ischemic attack or stroke had surgery delayed well beyond the period of maximum effectiveness. To enhance secondary stroke prevention, greater efforts are needed to minimize delays to diagnosis and surgical treatment for patients with symptomatic carotid stenosis.

▶ The study examined compliance with the clinical practice guidelines for the timing of carotid endarterectomy (CEA) among patients with moderate (50%-69%) or severe (70%-99%) symptomatic stenoses treated at designated stroke centers. According to cited guidelines, CEA "should be performed without delay, preferably 2 weeks"[1] or "as soon as the patient is fit for the procedure, preferably within 2 weeks."[2] Somewhat surprisingly, the authors reported that the median time from index to CEA was 30 days and that only one-third of the procedures were performed within the 2-week window. Although there were multiple problems with the study design (eg, small sample size, retrospective design, administrative database, and hospital-based cohort), the results suggest that CEA was performed outside of the period of maximal effectiveness in most patients. This suggests that there are opportunities within the care delivery system for improvement, including early recognition of the neurologic event, prompt investigation with the appropriate carotid-focused imaging, and timely referral to a vascular surgeon for definitive treatment. Although it was not possible to determine where the source of delay occurred in this study, it is worthwhile to note that median time to surgery was 14 and 46 days, respectively, for patients with a transient ischemic attack (TIA) and ischemic stroke. These delays suggest that the timing was partially dictated by the clinical presentation. Indeed, the timing for CEA after an ischemic stroke has been debated for a long time despite the clinical practice guidelines cited. It is clear that the likelihood of a recurrent carotid-based event is highest around the time of the sentinel event and that this risk decreases with time, approaching that of an asymptomatic lesion by approximately 120 days. It is also clear that performing a CEA on patients with an acute stroke is associated with an increased perioperative stroke rate, oftentimes an exacerbation of the initial event. In our own practice, we have delayed CEA after ischemic stroke until the neurological symptoms have improved to a stable point (ie, plateau) or at least until the brain edema has resolved on CT or MR scan. This study and the newer practice guidelines argue for a more aggressive approach or earlier intervention provided that "the patient is fit for the procedure."

T. S. Huber, MD, PhD

References

1. Chaturvedi S, Bruno A, Feasby T, et al. Carotid endarterectomy - an evidence-based review: report of the Therapeutics and Technology Assessment Subcommittee of the American Academy of Neurology. *Neurology.* 2005;65:794-801.
2. Canadian Stroke Network. *Canadian Best Practice Recommendations for Stroke Care: 2006.* Ottawa: Canadian Stroke Network; 2006.

Miscellaneous

Endovascular treatment of spontaneous dissections of the superior mesenteric artery

Gobble RM, Brill ER, Rockman CB, et al (New York Univ Langone Med Ctr)
J Vasc Surg 50:1326-1332, 2009

Background.—Spontaneous dissection of the superior mesenteric artery (SMA) is exceedingly rare. Treatment options range from observation to anticoagulation to open surgery or endovascular repair. We present our experience to date in the management of isolated SMA dissections.

Methods.—A retrospective review of the vascular surgery and radiology databases from 1998 to 2008 was performed. In general, incidental radiologic findings of a dissection were managed expectantly. The decision to intervene was based on anatomic suitability, patient comorbidities and symptoms, and physician preference. Endovascular stents were placed using a brachial approach, with the choice of stent determined by physician preference. Patients who underwent endovascular stent placement (ESP) were maintained on antiplatelet therapy for 6 months postoperatively. Follow-up consisted of yearly office visits and adjunctive computerized tomography (CT) or magnetic resonance imaging (MRI) when clinically indicated.

Results.—CT or MRI imaging identified nine patients (7 men, 2 women) with an isolated SMA dissection. One patient also had a concomitant celiac artery dissection. Median age was 70 years (range, 46-73 years). Median follow-up time was 32 months (range, 13.8-62.5 months). Presentations included an incidental radiologic finding in three patients and acute onset abdominal pain in six. Treatment included expectant management in four patients, anticoagulation in two, and ESP in three. ESP was performed primarily in two patients and in a third patient after initial management with anticoagulation failed. The reduction in the diameter of the true lumen was significantly greater in patients treated with ESP vs patients who were successfully managed expectantly or with anticoagulation ($F = 15.59$, $P < .005$). No procedural complications were associated with ESP.

Conclusions.—An isolated SMA dissection is a rare entity that may be managed successfully in a variety of ways based on clinical presentation. Endovascular stenting can be performed with good results and may be the preferred treatment in patients with symptomatic isolated SMA dissections.

▶ This article and an article by Takach et al[1] contribute to our understanding of the natural history and the treatment strategies for patients with spontaneous, isolated dissections of the mesenteric vessels. With the rapid progression of CT arteriography and the low threshold for its application, it has become apparent that spontaneous dissections of the celiac and superior mesenteric vessels are uncommon but not rare. Indeed, most vascular surgeons will see a couple of such cases over the course of the year. As emphasized in the Gobble et al's article and Takach et al's article,[1] the clinical presentation may range from acute abdominal pain to an incidental finding at the time of imaging obtained for other reasons. The etiology of these dissections remains unclear, but a variety of causes have been implicated. Given the limited number of reports and follow-up, it is not surprising that the treatment strategies remain unresolved. However, Gobble et al's article and Takach et al's article[1] do suggest that the natural history of these dissections is similar to dissections in other vessels (ie, cervical and aortic) and that the dissection or the dissection channel can regress, thrombose, or become aneurysmal. Both open and endovascular treatments have been effective for patients having complications associated with the dissection (ie, malperfusion, aneurysm, refractory pain), with the endovascular approach generally being the initial option. Medical management appears to be appropriate for asymptomatic patients, although the exact definition of what medical management entails is debatable. The experience with spontaneous cervical dissections suggests that a 3- to 6-month course of anticoagulation may be appropriate, but the incremental benefit between anticoagulation and antiplatelet therapies remains unclear. Similarly, beta-blockade may be beneficial, as in the case of type B aortic dissections. It is clear that patients with spontaneous dissections merit long-term follow-up with serial imaging due to the potential for aneurysmal degeneration.

T. S. Huber, MD, PhD

Reference

1. Takach TJ, Madjarov JM, Holleman JH, et al. Spontaneous splanchnic dissection: application and timing of therapeutic options. *J Vasc Surg*. 2009;50:557-563.

Spontaneous splanchnic dissection: Application and timing of therapeutic options

Takach TJ, Madjarov JM, Holleman JH, et al (Carolinas Heart Inst, Charlotte, NC)

J Vasc Surg 50:557-563, 2009

Background.—Spontaneous splanchnic dissection (SSD) occurs infrequently and has a poorly defined natural history. Few studies address the application, timing, and consequences of therapeutic options. Our goal was to apply conservative (non-operative) management in the care of each patient, reserving interventions for specific indications that may be predictive of adverse outcomes.

Methods.—Between 2003 and 2008, 10 consecutive patients (mean age 54.7-years-old, 70.0% male) presented with 11 SSDs involving either the celiac artery (n = 6), superior mesenteric artery (n = 3), or both (n = 1). Each patient had acute, spontaneous onset of persistent abdominal pain and was diagnosed with SSD following multidetector row computed tomographic angiography (CTA). Non-operative management (anticoagulation, anti-impulse therapy, analgesics, and serial CTA examinations) was initially used in 9 patients. Endovascular (n = 2) or operative (n = 2) intervention was performed either immediately (n = 1) or following failed medical management (n = 3) in 4 patients for specific indications that included persistent symptoms (n = 3), expansion of false lumen (n = 3), and/or radiologic malperfusion (n = 3).

Results.—All patients were asymptomatic after successful non-operative management or following intervention. No morbidity occurred. Upon complete follow-up (mean 13.4 months, range, 2 to 36 months), all patients remained asymptomatic. Preservation of distal perfusion with either thrombosis or ongoing regression of false lumen was achieved in 5 patients who received only non-operative management and in 4 patients following intervention. A stable chronic dissection was present in 1 patient who had only non-operative management.

Conclusion.—Successful outcomes following SSD may be achieved with either non-operative therapy alone or intervention if persistent symptoms, expansion of false lumen, and/or malperfusion occur. The unpredictable response of the false lumen to conservative management mandates close, long-term follow-up. Endovascular and operative interventions produced similar outcomes in a small number of patients with limited follow-up. Although SSD is currently perceived as rare, the increasing use of CTA may prove that the true incidence has been underestimated.

▶ This article and an article by Gobble et al[1] contribute to our understanding of the natural history and the treatment strategies for patients with spontaneous, isolated dissections of the mesenteric vessels. With the rapid progression of CT arteriography and the low threshold for its application, it has become apparent that spontaneous dissections of the celiac and superior mesenteric vessels are uncommon but not rare. Indeed, most vascular surgeons will see a couple of such cases over the course of the year. As emphasized in Takach et al's article and Gobble et al's article,[1] the clinical presentation may range from acute abdominal pain to an incidental finding at the time of imaging obtained for other reasons. The etiology of these dissections remains unclear, but a variety of causes have been implicated. Given the limited number of reports and follow-up, it is not surprising that the treatment strategies remain unresolved. However, Takach et al's article and Gobble et al's article[1] do suggest that the natural history of these dissections is similar to dissections in other vessels (ie, cervical and aortic) and that the dissection or the dissection channel can regress, thrombose, or become aneurysmal. Both open and endovascular treatments have been effective for patients having complications associated with the dissection (ie, malperfusion, aneurysm, and refractory pain), with the endovascular approach generally being the initial option. Medical management appears to be appropriate for asymptomatic patients, although the exact definition of what medical management entails is debatable. The experience with spontaneous cervical dissections suggests that a 3- to 6-month course of anticoagulation may be appropriate, but the incremental benefit between anticoagulation and antiplatelet therapies remains unclear. Similarly, beta-blockade may be beneficial, as in the case of type B aortic dissections. It is clear that patients with spontaneous dissections merit long-term follow-up with serial imaging due to the potential for aneurysmal degeneration.

T. S. Huber, MD, PhD

Reference

1. Gobble RM, Brill ER, Rockman CB, et al. Endovascular treatment of spontaneous dissections of the superior mesenteric artery. *J Vasc Surg*. 2009;50:1326-1332.

Experience and Technique for the Endovascular Management of Iatrogenic Subclavian Artery Injury

Cayne NS, Berland TL, Rockman CB, et al (New York Univ Med Ctr)
Ann Vasc Surg 24:44-47, 2010

Background.—Inadvertent subclavian artery catheterization during attempted central venous access is a well-known complication. Historically, these patients are managed with an open operative approach and repair under direct vision via an infraclavicular and/or supraclavicular incision. We describe our experience and technique for endovascular management of these injuries.

Methods.—Twenty patients were identified with inadvertent iatrogenic subclavian artery cannulation. All cases were managed via an endovascular technique under local anesthesia. After correcting any coagulopathy, a 4-French glide catheter was percutaneously inserted into the ipsilateral brachial artery and placed in the proximal subclavian artery. Following an arteriogram and localization of the subclavian arterial insertion site, the subclavian catheter was removed and bimanual compression was performed on both sides of the clavicle around the puncture site for 20 min. A second angiogram was performed, and if there was any extravasation, pressure was held for an additional 20 min. If hemostasis was still not obtained, a stent graft was placed via the brachial access site to repair the arterial defect and control the bleeding.

Results.—Two of the 20 patients required a stent graft for continued bleeding after compression. Both patients were well excluded after endovascular graft placement. Hemostasis was successfully obtained with bimanual compression over the puncture site in the remaining 18 patients.

There were no resultant complications at either the subclavian or the brachial puncture site.

Conclusion.—This minimally invasive endovascular approach to iatrogenic subclavian artery injury is a safe alternative to blind removal with manual compression or direct open repair.

▶ The proliferation of the endovascular approach with the evolution of the various wires, catheters, and stent technologies has significantly impacted the management of trauma to the great vessels. Indeed, the endo-first approach is probably most beneficial in this setting, given the inaccessibility of the vessels for open repair and the associated morbidity and mortality. This article and articles by Tran et al[1] and Pikwer et al[2] describe novel, endovascular approaches for treatment of iatrogenic trauma to the great vessels from attempted placement of central venous lines or catheters. Inadvertent injury to these vessels is quite common during line placement but usually recognized before the introduction of the catheter due to the pulsatile bleeding. This can be usually remediated by simple withdrawal of the finder needle and local compression. However, introduction of a catheter into the artery itself is a bit more problematic, albeit quite rare. The articles describe a variety of definitive endovascular techniques, including the use of a closure device, coil embolization, and placement of a covered stent; all are within the skill set of a modern vascular surgeon. Furthermore, temporary control of the great vessels can be obtained with an angioplasty or a thromboembolectomy balloon before open repair. The specific endovascular approach is usually dictated by the site of the vessel injury, and the procedures are best performed in the operating room or at least in an imaging suite. A nice treatment algorithm for inadvertent subclavian artery catheterization is provided in the report by Cayne et al. Briefly, the brachial artery is catheterized with a 4-French sheath, and an arteriogram is obtained using a 4-French catheter. The inadvertent subclavian artery catheter is then removed and pressure is applied both above and below the clavicle. A covered stent is placed across the puncture site in the presence of persistent bleeding and is facilitated by upsizing the brachial sheath. Although these approaches represent a novel application of standard endovascular techniques, the best treatment for iatrogenic arterial injuries is prevention using ultrasound guidance to facilitate placement of the initial central venous catheter.

T. S. Huber, MD, PhD

References

1. Tran V, Shiferson A, Hingorani AP. Use of the StarClose device for closure of inadvertent subclavian artery punctures. *Ann Vasc Surg*. 2009;23:688.e11-688.e13.
2. Pikwer A, Acosta S, Kölbel T, Malina M, Sonesson B, Akeson J. Management of inadvertent arterial catheterisation associated with central venous access procedures. *Eur J Vasc Endovasc Surg*. 2009;38:707-714.

Long-Term Outcome of Prophylactic Coronary Revascularization in Cardiac High-Risk Patients Undergoing Major Vascular Surgery (from the Randomized DECREASE-V Pilot Study)

Schouten O, for the DECREASE Study Group (Erasmus MC, Rotterdam, The Netherlands; et al)

Am J Cardiol 103:897-901, 2009

Prophylactic coronary revascularization in vascular surgery patients with extensive coronary artery disease was not associated with an improved immediate postoperative outcome. However, the potential long-term benefit was unknown. This study was performed to assess the long-term benefit of prophylactic coronary revascularization in these patients. Of 1,880 patients scheduled for major vascular surgery, 430 had ≥3 risk factors (age >70 years, angina pectoris, myocardial infarction, heart failure, stroke, diabetes mellitus, and renal failure). All underwent cardiac testing using dobutamine echocardiography or nuclear stress imaging. Patients with extensive stress-induced ischemia (≥5 segments or ≥3 walls) were randomly assigned to additional revascularization. In total, 101 patients showed extensive ischemia and were assigned to revascularization (n = 49) or no revascularization (n = 52). After 2.8 years, the overall survival rate was 64% for patients randomly assigned to no preoperative coronary revascularization versus 61% for patients assigned to preoperative coronary revascularization (hazard ratio [HR] 1.18, 95% confidence interval [CI] 0.63 to 2.19, p = 0.61). Rates for survival free of all-cause death, nonfatal myocardial infarction, and coronary revascularization were similar in both groups at 49% and 42% for patients allocated to medical treatment or coronary revascularization, respectively (HR 1.51, 95% CI 0.89 to 2.57, p = 0.13). Only 2 patients assigned to medical treatment required coronary revascularization during follow-up. Also, in patients who survived the first 30 days after surgery, there was no apparent benefit of revascularization on cardiac events (HR 1.35, 95% CI 0.72 to 2.52, p = 0.36). In conclusion, preoperative coronary revascularization in high-risk patients undergoing major vascular surgery was not associated with improved postoperative or long-term outcome compared with the best medical treatment.

▶ The long-term results (median follow-up 2.8 yrs) from the Dutch Echocardiographic Cardiac Risk Evaluation Applying Stress Echocardiography (DECREASE)-V Pilot study help further define the role of coronary revascularization before major vascular surgery. Preoperative coronary revascularization was not associated with either a survival (revascularization—64% vs no revascularization—61%) or event-free survival (revascularization—49% vs no revascularization—42%) benefit. This is particularly notable since the inclusion criteria included > 3 cardiovascular risk factors (age > 70 years, angina, myocardial infarction, heart failure, stroke, diabetes, and renal failure) and extensive stress-induced ischemia on noninvasive testing. Admittedly, the sample size was small and somewhat underpowered, but the findings corroborate those of the Coronary Artery Revascularization Prophylaxis (CARP) study[1] that reached similar conclusions. Notably, coronary artery revascularization before elective vascular surgery among patients with stable cardiac symptoms does not appear to improve perioperative or long-term mortality. These findings are reflected in the most recent version of the ACC/AHA guidelines.[2] In their algorithm, patients with stable cardiac symptoms who can generate 4 metabolic equivalents (METs) can undergo their vascular surgical procedures without further testing. In the subset of patients who cannot generate 4 METS for whatever reason (eg, amputation and COPD), noninvasive testing may be indicated if the results would change their management. Notably, preoperative cardiac consultation and further testing are indicated for patients with unstable cardiac conditions, including unstable angina, decompensated congestive heart failure, severe valvular disease, and uncontrolled arrhythmias. In their discussion, the authors emphasize that the annual mortality in CARP and the DECREASE V trial (6.8% and 8.2%, respectively) exceeds that of similar trials of nonsurgical patients with multivessel coronary artery disease, thereby suggesting that patients with polyvascular disease have worse outcomes. This serves to emphasize the severity of the associated comorbidities in our vascular surgery patient population and the importance of optimizing their medical care and reducing their atherosclerotic risk factors.

T. S. Huber, MD, PhD

References

1. McFalls EO, Ward HB, Mortiz TE, et al. Coronary-artery resvascularization before elective major vascular surgery. *N Engl J Med.* 2004;351:2795-2804.
2. Fleisher LA, Beckman JA, Brown KA, et al. ACC/AHA 2007 Guidelines on Perioperative Cardiovascular Evaluation and Care for Noncardiac Surgery: Executive Summary: A Report of the American College of Cardiology/American Heart Association Task Force on Practice Guidelines. *Circulation.* 2007;116:1971-1996.

Revascularization versus Medical Therapy for Renal-Artery Stenosis

The ASTRAL Investigators (Univ of Birmingham, UK; et al)
N Engl J Med 361:1953-1962, 2009

Background.—Percutaneous revascularization of the renal arteries improves patency in atherosclerotic renovascular disease, yet evidence of a clinical benefit is limited.

Methods.—In a randomized, unblinded trial, we assigned 806 patients with atherosclerotic renovascular disease either to undergo revascularization in addition to receiving medical therapy or to receive medical therapy alone. The primary outcome was renal function, as measured by the reciprocal of the serum creatinine level (a measure that has a linear relationship with creatinine clearance). Secondary outcomes were blood pressure, the time to renal and major cardiovascular events, and mortality. The median follow-up was 34 months.

Results.—During a 5-year period, the rate of progression of renal impairment (as shown by the slope of the reciprocal of the serum creatinine level) was -0.07×10^{-3} liters per micromole per year in the revascularization group, as compared with -0.13×10^{-3} liters per micromole per year in the medical-therapy group, a difference favoring revascularization of 0.06×10^{-3} liters per micromole per year (95% confidence interval [CI], −0.002 to 0.13; P = 0.06). Over the same time, the mean serum creatinine level was 1.6 μmol per liter (95% CI, −8.4 to 5.2 [0.02 mg per deciliter; 95% CI, −0.10 to 0.06]) lower in the revascularization group than in the medical-therapy group. There was no significant between-group difference in systolic blood pressure; the decrease in diastolic blood pressure was smaller in the revascularization group than in the medical-therapy group. The two study groups had similar rates of renal events (hazard ratio in the revascularization group, 0.97; 95% CI, 0.67 to 1.40; P = 0.88), major cardiovascular events (hazard ratio, 0.94; 95% CI, 0.75 to 1.19; P = 0.61), and death (hazard ratio, 0.90; 95% CI, 0.69 to 1.18; P = 0.46). Serious complications associated with revascularization occurred in 23 patients, including 2 deaths and 3 amputations of toes or limbs.

Conclusions.—We found substantial risks but no evidence of a worthwhile clinical benefit from revascularization in patients with atherosclerotic renovascular disease. (Current Controlled Trials number, ISRCTN59586944.)

▶ The Angioplasty and Stenting for Renal Artery Lesions (ASTRAL) trial further defines the role (or lack thereof) for endovascular revascularization in patients with atherosclerotic renal artery occlusive disease. In this well-performed study, patients with clinical findings consistent with atherosclerotic renovascular disease and a significant lesion were randomized to revascularization (angioplasty ± stenting) or medical therapy alone. Although the progression of renal impairment (as measured by the slope of the reciprocal of the serum creatinine level) and the serum creatinine levels favored revascularization, the differences were not clinically relevant. Furthermore, there were no significant differences in systolic blood pressure, renal events (ie, acute kidney injury, initiation of dialysis, transplantation, nephrectomy, and death from renal failure), cardiovascular events, or survival. Simply, revascularization did not improve blood pressure control or salvage renal function, but it was associated with a moderate risk (ie, 9% complication rate and 2 deaths). These results corroborate several other smaller randomized trials. Notably, the technical success rates for the revascularization were excellent (95%) and almost all of the patients had concomitant angioplasty and stent. It is certainly conceivable that there may be some role for revascularization in this setting, as the authors concede in their discussion. Patients were referred for enrollment only if there was uncertainty about the need for revascularization (ie, clinical equipoise). Furthermore, the optimal medical therapy may have further obscured a benefit for revascularization in comparison to the more real-world setting in which medical treatment may not be as conscientious. However, the role for revascularization (both open and endovascular) in this setting is diminishingly small, given the available medical therapies and the pathophysiology of the underlying disease process. In our own practice, we have limited its application to patients with severe hypertension truly refractory to multimedical therapies. It is not surprising that renal angioplasty and stenting has made it on the proverbial radar screen at the Centers for Medicare and Medicaid Services (CMS), given its widespread application, cost, and limited utility.

T. S. Huber, MD, PhD

Peripheral Arterial Occlusive Disease

Clinical success using patient-oriented outcome measures after lower extremity bypass and endovascular intervention for ischemic tissue loss

Taylor SM, York JW, Cull DL, et al (Univ of South Carolina School of Medicine, Greenville)

J Vasc Surg 50:534-541, 2009

Introduction.—Successful outcome after lower extremity revascularization is usually measured by physician-oriented terms such as graft patency and amputation-free survival. It has been increasingly appreciated that these criteria do not necessarily translate into success from the perspective of the patient. The purpose of this study, therefore, is to retrospectively examine success after lower extremity revascularization for tissue loss using patient-oriented measures and to include patients who underwent both open surgical bypass and endovascular therapy.

Methods.—Between 1998 and 2005, 677 patients (316 endovascular and 361 open surgery) underwent revascularization for ischemic tissue loss. The method of revascularization (endovascular or open surgery) was left to the discretion of the surgeon. Revascularization was considered to be clinically successful if each of the following occurred: reconstruction patency until wound healing, limb salvage for 1 year, maintenance of ambulation for 1 year, and survival for 6 months. The influence of 20 intrinsic patient factors, including type of revascularization (open vs endo) was examined using the χ^2 test. Significant factors in bivariate analysis were included in a logistic regression model to determine independent predictors and probability of failure.

Results.—Overall clinical success was achieved in 277 (40.9%) patients. Success for open surgical and endovascular cohorts was 44.3% and 37.0%, respectively ($P = .06$). Type of intervention was not a significant factor in either bivariate or logistic regression analysis. Independent predictors of failure (odds ratio [OR]; 95% confidence interval [CI]) regardless of treatment type included impaired ambulatory status at the time of presentation (OR 3.24; CI 2.14, 4.90), diabetes (OR 1.62; CI 1.14, 2.32), endstage renal disease (ESRD) (OR 1.55; CI 1.07, 2.23), presence of gangrene (OR 2.0; CI 1.42, 2.82), and prior vascular intervention (OR 1.46; CI 1.02, 2.10). Paradoxically, hyperlipidemia (OR 0.70; CI 0.50, 0.98) was a predictor for success. Probability of failure was

35.4% (OR 1.0) if no independent predictors were present and increased with the addition of each adverse predictor. For instance, diabetic patients with impaired ambulatory status and gangrene had an 85.2% (OR 10.5) probability of failure. In the worst case scenario, a diabetic patient with ESRD, impaired ambulatory status, gangrene, and a prior vascular intervention was considered, probability of failure was a dismal 92.8% (OR 23.7).

Conclusion.—Clinical success after lower extremity revascularization for ischemic tissue loss is determined by intrinsic patient factors and not by method of revascularization. These data reiterate that future investigation efforts should be focused less on the method of revascularization and more on identification of patient cohorts at risk for failure regardless of treatment.

▶ The study documents the sobering outcomes after lower extremity revascularization for ischemic tissue loss from a patient perspective. As noted by the authors, the traditional foci after revascularization have been bypass graft patency and amputation-free survival. However, these outcome measures are not important from a patient standpoint, and I would contend that it is irrelevant to our patients whether their bypass graft is patent if their rest pain or tissue loss persists. The authors have identified 4 patient-relevant outcome measures, including patent revascularization until wound healing, limb salvage for 1 year, independent ambulation for 1 year, and survival to 6 months. Although collectively these outcomes do not seem too difficult (ie, the bar does not seem too high), it was disheartening that only 41% of the patients had a successful outcome or met all of the criteria. Clearly, this reflects the debilitated state of the patient population with ischemic tissue loss and emphasizes the point that these patients are at the end of their lives. It is interesting to note that the patent revascularization until wound healing was the most discriminating of the measures and associated with only a 44% success rate. The authors identified 5 predictors of adverse outcome (impaired ambulation at presentation, end-stage renal disease, diabetes, gangrene, and previous revascularization that merit further emphasis) that should likely be committed to memory. Predictably, as the number of these factors increased, the likelihood of a successful outcome decreased, and the combination of all the 5 predictors was associated with a 7% success rate. This is particularly enlightening for our own practice because it is not unusual to see patients with tissue loss and this combination of clinical factors. Despite the study design and selection bias, it was very interesting to see that the means of revascularization (ie, open vs endovascular) did not appreciably impact clinical success. The application of these endovascular therapies has been one of the major foci of our discipline, but the current report suggests the ongoing arguments about less invasive (endovascular) versus more invasive, better long-term outcome (open) are really secondary to the underlying disease process. Perhaps the biggest challenge that this study poses is how to incorporate the data into our own practices. Although the defined clinical success rate was quite low, there are not a lot of treatment options for patients with ischemic tissue loss, and few patients are excited about the prospect of a major amputation. The data should challenge us all to rethink our approach to ischemic tissue loss and limb-threatening ischemia. Despite aggressive approaches at revascularization, the outcomes for many of our patients are dismal and primary amputation may be a better option, given the fact that it is oftentimes inevitable. I agree with the Greenville group's recurring theme that claudication and limb-threatening ischemia are clearly different problems and that we should, probably, be more aggressive with claudicants and less aggressive with those patients with limb-threatening ischemia, particularly tissue loss.

T. S. Huber, MD, PhD

Perioperative outcomes and amputation-free survival after lower extremity bypass surgery in California hospitals, 1996-1999, with follow-up through 2004

Feinglass J, Sohn M-W, Rodriguez H, et al (Northwestern Univ Feinberg School of Medicine, Chicago, IL)
J Vasc Surg 50:776-783, 2009

Objective.—There are very few population-based studies of long-term outcomes after lower extremity (LE) bypass graft surgery. This study analyzes perioperative and long-term limb salvage and amputation-free survival outcomes for patients undergoing initial aortoiliac or femoropopliteal bypass graft surgery in California hospitals from 1996 to 1999.

Methods.—Administrative data with encrypted identifiers were used to identify a chronologically first, index admission of all patients undergoing LE bypass procedures for occlusive disease from 1996 to 1999. A 1993 to 1995 look-back period was used to exclude patients who had undergone prior bypass surgery or amputation procedures. Patients with incident procedures were then followed forward to determine subsequent hospitalizations and vital status through 2004. The study comprised 28,128 patients discharged from 345 California hospitals with a median 61.5-month follow-up. Risk factors included demographic characteristics, comorbid conditions, admission type, gangrene or ulceration, operation level, hospital LE bypass surgery volume, and year of discharge. Logistic regression was used to analyze 30-day outcomes, and Kaplan-Meier analysis and Cox proportional hazard models were used to analyze amputation-free survival.

Results.—Overall 30-day mortality was 4.3, and the 30-day major amputation rate was 2.6%. Limb salvage was 81.9% at 5 years and 76.4% at 9 years. Amputation-free survival was 51.5% at 5 years and 34.1% at 9 years. Risk factors were generally similar for both perioperative and late outcomes. Advanced age, higher comorbidity level, gangrene, and emergency or nursing home admission conferred significantly greater risk. Hospital volume was associated with both perioperative and late outcomes. African American and Hispanic patients had much higher amputation rates but did not have higher mortality risk after controlling for baseline severity of illness.

Conclusions.—Long-term outcomes of LE bypass surgery were superior for high-volume hospital patients. Graft surveillance and risk factor follow-up care provide a major opportunity for quality improvement efforts. The contrast between traditional limb salvage and amputation-free survival outcomes raises questions about the value of surgical treatment, particularly for patients with limited life expectancy and without coding of tissue loss or critical limb ischemia.

▶ The study has attempted to define the long-term outcome for patients undergoing aortoiliac or femoropopliteal bypass using the California statewide administrative database. Notably, the authors reported a perioperative mortality rate of 4%, remedial bypass/revision rate of 29%, and a 5-year amputation-free survival rate of 52%. These numbers are consistent (or worse) with most single-institution series and serve to define the outcome of these select patients/procedures, given the overall size of the sample and the longitudinal nature of the study that linked the index procedure with subsequent hospitalizations/procedures. The data emphasize the fairly poor long-term outcome for patients undergoing surgical bypass for peripheral arterial occlusive disease and provide some frame of reference for counseling patients. Indeed, this is appropriate, given the shift in the focus of reporting outcomes after lower extremity revascularization from traditional measures of graft patency and limb salvage to more patient-centric assessments (eg, amputation-free survival, independent ambulation, and wound healing). Notably, the reported outcomes are likely better than those for patients undergoing infrageniculate bypass, and they may represent a best-case scenario for patients with lower extremity arterial occlusive disease because a large percentage of the aortoiliac or femoropopliteal bypasses were likely performed for claudication (as opposed to rest pain or tissue loss). The findings are also noteworthy because they reflect the outcomes of open surgical treatment before the widespread implementation of the endovascular therapies. Despite my enthusiasm for the study, the data must be interpreted with some caution, given the limitations of the study design and the administrative database that include no indication for the surgical procedure and potential inaccuracies identifying the index procedure, subsequent procedures/admissions, and care provided outside of California.

T. S. Huber, MD, PhD

Reliability of Preoperative Duplex Scanning in Designing a Therapeutic Strategy for Chronic Lower Limb Ischemia

Fontcuberta J, Flores A, Orgaz A, et al (Hosp Virgen de la Salud, Toledo, Spain)
Ann Vasc Surg 23:577-582, 2009

The objective of this study was to compare the treatment plan designed on the basis of preoperative duplex scanning evaluation of the critical limb ischemia with the treatment plan finally carried out, after assessing the findings obtained during surgical or endovascular treatment. Over a period of 51 months a preoperative duplex scanning study was carried out in 335 consecutive patients with chronic critical ischemia, to design the best therapeutic strategy. Agreement between both plans were as follows: 80%, 82,7% and 59% in the examinations of the iliac arteries, femoropopliteal or tibial arteries respectively. The operation plan was more frequently modified due to a duplex scanning failure in procedures involving the the distal vessels(10 of 44 [22.7%], $p < 0.01$). In conclusion, duplex scanning evaluation of patients with occlusive arterial disease of the lower limbs permits the design of both a medical and a surgical or endovascular treatment plan with a high level of agreement with the findings obtained during the revascularization procedure.

▶ The study emphasizes the utility of preoperative arterial duplex scanning in patients with critical limb ischemia. Notably, patients underwent duplex scanning examination before open or endovascular treatment, and the actual treatment was compared with the plan based upon the duplex scanning. Not surprisingly, the agreement between the treatment and plans was quite good and varied by anatomic level (aortoiliac—80%, femoropopliteal—82%, and crural—59%). The corresponding sensitivity, specificity, and predictive values varied similarly, with better values reported for the more proximal vessels (ie, aortoiliac and femoropopliteal). The authors make the important point that the goal of the preoperative imaging is to identify lesions that are potentially amenable to treatment and that the gold standard for comparison is the short- and immediate-term results after revascularization. Notably, this is different than the ability of the techniques to simply identify the anatomy of the various vascular beds. These results mirror our own experience and clinical practice. We have been pleasantly pleased with our ability to image the aortoiliac segment and concede that some of the measures are indirect. We would also concede that our success in this anatomic location likely reflects the experience and commitment of our vascular technologists more than anything else. Arterial duplex scanning has emerged as our preferred imaging technique before endovascular treatment and has essentially replaced diagnostic catheter-based arteriography. CT arteriography has also been helpful in this setting but limited by the obvious expense, contrast load, and radiation exposure. The goals of the arterial duplex scanning study in our own practice are to outline the arterial tree from the aorta to the foot, identify the potential lesions that can be treated, and help plan the site of arterial access (ie, ipsilateral femoral, contralateral femoral, and left brachial). This allows us to articulate the plan to the patients quite well, and, similar to the authors' experience, the actual treatment rarely diverges from the preoperative plan.

T. S. Huber, MD, PhD

Venous

Characterizing resolution of catheter-associated upper extremity deep venous thrombosis

Jones MA, Lee DY, Segall JA, et al (Utah Vascular Ctr, Provo; Oregon Health Sciences Univ, Portland; Kaiser Permanente, Clackamas, OR)
J Vasc Surg 51:108-113, 2010

Objective.—Catheter-associated upper extremity deep venous thrombosis (CAUEDVT) is well known; however, resolution rates and factors affecting resolution of CAUEDVT are not well characterized. This study determined resolution rates and factors associated with resolution of CAUEDVT.

Methods.—From January 1, 2002, to June 30, 2006, 1761 upper extremity venous duplex ultrasound (DU) studies were performed, and a new UEDVT was found in 253 (14.4%). Of these, 150 patients had routine follow-up and 101 had CAUEDVT. Demographics, follow-up DU results, and risk factors for venous thrombosis were recorded in the patients with follow-up studies and CAUEDVT. Univariate analysis and multivariate logistic regression analysis was performed to determine independent risk factors for complete thrombus resolution.

Results.—There were 49 men (49%) and 52 women (51%) with CAUEDVT and follow-up studies. Mean age was 49 years (range, 5 months-80 years). Patients with CAUEDVT had risk factors for venous thrombosis that included malignancy in 34%, recent surgery/trauma in 34%, known hypercoagulable state in 11%, concomitant lower extremity DVT in 21%, and pulmonary embolism in 5%. Complete resolution of DVT on follow-up was documented in 46%. Thrombosis resolved in only 25% (6 of 24) when the catheter was not removed ($P \leq .05$). Anticoagulation did not improve the rate of thrombus resolution ($P \leq 1.0$) compared with catheter removal alone. Of the patients who had thrombus resolution, 75% resolved by 100 days (range, 1-914 days) after catheter removal ≤48 hours of diagnosis. In multivariate analysis, only catheter removal predicted the likelihood of thrombus resolution (odds ratio, 3.25; 95% confidence interval, 1.16-9.09; $P = .025$). New-site UEDVT developed in 86% of patients with CAUEDVT who underwent catheter removal and immediate catheter placement in a new site. Pulmonary embolism developed in five patients with CAUEDVT. Of these, three had documented lower extremity DVT as well. No pulmonary emboli were fatal.

Conclusions.—More than half of CAUEDVT resolve ≤113 days when the catheter is removed ≤48 hours of diagnosis. New-site catheter placement has a high rate of new associated UEDVT. Anticoagulation does not appear to augment resolution of UEDVT.

▶ In contrast to the more common lower extremity deep venous thrombosis (DVT), the appropriate management of upper extremity DVT remains unresolved, particularly for catheter-associated thromboses. The critical, unresolved issues include the management of the catheter, the natural history of the thrombus, and the role for anticoagulation therapy. In this study, the authors have attempted to elucidate the natural history of catheter-associated DVTs in a subset of patients that had serial or follow-up ultrasound studies. The authors reported that the thrombus resolved in 46% of the patients and that the incidence was greater among those patients who had their catheter removed (52% vs 25%). Indeed, multivariate analysis demonstrated that only removal of the catheter was associated with thrombus resolution; neither anticoagulation nor the duration of time that the catheter was present affected the incidence of resolution. Interestingly, catheter removal and replacement were associated with an 86% incidence of another catheter-associated DVT while the overall incidence of pulmonary embolus was low (5%), and none were fatal. Although I think the study has several limitations (ie, retrospective design, small sample size, lack of surveillance ultrasound protocol, lack of imaging protocol for pulmonary embolus, lack of anticoagulation protocol, utility of diagnostic ultrasound in the thoracic cavity, and no long-term outcome), I think it illustrates several important points regarding the management of upper extremity catheter-associated DVTs. Specifically, catheter removal is often associated with thrombus resolution, anticoagulation may not be necessary, the likelihood of pulmonary embolus is quite low, and resisting the catheter is oftentimes associated with the same outcome. I was struck by the prevalence of DVT risk factors (malignancy—34%, surgery/trauma—34%, and hypercoagulable condition—11%) among the patients and the number of DVTs associated with the percutaneous inserted central catheter (PICC). Indeed, the presence of a hypercoagulable state and intimal injury (ie, catheter) comprise 2 of the components in Virchow's triad. In our own institution, PICC lines are overused and have become more of a convenience item for patients and health care providers rather than a true medical necessity. I do not quite share the authors' conclusions that the management of catheter-associated DVTs can be simplified by eliminating the use of anticoagulation and the practice of replacing the catheter at a new site, although I would concur that future studies are needed to confirm their findings.

T. S. Huber, MD, PhD

High prevalence of right-to-left shunt in patients with symptomatic great saphenous incompetence and varicose veins

Wright DD, Gibson KD, Barclay J, et al (BTG International Ltd in London, UK; Lake Washington Vascular and Overlake Hosp, Bellevue; BTG International Ltd in Conshohocken, PA; et al)

J Vasc Surg 51:104-107, 2010

Background.—Varicose veins are common and increasingly are being treated by less invasive endoscopic methods such as foam sclerotherapy. Patent foramen ovale (PFO) is also common, present in approximately one-quarter of adults. PFO allows bubbles introduced by foam sclerotherapy to cross into the general circulation, potentially causing cerebral artery gas embolization with unevaluated consequences.

Methods.—Men and women aged 18 to 60 years with symptomatic varicose veins (CEAP $C_{3\text{-}5}$) responded to an advertisement to recruit volunteers for a study on endovenous microfoam ablation (EMA). Participants' veins were screened by duplex ultrasound imaging, and those with isolated great saphenous vein (GSV) incompetence were tested for right-to-left (R-L) vascular shunt using transcranial Doppler (TCD) of the middle cerebral artery to detect the presence of bubble emboli after an injection of an agitated saline, blood, and air mixture as a contrast at rest and with the Valsalva maneuver.

Results.—Of 221 participants tested for R-L shunt, 85 (38.5%) were positive at rest (95% confidence interval [CI], 32.5-45.2) and 114 (51.8%) were positive after the Valsalva maneuver (95% CI, 45.4-58.5). A total 130 patients (58.8%) were positive for R-L shunt at rest or after Valsalva (95% CI, 52.5%-65.1%). This is significantly higher than the reported 26% prevalence of PFO in the general population (95% CI, 24.4-30.1).

Conclusions.—The prevalence of R-L shunt in patients with GSV incompetence CEAP $C_{3\text{-}5}$ in this study was higher than expected in the general population. TCD does not differentiate between intracardiac shunts and intrapulmonary shunts, so this observation needs further investigation. This link between R-L shunt and varicose veins is novel and, whether etiologic or functional, may improve the understanding of both conditions. The findings have importance in the treatment of varicose veins with foam sclerotherapy and EMA.

► This study documented that 39% of patients with symptomatic varicose veins (CEAP C3-5; C3-5—clinical [3—edema, 4—skin changes, and 5—healed ulcer]; E—etiology, A—anatomy, and P—pathology) undergoing endovenous microfoam ablation had evidence of a right-to-left shunt (ie, venous to arterial) at rest, with 51% demonstrating a shunt after a Valsalva maneuver. Although the number of embolic events detected by transcranial Doppler was likely insignificant for most of the patients, a remarkable 13% had evidence of severe shunting (>150 events) after Valsalva, thereby demonstrating the potential for the foam particles to enter the cerebral circulation (and potentially cause neurologic events). Indeed, neurologic events have been reported after foam ablation and are particularly disconcerting in the healthy patient population undergoing treatment of their symptomatic varicose veins. It is noteworthy that none of the patients developed any clinical sequelae after microfoam ablation in this study. Although disturbing, it is not clear how these findings should be incorporated into clinical practice. They suggest that the potential for a right-to-left shunt is a real potential for patients with varicose veins and that the prevalence of a patent foramen ovale may be greater than the 26% traditionally quoted. The findings clearly merit further validation with an appropriate control group and may justify screening for a patent foramen ovale before foam injection.

Furthermore, they may temper some enthusiasm for the technique, one that has been somewhat slow to proliferate in the United States.

T. S. Huber, MD, PhD

Results of Surgical Treatment Compared with Ultrasound-Guided Foam Sclerotherapy in Patients with Varicose Veins: A Prospective Randomised Study

Figueiredo M, Araújo S, Barros N Jr, et al (Universidade Federal de São Paulo [UNIFESP], Brazil; Sociedade Brasileira de Angiologia e Cirurgia Vascular, Brazil)

Eur J Vasc Endovasc Surg 38:758-763, 2009

Objective.—This study aims to compare venous clinical severity scores in patients with healed venous ulcers due to varicose veins of the lower limbs (the clinical, etiologic, anatomic, and pathophysiologic data (CEAP) classification: C_5 EpAsPr) treated by saphenous stripping and phlebectomy or by ultrasound-guided foam sclerotherapy.

Method.—Sixty patients were included: 29 underwent saphenous stripping and phlebectomy for varices in saphenous tributaries and 27 were treated by ultrasound-guided foam sclerotherapy; four cases were lost to follow-up. The main outcome measure was venous clinical severity scores (pain, oedema, inflammation, hyperpigmentation and lipodermatosclerosis). An ultrasound examination was carried out prior to treatment and 30, 60 and 180 days after the procedure to assess the relative efficacy of the methods in obliterating the saphenous trunk.

Results.—The mean venous clinical severity scores measured before and after 180 days were as follows: Surgery group – pain: before 1.97 standard deviation (SD) 0.19, 180 days 0.72 SD 0.53; oedema: before 1.66 SD 0.48, 180 days 0.55 SD 0.63; inflammation: before 1.55 SD 0.63, 180 days 0.72 SD 0.45. Foam sclerotherapy group – pain: before 1.81 SD 0.40, 180 days 0.56 SD 0.51; oedema: before 1.70 SD 0.47, 180 days 0.48 SD 0.64; inflammation: before 1.67 SD 0.68, after 0.89 SD 0.32. All scores showed statistically significant reductions in both patient groups. The saphenous vein had been obliterated, 180 days after treatment, in 78% of the surgery group, compared with 90% in the foam sclerotherapy group.

Conclusions.—Ultrasound-guided foam sclerotherapy is a safe and effective option for patients with chronic venous disorders.

▶ The authors have performed a nice randomized controlled trial comparing open surgical treatment and ultrasound-guided foam sclerotherapy for patients with varicose veins (C5—clinical, healed ulcer; Ep—etiology, primary; As—anatomy, superficial; Pr —pathology, reflux [C5EpAsPr]). The surgical treatment encompassed saphenofemoral/saphenopopliteal ligation, saphenous vein stripping, phlebectomy, and/or ligation of incompetent perforators. The sclerotherapy was performed by injecting the saphenous, accessory, and/or perforator veins with polidocanol foam with a total volume not exceeding

10 mL per session. The main outcome measure was clinical severity (pain, edema, inflammation, pigmentation, and lipodermatosclerosis) assessed with a validated venous scoring system (0—absent, 1—mild, 2—moderate, and 3—severe),[1] and patency of the saphenous system was assessed with ultrasound at 180 days. Not surprisingly, both treatments resulted in clinical improvement and obliteration of the saphenous vein although there were no differences between the treatments themselves. Notably, the sclerotherapy approach required a mean of 2.1 sessions per patient. These findings are significant, given the homogenous patient population demonstrated by the CEAP classification and the study design. However, they are limited by the relatively small sample size, likely underpowered, and the relatively short period of follow-up. Indeed, the long-term recurrence rate for foam sclerotherapy may be higher than varicose vein stripping as suggested by other types of sclerosants. Regardless, the approach merits consideration and affords a less invasive alternative to surgical stripping that can be easily repeated. The application of the approach has been somewhat limited in the United States relative to Europe and may be related to potential for neurologic events (albeit small) from embolization of the foam particles into the cerebral circulation (presumably from a patent foramen ovale).

T. S. Huber, MD, PhD

Reference

1. Rutherford RB, Padberg FT Jr, Comerota AJ, Kistner RL, Meissner MH, Moneta GL. Venous severity scoring: an adjunct to venous outcome assessment. *J Vasc Surg*. 2000;31:1307-1312.

To Wear or not to Wear Compression Stockings after Varicose Vein Stripping: A Randomised Controlled Trial

Houtermans-Auckel JP, van Rossum E, Teijink JAW, et al (Atrium Med Centre Parkstad, Heerlen, The Netherlands; Zuyd Univ of Applied Sciences, Heerlen, The Netherlands; Catharina Hosp, Eindhoven, The Netherlands)
Eur J Vasc Endovasc Surg 38:387-391, 2009

Objectives.—To assess the need to wear compression stockings for 4 weeks after inversion stripping of the great saphenous vein (GSV) from the groin to the level of the knee.

Design.—Randomised controlled trial.

Patients.—A total of 104 consecutive patients with primary complete incompetence of the GSV treated by inversion stripping of the GSV.

Methods.—Postoperatively treated limbs underwent elastic bandaging for 3 days. Volunteers were randomised to wear a compression stocking for additional 4 weeks (intervention group) or no compression stocking (control group). The primary outcome was limb oedema as assessed by photoelectric leg volume measurement. Secondary outcome measures were pain scores, postoperative complications and return to full work.

Results.—The control leg volume was 3657 ml (standard deviation, SD 687) preoperatively and 3640 ml (SD 540) 4 weeks postoperatively (non significant, N.S.). The stocking leg volume was 3629 ml (SD 540) preoperatively, falling to 3534 ml (SD 543) ($P < 0.01$) 4 weeks postoperatively. The difference in leg volume between both the groups was not statistically significant. Patients in the control group resumed work earlier (control 11 days, stocking 15 days, $P = 0.02$, Mann–Whitney test). No difference was observed in the number and type of complication and in pain scores during the 4-week follow-up period.

Conclusions.—Wearing an elastic compression stocking has no additional benefit following elastic bandaging for 3 days in postoperative care after stripping of the great saphenous vein as assessed by control of limb oedema, pain, complications and return to work.

▶ In this simple elegant study, the authors ask the question whether it is worthwhile to wear compression stockings after open surgical varicose vein stripping. Notably, only patients with primary varicose veins (clinical, etiologic, anatomic, and pathophysiologic [CEAP] classification C2, C3) were included in the study, and the surgical procedure involved flush ligation of the saphenofemoral junction and stripping of the great saphenous vein (GSV) in the thigh. Patients were randomized to elastic bandages for 3 days (control) or bandages plus compression stockings (23-32 mm Hg) that they were supposed to wear both day and night for the first 2 weeks and then just during the day for the next 2 weeks. The authors demonstrated that there was neither a significant difference in the degree of edema (ie, measured volume of the leg) between the 2 groups at 4 weeks (primary outcome measure) nor in the pain scores or incidence of complications. Somewhat surprisingly, the patients in the control group returned to work significantly sooner (11 vs 15 days). These findings are unexpected and contradict the surgical dogma, including the practice guidelines from the authors' native country (ie, Dutch Society for Surgery). They demonstrate the value of well-performed randomized trials to ask fundamental questions. Indeed, one of my colleagues has the 50-20 rule in that every 20 years we realize that 50% of the things in medicine that we thought were absolute gospel truths are just plain wrong. Despite the small sample size in this study, the evidence is fairly convincing and should change practice patterns in this select group of patients (ie, those that would meet the enrollment criteria for the study). In our own practice, we have a great deal of difficulty getting patients to wear their stockings, particularly during the warmer months of the year. Furthermore, they are expensive, usually not covered by insurance, and somewhat difficult to put on, particularly for our older patients.

T. S. Huber, MD, PhD

Volume associated dynamic geometry and spatial orientation of the inferior vena cava

Murphy EH, Arko FR, Trimmer CK, et al (Univ of Texas Southwestern Med Ctr, Dallas)

J Vasc Surg 50:835-843, 2009

Background.—The geometry and dynamics of the vena cava are poorly understood and current knowledge is largely based on qualitative data. The purpose of this study is to quantitate the dimensional changes that occur in the infrarenal inferior vena cava (IVC), in response to changes in intravascular volume.

Methods.—IVC dimensions were measured at 1 cm and 5 cm below the renal veins, on serial contrasted computed tomographic (CT) scans, in 30 severely injured trauma patients during hypovolemic (admission) and fluid resuscitated (follow-up) states. Changes in volume of the infrarenal segment were calculated and correlated with changes in IVC diameter and orientation. The orientation of the infrarenal caval segment was quantified as the angulation of the major axis from the horizontal. A representation of the IVC diameter, as would be seen on standard anterior-posterior venographic imaging, was determined by projecting the CT image of the major axis onto a coronal plane. CT representations of venographic diameters were compared with measurements of the true major axis to assess accuracy of venograms for caval sizing and filter selection.

Results.—All patients had evidence of a collapsed IVC (<15 mm minor axis dimension) on admission. Mean time between admission and follow-up CT was 49.5 (range: 1-202) days. The volume of the infrarenal segment increased more than twofold with resuscitation, increasing from 6.9 ± 2.2 (range: 3.1-12.4) mL on admission, to 15.7 ± 5.0 (range: 9.2-28.5) mL on follow-up ($P < .01$). At both 1 and 5 cm below the renal veins, the IVC expanded anisotropically such that the minor axis expanded up to five times its initial size accommodating 84% of the increased volume of the segment, while only small diameter changes were observed in the major axis accounting for less than 5% of the volume increase ($P < .001$). Further, the IVC was left-anterior-oblique in all patients, with the major axis 26 degrees off the horizontal on average. This orientation did not change significantly with volume resuscitation ($P > 0.5$). The obliquity of the IVC resulted in significant underestimation of caval size of up to 6.8 mm, when using the venographic representation for sizing instead of the true major axis ($P < 0.001$).

Conclusions.—In response to changes in intravascular volume, the IVC undergoes profound anisotropic dimensional changes, with greater displacement seen in the minor axis. In addition, the IVC is oriented left-anterior oblique and caval orientation is not altered by changes in volume status. IVC obliquity may result in underestimation of caval size by anterior-posterior venogram.

▶ The authors have demonstrated the impact of circulating volume on the dimensions of the inferior vena cava (IVC) and underscored the fact that it is a dynamic capacitance vessel. In their study, the quantitative changes in the IVC were analyzed among trauma patients (mean trauma severity score 20) using serial CT scans performed before and after resuscitation. Several important physiologic changes with clinical relevance were identified. First, the calculated volume of the IVC changes significantly in response to the circulating volume with an observed increase of more than 2-fold. Second, the geometric changes in response to volume are anisotropic (ie, unequal changes along the minor and major axes), with the largest increase in the minor axis. Notably, the minor axis of the IVC (measured 1 cm below the renal veins) increased almost 2-fold, with the largest increase being almost 3.5-fold, while the major axis at the same location increased only 7%. Third, the major axis of the IVC is located in a left-anterior-oblique (LAO) configuration with a mean value of 26° from the horizon (range up to 44°), and this obliquity did not appear to change with volume or the placement of a filter. These findings are clinically relevant for the placement of IVC filters below the renal veins, particularly in trauma patients who may be under resuscitation. The IVC diameter should be measured using the major axis in the appropriate orientation or obliquity. A cavogram in an anteroposterior orientation is not appropriate and potentially leads to undersizing. The cavogram should be performed in a right anterior oblique (RAO) projection to optimize visualization of the major axis (LAO orientation). Alternatively, the IVC can be sized using either transabdominal or intravascular ultrasound (IVUS). In our own practice, we place most of our IVC filters at the bedside using IVUS. In preparation, we review any preoperative CT scans to determine the orientation and length of the major axis to confirm that the cava is the appropriate size for the commercially available filters, and then we finalize the size measurements during the procedure with IVUS.

T. S. Huber, MD, PhD

13 General Thoracic Surgery

Benign Esophageal Disease

Radiofrequency Ablation of Barrett's Esophagus: Short-Term Results

Eldaif SM, Lin E, Singh KA, et al (Emory Univ School of Medicine, Atlanta, GA)

Ann Thorac Surg 87:405-410, 2009

Background.—The presence of Barrett's esophagus (BE) increases the risk of esophageal cancer. Total regression of BE is uncommon with medication or laparoscopic fundoplication, and endoscopic techniques to obliterate BE have varied results. This study evaluated the early results of a balloon-based catheter radiofrequency ablation (RFA) system in patients with medically refractory reflux symptoms and biopsy-proven BE.

Methods.—The medical records of 27 consecutive patients who underwent RFA for BE from March 2005 through January 2007 were reviewed. Esophagogastroduodenoscopy was performed before ablation to document presence of BE and no cancer and at 8 weeks after the RFA to assess the presence of residual BE.

Results.—Mean patient age was 53.6 ± 12.5 years; 16 (59%) were men. The average length of the Barrett segment treated was 4.6 ± 4.7 cm. Two patients (7.4%) had low-grade dysplasia. No patient had high-grade dysplasia and cancer. There was no periprocedural morbidity or at follow-up, no postprocedure dysphagia or stricture. In all patients, the BE was completely replaced with normal squamous epithelium. Symptoms regressed in 16 patients (60%) with RFA and proton pump inhibitor therapy. Eleven required an antireflux procedure for persistent symptoms.

Conclusions.—Short-term results show that RFA for BE is safe and achieves 100% replacement of intestinal metaplasia. RFA of BE combined with fundoplication may be offered to patients with BE and medically refractory reflux symptoms. Long-term endoscopic surveillance is needed

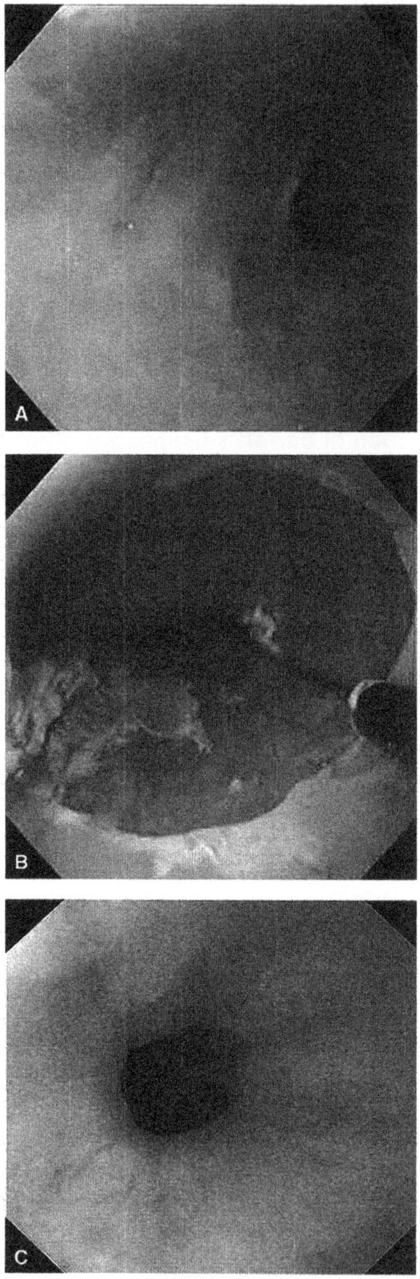

FIGURE 1.—Endoscopic view at (A) initial presentation of a patient with Barrett's esophagus, (B) immediately after ablation with the circumferential radiofrequency ablation balloon and sloughing of the mucosa, and (C) at 8 weeks showing normal distal esophageal mucosa. (Reprinted from Eldaif SM, Lin E, Singh KA, et al. Radiofrequency ablation of Barrett's esophagus: short-term results. *Ann Thorac Surg*. 2009;87:405-410, with permission from The Society of Thoracic Surgeons.)

to determine if the risk of cancer is reduced with this bimodality therapy (Fig 1).

▶ It is well established that Barrett's esophagus is a principal risk factor for the development of adenocarcinoma of the esophagus. Currently, surveillance endoscopy with biopsy is recommended for patients with Barrett esophagus. Management strategies for Barrett's esophagus have improved with medication and antireflux procedures. With either of these strategies it is uncommon for Barrett epithelium to complete regress. Therefore, endoscopic ablative techniques such as radiofrequency ablation (RFA) are being evaluated to ascertain whether or not they can completely obliterate Barrett's epithelium.

This single-institution, retrospective study was performed at Emory University on 27 patients who had Barrett's epithelium without the evidence of high-grade dysplasia. Only 2 patients had low-grade dysplasia–the remainder had Barrett's metaplasia only. The length of Barrett's epithelium ranged from 1 cm to greater than 6 cm with 48% of patients having a relatively short segment of Barrett's of 1 to 3 cm. The results of this study demonstrate that RFA can be performed safely with no perioperative morbidity and no post-procedure dysphagia. Manometric studies were done in 11 (41%) of the 27 patients before and after RFA, and there was no change in esophageal manometry findings.

This study emphasizes the importance of having surgeons involved in endoscopic therapies for esophageal diseases. The findings that RFA is safe corroborate what other groups have found when using it for management of Barrett's epithelium. Unfortunately, the study has a very short-term follow-up, which is a limitation. Thus, it is still possible that the true eradication of Barrett's epithelium and/or the development of complications may be different than postulated by the authors, in that patients could develop a delayed esophageal stricture or other sequelae related to the RFA.

The issue of managing the continued acidic and alkaline insults to the esophagus also needs to be addressed. The authors attempted to do this by performing antireflux procedures in a number of patients with resolution of their symptoms. Unfortunately, very few of the patients had post-antireflux procedure pH probes to document that. In summary, this is a nice study confirming that RFA of Barrett's esophagus is safe and effective at short-term intervals. Additional longer follow-up studies will be needed, but these results are encouraging and again highlight the importance of having surgeons involved in the endoscopic management of Barrett's esophagus.

D. R. Jones, MD

Esophageal Cancer

Mature Results from a Phase II Trial of Postoperative Concurrent Chemoradiotherapy for Poor Prognosis Cancer of the Esophagus and Gastroesophageal Junction

Adelstein DJ, Rice TW, Rybicki LA, et al (Cleveland Clinic Taussig Cancer Inst, OH)

J Thorac Oncol 4:1264-1269, 2009

Introduction.—Mature results are presented from a phase II trial of postoperative concurrent chemoradiotherapy in patients with poor-prognosis cancer of the esophagus and gastroesophageal junction after primary surgical resection.

Methods.—Resected patients with a pathologic stage of T3, N1, or M1a were eligible for this trial. Concurrent chemoradiotherapy was begun between 6 and 10 weeks after surgery and consisted of radiotherapy (1.8 Gy/d to a planned dose of 50.4–59.4 Gy), concurrent with two cycles of 5-fluorouracil (1000 mg/m^2/d) and cisplatin (20 mg/m^2/d), both given as 4-day continuous intravenous infusions during the first and fourth weeks of the radiation.

Results.—Between 1995 and 2006, 50 patients were enrolled. The median age was 59 (range, 33–76) years, and most patients were male (86%), Caucasian (96%), and had undergone a transthoracic esophago-gastrectomy (74%) for what proved to be a node positive (86%) adenocarcinoma (86%). Postoperative concurrent chemoradiotherapy was accompanied by neutropenia requiring hospitalization for fever in only four patients (8%) and no toxic deaths. With a median follow-up of 47 (range, 36–124) months, the Kaplan-Meier 4-year projected overall survival is 51%, freedom from recurrence 50%, distant metastatic control 56%, and locoregional control 86%. An earlier pathologic stage was the only predictor for a better outcome.

Conclusions.—This schedule of postoperative concurrent chemoradiotherapy has acceptable toxicity for patients with poor-prognosis esophageal and gastroesophageal junction cancer after surgery. Outcomes are better than historical results after surgery alone and justify further investigation of this approach.

▶ Despite appropriate staging modalities, patients with esophageal carcinoma who undergo resection can still have N1 or M1a disease at their final pathologic diagnosis. The role of adjuvant chemoradiation in these patients has been poorly studied. Furthermore, the results of such adjuvant strategies have been mixed without a true consensus defining the optimal approach. In this study, patients with T3N1 or M1a disease found at the time of surgery underwent a course of adjuvant concurrent chemoradiotherapy. This study was a prospective phase II trial of postoperative concurrent chemoradiotherapy. A total of 50 patients were accrued over 12 years. The most important point of this study is that there was a 51% freedom from recurrence with a projected 4-year survival of 51%. In addition, locoregional control was 86% in this small study. One of the most difficult aspects of adjuvant chemoradiation for patients undergoing esophageal resection is the difficulty in the radiation planning fields as well as toxicity related to the treatment. Important observations in this study are that no patient died due to toxicity and the toxicity attributable to chemoradiotherapy was quite manageable. Bone marrow suppression and mucitis and dysphagia were the more common complications. Thus, treatment toxicity is certainly acceptable and when combined with median overall survival of 53 months with a 4-year overall survival of 51%, there should be some excitement about this regimen. Another reason why adjuvant concurrent chemotherapy is an attractive option is that it allows treatment to be based on a true pathologic stage rather than what can often be a relatively inaccurate clinical stage. In addition, preoperative dysphagia and issues of nutritional support often compromise a patient's tolerance of induction chemoradiotherapy. In delivering this therapy in an adjuvant setting, dysphagia has been relieved and postoperative alimentation can be supported by a surgically placed feeding tube. This is the most recent and comprehensive study examining the specific role of adjuvant chemoradiotherapy after an esophagectomy and should be incorporated into the practicing surgeons' knowledge base when discussing treatment strategies and algorithms with their nonsurgical oncology colleagues.

D. R. Jones, MD

Predictors of major morbidity and mortality after esophagectomy for esophageal cancer: A Society of Thoracic Surgeons General Thoracic Surgery Database risk adjustment model

Wright CD, Kucharczuk JC, O'Brien SM, et al (Massachusetts General Hosp, Boston; Univ of Pennsylvania, Philadelphia; Duke Univ, Durham, NC; et al)

J Thorac Cardiovasc Surg 137:587-596, 2009

Objective.—To create a model for perioperative risk of esophagectomy for cancer using the Society of Thoracic Surgeons General Thoracic Database.

Methods.—The Society of Thoracic Surgeons General Thoracic Database was queried for all patients treated with esophagectomy for esophageal cancer between January 2002 and December 2007. A multivariable risk model for mortality and major morbidity was constructed.

Results.—There were 2315 esophagectomies performed by 73 participating centers. Hospital mortality was 63/2315 (2.7%). Major morbidity (defined as reoperation for bleeding [n = 12], anastomotic leak [n = 261], pneumonia [n = 188], reintubation [n = 227], ventilation beyond 48 hours [n = 71], or death [n = 63]) occurred in 553 patients (24%). Preoperative spirometry was obtained in 923/2315 (40%) of patients. A forced expiratory volume in 1 second <60% of predicted was associated with major morbidity (P =.0044). Important predictors of major morbidity are: age 75 versus 55 (P =.005), black race (P =.08), congestive heart failure (P =.015), coronary artery disease (P =.017), peripheral vascular

TABLE 2.—Frequency of Intraoperative and Postoperative Events in Patients After Esophagectomy for Cancer with and without Morbidity

Type of Event	All Patients	Patients Without Major Morbidity	Patients With Major Morbidity	P Value
Pulmonary embolus	0.9% (22/2315)	0.5% (8/1762)	2.5% (14/553)	<.001
DVT	2.0% (47/ 2315)	1.3% (23/1762)	4.3% (24/553)	<.001
Tracheostomy	4.0% (92/2315)	0.3% (6/1762)	15.6% (86/553)	<.001
Atrial fibrillation	17.5% (406/2315)	14.9% (262/1762)	26.0% (144/553)	<.001
MI	0.7% (15/2315)	0.3% (6/1762)	1.6% (9/553)	<.001
Intraoperative blood transfusion*	7.2% (138/1926)	6.3% (91/1446)	9.8% (47/480)	.131
Postoperative blood transfusion*	15.9% (306/1926)	11.8% (171/1446)	28.1% (135/480)	<.001
RLN paralysis	2.3% (52/2315)	1.5% (27/1762)	4.5% (25/553)	<.001
Renal failure	2.6% (60/2315)	0.7% (13/1762)	8.5% (47/553)	<.001
Sepsis	3/2% (75/2315)	0.7% (12/1762)	11.4% (63/553)	<.001
Chylothorax	1.9% (45/2315)	1.9% (33/1762)	2.2% (12/553)	.988

DVT, Deep venous thrombosis; *MI*, myocardial infarction; *RLN*, recurrent laryngeal nerve.
*Only available in STS data version 2.07.

disease ($P = .009$), hypertension ($P = .029$), insulin-dependent diabetes ($P = .009$), American Society of Anesthesiology rating ($P = .001$), smoking status ($P = .022$), and steroid use ($P = .026$). A strong volume performance relationship was not observed for the composite measure of morbidity and mortality in this patient cohort.

Conclusions.—Thoracic surgeons participating in the Society of Thoracic Surgeons General Thoracic Database perform esophagectomy with a low mortality. We identified important predictors of major morbidity and mortality after esophagectomy for esophageal cancer. Volume alone is an inadequate proxy for quality assessment after esophagectomy (Table 2).

► Patients with esophageal cancer who require an esophagectomy have multiple comorbid conditions, and many have undergone preoperative therapies. It is known that the risk of complications, particularly pulmonary complications, is very high in this group. There has been only one large multi-institutional prospective study of perioperative risk factors for esophagectomy for cancer. This was a Veterans Administration system study, which is not representative of the general United States patient population. Using the Society of Thoracic Surgeon's (STS) General Thoracic Database, the authors provide the reader with the risk-adjusted model assessing major predictors of morbidity and mortality following esophagectomy.

It is important to note the limitations of using the STS database. First, the database is entirely voluntary, and currently there is no internal or external auditing to assess data accuracy. Although these shortcomings are significant and are being addressed by the STS, their presence does cloud any result from the STS database.

Notwithstanding these limitations, the authors examine more than 2300 esophagectomies performed by 73 participating centers. The overall mortality was 2.7%, but major morbidity occurred in a significant number of patients. Important predictors for major morbidity include advanced age (age >75 years), black race, congestive heart failure, coronary artery disease, peripheral vascular disease, hypertension, and insulin-dependent diabetes. Interestingly, the authors did not find induction therapy to be predictive of increased measured morbidity. A strong volume performance relationship was not observed for the composite measure of morbidity and mortality in this patient population. The utility of knowing a priori prognostic variables before an esophagectomy is limited. Certainly, one can make an argument to more thoroughly investigate cardiovascular disease processes, particularly in elderly patients who are being considered for this operation.

D. R. Jones, MD

Recurrence after neoadjuvant chemoradiation and surgery for esophageal cancer: Does the pattern of recurrence differ for patients with complete response and those with partial or no response?

Meguid RA, Hooker CM, Taylor JT, et al (Johns Hopkins School of Medicine, Baltimore, MD; et al)

J Thorac Cardiovasc Surg 138:1309-1317, 2009

Objective.—We hypothesized that most relapses in patients with esophageal cancer having neoadjuvant chemoradiation therapy would occur outside of the surgical and radiation fields.

Methods.—Recurrence patterns, time to recurrence, and median survival were examined in 267 patients who had esophagectomy after neoadjuvant chemoradiation therapy at Johns Hopkins over 19 years.

Results.—Of 267 patients, 82 (30.7%) showed complete response to neoadjuvant therapy, with 108 (40.4%) and 77 (28.8%) showing partial response or no response, respectively. Recurrence developed in 84 patients (patients with complete response 18/82, 21.4%; patients with partial response 39/108, 36.1%; patients with no response 27/77, 35.1%; $P = .055$, respectively). Most patients had recurrences at distant sites (65/84;77.4%) regardless of pathologic response, and subsequent survival was brief (median 8.37 months). Median disease-free survival was short (10 months) and did not differ based on recurrence site for patients with partial response or no response, but was longer for patients with complete response with distant recurrence, whose median disease-free survival was 27.3 months ($P = .008$). By multivariate analysis, no other factor except for pathologic response to neoadjuvant therapy was associated with disease recurrence or death. Patients with partial response or no response were 1.97 and 2.23 times more likely to have recurrence than patients with complete response ($P = .024$ and $P = .012$, respectively).

Conclusions.—Most esophageal cancer recurrences after neoadjuvant therapy and surgery are distant, and survival time after recurrence is

TABLE 2.—First Tumor Recurrence Site According to Pathologic Response Status to Neoadjuvant Therapy (n = 84)

	Proportion of Patients with Recurrence from Total Cohort						
	Complete Response (n = 82)		Partial Response (n = 108)		No Response (n = 77)		
	n	%	n	%	n	%	*P* Value
Overall recurrence	18	22.0	39	36.1	27	35.1	.055
Tumor site							
Esophagus and mediastinum	5	27.2	8	20.5	6	22.2	
Lung and pleura	4	22.2	7	17.9	4	14.8	
Abdomen	5	27.7	9	23.0	4	14.8	
Liver	1	5.5	6	15.3	6	22.2	
Brain	1	5.5	2	5.1	2	7.4	
Bone	2	11.1	7	17.9	5	18.5	

short regardless of pathologic response. Fewer patients achieving complete response had recurrences, and distant recurrences in these patients manifest later than in patients showing partial response and those showing no response. Only pathologic response is significantly associated with disease recurrence, suggesting that tumor biology and chemosensitivity are critical in long-term patient outcome (Table 2).

► Approximately 25% to 30% of patients who undergo induction therapy achieve a pathologic complete response. The most common induction regimen is concurrent chemoradiation, although other groups use chemotherapy alone. Importantly, no restaging studies have been shown to accurately predict which patient has a complete pathologic response before performing an esophagectomy. In this article from Johns Hopkins Hospital, 267 patients underwent induction therapy. The pathologic complete response rate was 31%, with 40% of patients having a partial response and 29% having no demonstrable response. Characteristics of the study population by pathologic response showed that overall recurrence trended toward significance ($P = .055$) for patients who had a complete pathologic response. Despite having a complete pathologic response, 22% of patients still developed a recurrence. The recurrence rate was 35% in patients whose tumors had no histopathologic response. The most common site of tumor recurrence remains locoregional for those patients who have had a complete response. Interestingly, those patients who did not have a response had a significantly higher incidence of distant metastatic disease compared with the pathologic complete responders.

This article demonstrates that recurrence-free survival appears to only be affected by complete pathologic response. Patients with a partial pathologic response have an almost identical rate of recurrence-free survival as those patients with no response. One of the strongest benefits of neoadjuvant chemoradiation is, in fact, in locoregional control. The locoregional failure rate was 23% for those patients having neoadjuvant chemoradiation. It is important to remember that in the randomized clinical trial from the University of Michigan and a large randomized United States G-I intergroup trial, locoregional disease recurrence rates for the surgery alone control arms were 42% and 58%, respectively. Thus, induction chemoradiation combined with surgery decreases the locoregional recurrence rates significantly compared with surgery alone. As thoracic surgeons we need to remember one of the most important things we can achieve with an esophagectomy is to do everything possible to obtain an R0 resection and to decrease the chances of locoregional failure.

D. R. Jones, MD

The effect of volume on esophageal cancer resections: What constitutes acceptable resection volumes for centers of excellence?

Meguid RA, Weiss ES, Chang DC, et al (Johns Hopkins School of Medicine, Baltimore, MD)

J Thorac Cardiovasc Surg 137:23-29, 2009

Objective.—Volume–outcome relationships for esophageal cancer resection have been well described with centers of excellence defined by volume. No consensus exists for what constitutes a "high-volume" center. We aim to determine if an objective evidence-based threshold of operative volume associated with improvement in operative outcome for esophageal resections can be defined.

Methods.—Retrospective analysis was performed on patients undergoing esophageal resection for cancer in the 1998 to 2005 Nationwide Inpatient Sample. A series of multivariable analyses were performed, changing the resection volume cutoff to account for the range of annual hospital resections. The goodness of fit of each model was compared by pseudo r^2, the amount of data variance explained by each model.

Results.—A total of 4080 patients underwent esophageal resection. The median annual hospital resection volume was 4 (range: 1–34). The mortality rate of "high-volume" centers ranged from 9.94% (≥2 resection/year) to 1.56% (≥30 resections/year). The best model was with an annual hospital resection volume greater than or equal to 15 (3.87% of data variance explained). The difference in goodness of fit between the best model and other models with different volume cutoffs was 0.64%, suggesting that volume explains less than 1% of variance in perioperative death.

Conclusion.—Our data do not support the use of volume cutoffs for defining centers of excellence for esophageal cancer resections. Although volume has an incremental impact on mortality, volume alone is insufficient for defining centers of excellence. Volume seems to function as an imperfect surrogate for other variables, which may better define centers of excellence. Additional work is needed to identify these variables.

▶ Volume-outcome relationships for a number of different procedures have been reported in the literature. Specific to esophageal cancer the Leapfrog Group has defined criteria for "evidenced-based hospital referral" for esophageal resections to hospitals performing a minimum of 13 resections annually.

This study is one of the first to determine if an objective evidence-based threshold of operative volume is truly associated with improved hospital outcomes following esophageal resection for cancer.

As with most studies of this nature, the authors used a retrospective administrative database (Nationwide Inpatient Sample). This database comprises discharge records of approximately 20% of the sample of hospital discharges in the United States. The authors found that out of a total of 4080 patients who underwent esophageal resection, the median annual hospital resection volume was 4. The mortality rate of high-volume centers range from 1.5% to 10%. Statistical modeling was performed that attempted to address the impact of hospital volume on outcome. Interestingly, the authors suggest that hospital volume explains less than 1% of the variance in perioperative death between institutions. This strongly suggests that volume alone is an imperfect surrogate for defining centers of excellence.

This study adds to an increasing body of literature that suggests volume alone is not a good indicator for quality. In our own experience, we found that processes of care, patient's safety initiatives, and use of multiple disciplinary teams and standardized clinical care pathways are all likely to be more important than volume alone. Usually these types of factors are also associated with high-volume centers — but not always. The importance of this article is that surgeons are beginning to be actively involved in helping define what constitutes a center of excellence and how to best measure "quality."

D. R. Jones, MD

Lung Transplantation

The Impact of Center Volume on Survival in Lung Transplantation: An Analysis of More Than 10,000 Cases

Weiss ES, Allen JG, Meguid RA, et al (The Johns Hopkins Med Insts, Baltimore, MD)

Ann Thorac Surg 88:1062-1070, 2009

Background.—Whether center volume influences outcomes in lung transplantation is unknown. We reviewed United Network for Organ Sharing data to examine the effect of center volume on short-term mortality.

Methods.—We reviewed United Network for Organ Sharing data (1998 through 2007) to identify 10,496 first-time adult lung transplantation recipients at 79 centers. Centers were stratified by quartiles of mean annual volume. Risk of 30-day mortality and 1- and 5-year mortality (censored for 30-day death) were assessed by multivariable Cox proportional hazards regression.

Results.—Mean center volume ranged from less than 1 to 58.2 (median, 9.4 cases/year; volume quartiles: 0 to 2.1, 2.2 to 9.4, 9.5 to 19.9, and 20 to 58.2 cases). Each 1 case/year decrease led to a 2% increase in 30-day mortality (hazard ratio, 1.02; 95% confidence interval, 1.01 to 1.02; $p < 0.001$). Centers of lowest quartile (performing ≤2.1 lung transplantations/year) had a 30-day cumulative mortality of 9.6% or 89% increase in the risk of death (hazard ratio, 1.89; 95% confidence interval, 1.01 to 3.44; $p = 0.05$) compared with the highest quartile centers despite fewer idiopathic pulmonary fibrosis patients (15.6% versus 25.8%; $p < 0.001$) and younger age (40.9 versus 51.5 years; $p < 0.001$). Low-volume centers had double the risk of 30-day censored 1-year mortality (hazard ratio, 1.95; 95% confidence interval, 1.30 to 2.92; $p = 0.001$). High-volume centers (≥20 lung transplantations/year) had the lowest 30-day mortality (4.1%).

Conclusions.—We provide an initial examination of the relationship of volume and lung allocation score to outcomes for lung transplantation. Low center volume is associated with increased short-term and cumulative mortality despite fewer idiopathic pulmonary fibrosis patients and younger patients.

▶ It is not well established whether center volume influences outcome in lung transplantation. In this study, the authors examined the United Network for Organ Sharing database between 1998 and 2007. There were over 10 000 lung transplants performed in 79 centers during this time. The authors show that low-volume centers had double the risk of 30-day censored 1-year mortality, and high-volume centers had the lowest 30-day mortality. This occurs despite fewer idiopathic pulmonary fibrosis patients and younger patients in lower center volume hospitals compared with higher center volume hospitals.

The relationship between center volume and outcomes in complex surgical procedures such as lung transplantation is unclear and is likely multifactorial. Other groups examining heart transplants have identified a center effect where increasing volume leads to decreased mortality. The cumulative risk of mortality in this study at 30 days, 1 year, and 5 years is highly dependent on volume. These relationships persisted after censoring for 30-day mortality, indicating that the protective effect of volume was confined to the prevention of early mortality alone. However, an important caveat from this study is that not all low-volume centers had high rates of mortality. In addition, further statistical modeling indicates that the predictive power of 30-day mortality and 1- and 5-year censored mortality is not substantially influenced by volume alone. This fact coupled with the wide variance of survival in low-volume centers underscores the point that volume is insufficient in and of itself to explain lung transplantation mortality. This study suggests that volume likely has some effect on mortality, but other factors also play an important role.

D. R. Jones, MD

Malignant Mesothelioma

Extrapleural pneumonectomy followed by intracavitary intraoperative hyperthermic cisplatin with pharmacologic cytoprotection for treatment of malignant pleural mesothelioma: A phase II prospective study

Tilleman TR, Richards WG, Zellos L, et al (Brigham and Women's Hosp, Boston, MA; et al)

J Thorac Cardiovasc Surg 138:405-411, 2009

Objective.—We sought to prospectively determine the feasibility and safety of hyperthermic intraoperative intracavitary cisplatin perfusion immediately after extrapleural pneumonectomy in the treatment of malignant pleural mesothelioma.

Methods.—Patients with malignant pleural mesothelioma who were surgical candidates underwent extrapleural pneumonectomy followed by hyperthermic intraoperative intracavitary cisplatin perfusion, consisting of a 1-hour lavage of the chest and abdomen with cisplatin (42°C) at 225 mg/m^2. Pharmacologic cytoprotection consisted of intravenous sodium thiosulfate with or without amifostine. Morbidity and mortality were recorded prospectively.

Results.—Ninety-six (79%) of 121 enrolled patients underwent extrapleural pneumonectomy, of whom 92 (76%) received hyperthermic intraoperative intracavitary cisplatin perfusion after extrapleural pneumonectomy. Fifty-three (58%) patients had epithelial tumors, and 39 (42%) had nonepithelial histology. Hospital mortality was 4.3%. Morbidity (grade 3 or 4, 49%) included atrial fibrillation in 22 (23.9%) patients, venous thrombosis in 12 (13%) patients, and laryngeal nerve dysfunction in 10 (11%) patients. Nine patients had renal toxicity, which was attributable to cisplatin in 8 of them. Among the 27 patients who also received amifostine (910 mg/m^2), 1 patient had grade 3 renal toxicity attributable to cisplatin. Recurrence of malignant pleural mesothelioma was documented in 47 (51%) patients, with ipsilateral recurrence in 17.4% of patients. The median survival of the 121 enrolled patients was 12.8 months.

TABLE 4.—Sites of Pleural Mesothelioma Recurrence

Site	No.	Recurrences (%), Tilleman and Coworkers, 2009*	Recurrences (%), Baldini and Coworkers, 1997[14]
Ipsilateral hemithorax	16	34	67
Contralateral hemithorax	29	62	33
Abdomen	24	51	50
Distant	4	9	8

Editor's Note: Please refer to original journal article for full references.
*Current article.

Conclusions.—Hyperthermic intraoperative intracavitary cisplatin perfusion following extrapleural pneumonectomy can be performed with acceptable morbidity and mortality. The use of amifostine in addition to sodium thiosulfate might reduce cisplatin-associated renal toxicity. Hyperthermic intraoperative intracavitary cisplatin perfusion following extrapleural pneumonectomy might enhance local control in the chest (Table 4).

► Malignant mesothelioma remains one of the most deadly diseases of the thorax. Traditional therapies, such as an extrapleural pneumonectomy, and cytoreductive strategies, such as pleurectomy/decortication, have been the 2 primary local treatment strategies for this disease. Despite these locally aggressive resectional strategies, microscopic residual disease is frequently present such that there is a need for adjuvant therapies. Unfortunately, even with the addition of adjuvant radiation and chemotherapy, most patients experience eventual recurrence of their mesothelioma, which results in death.

In this study from the Brigham's and Women's Hospital, the authors build on a previous phase I study examining the role of hyperthermic intraoperative chemotherapy lavage as a means of delivering high-dose regional therapy to both the affected hemithorax and abdomen. These locations have the highest incidence of recurrence for malignant mesothelioma. Of the patients (N = 121) enrolled in this study, 92 completed hyperthermic intraoperative chemotherapy according to protocol. The overall mortality for the study was 4.3%. Radiographic or pathologic studies confirm recurrence occurred in 50% of patients with the most common site of recurrence being in the contralateral hemithorax and abdomen.

This prospective phase II study establishes both the safety and feasibility of administering hyperthermic intraoperative chemotherapy after extrapleural pneumonectomy. Issues related to this therapy include the small but very real renal toxicity attributed to this approach. Immediate survival of 13.1 months in the entire treatment cohort is encouraging but still reflects the dismal prognosis of this disease. Perhaps the most important aspect of this study is that surgeons are leading and performing important phase II studies, which are generating new knowledge in disease states where many others have adapted a very nihilistic approach. The authors are to be highly commended for undertaking such an important study and for completing it in extraordinarily quick time. Although the results of this study are similar to those observed in older, nonhyperthermic intrapleural chemotherapy trials, an important point of this trial is that intraoperative intracavitary chemotherapy did reduce overall local recurrences from 67% to 34% (see Table 4). Unfortunately, abdominal recurrences did not change despite adding the chemotherapy.

D. R. Jones, MD

Miscellaneous

Comparison of patterns of relapse in thymic carcinoma and thymoma

Huang J, Rizk NP, Travis WD, et al (Memorial Sloan-Kettering Cancer Ctr, NY)

J Thorac Cardiovasc Surg 138:26-31, 2009

Objective.—Thymic carcinomas are considered to be more aggressive than thymomas and carry a worse prognosis. We reviewed our recent experience with the surgical management of thymic tumors and compared the outcomes and patterns of relapse between patients with thymic carcinoma and those with thymoma.

Methods.—We performed a single-institution retrospective cohort study. Data included patient demographics, stage, treatment, pathologic findings, and postoperative outcomes.

Results.—During the period 1995–2006, 120 patients with thymic tumors underwent surgical intervention, including 23 patients with thymic carcinoma and 97 patients with thymoma, as classified according to the World Health Organization 2004 histologic classification. The overall 5-year survival was significantly different between patients with thymic carcinoma and those with thymoma (thymic carcinoma, 53%; thymoma, 89%; $P = .01$). Data on relapse were available for 112 patients. The progression-free 5-year survival was also significantly different between patients with thymic carcinoma and those with thymoma (thymic carcinoma, 36%; thymoma, 75%; $P < .01$). Using multivariate analysis, thymic carcinoma and incomplete resection were found to be independent predictors of progression-free survival. Relapses in patients with thymic carcinoma tended to occur earlier, and occurred significantly more frequently at distant sites than in patients with thymoma (60% vs 13%, $P = .01$).

Conclusions.—Patterns of relapse differ significantly between patients with thymic carcinoma and those with thymoma, with lower progression-free survival, earlier onset, and more distant relapses in patients with thymic carcinoma. Given the greater propensity for distant failures, the inclusion of systemic therapy in the treatment of thymic carcinoma might take on greater importance. Despite significantly higher rates of distant relapse, good overall survival in patients with thymic carcinoma can be achieved (Table 3).

▶ This single-institution, retrospective cohort study examines a large database of 120 patients with thymic tumors who underwent surgical resection from 1995 to 2006. Twenty-three of these patients had thymic carcinoma and 97 had thymoma. This article confirms that the tumor biology and clinical course of thymic carcinomas are significantly different from thymomas. The authors find on multivariate analysis the best estimates of progression-free survival include performing a complete R0 resection and not having thymic carcinoma. The addition of preoperative therapy (usually chemotherapy) or postoperative therapy had no significant effect on progression-free survival in either thymic carcinoma or thymoma patient populations.

TABLE 3.—Multivariate Analysis of Progression-Free Survival

Variable	Hazard Ratio	95% CI	*P* Value
Thymic carcinoma	4.1	1.5–11.3	.006
Incomplete Resection	22.9	4.0–133	<.001
Stage			
III	1.4	0.2–10.5	.77
IVA	1.0	0.1–8.2	.97
Preoperative therapy	0.5	0.1–3.9	.52
Postoperative therapy	0.5	0.1–1.6	.22

CI, Confidence interval.

Management of the anterior mediastinal mass can be challenging for even the most experienced thoracic surgeon. Most thoracic surgeons will offer surgical resection for a well-circumscribed thymic lesion without obtaining a preoperative tissue diagnosis. In cases where the mass is not well circumscribed or there is a question of invasion of adjacent structures, it is reasonable to obtain a tissue diagnosis, particularly if one is entertaining the use of induction chemotherapy. As thoracic oncologic surgeons we can never hear the message too often that a complete R0 resection is the most important thing we can do for our patients. This study highlights this point very well. Despite an aggressive surgical approach, the authors were able to obtain an R0 resection in only 52% of patients with a thymic carcinoma compared with 76% of patients with a thymoma. The most common reason why one does not achieve an R0 resection is involvement of the tumor with continuous structures that are not amendable to resection. This includes the heart, aorta, and bilateral pleural disease, which cannot be completely excised with either an isolated resection or extrapleural pneumonectomy.

The last important point made in this article is that thymic tumors tend to recur more frequently, at distant sites, and earlier than recurrences from primary thymomas. These observations should be taken into consideration in designing follow-up radiographic surveillance strategies for patients undergoing resection for thymic carcinoma.

D. R. Jones, MD

Long-Term Follow-Up of the Functional and Physiologic Results of Diaphragm Plication in Adults With Unilateral Diaphragm Paralysis

Freeman RK, Van Woerkom J, Vyverberg A, et al (St Vincent Hosp Indianapolis, IN)

Ann Thorac Surg 88:1112-1117, 2009

Background.—Patients with lifestyle-limiting dyspnea attributable to unilateral diaphragm paralysis have been shown to experience a decrease in their dyspnea and an improvement in their pulmonary spirometry and functional status with diaphragm plication acutely after surgery. This investigation summarizes these patients' outcomes with long-term follow-up.

Methods.—Adult patients undergoing plication of the hemidiaphragm for lifestyle-limiting dyspnea secondary to unilateral diaphragm paralysis were assessed preoperatively, 6 months after surgery and then annually using the Medical Research Council dyspnea score, pulmonary spirometry, activities of daily living questionnaire, and a chest radiograph. Patients with at least 48 months of follow-up were included in this investigation.

Results.—Forty-one patients underwent plication of the hemidiaphragm through video-assisted thoracoscopy (30) or thoracotomy (11). Mean follow-up was 57 ± 10 months. Mean forced vital capacity, forced expiratory volume at 1 second, functional residual capacity, and total lung capacity all improved by 19%, 23%, 21%, and 19% ($p < 0.005$), respectively, when measured 6 months after surgery, as were mean Medical Research Council dyspnea scores ($p < 0.0001$). These mean values remained constant over the follow-up period. Four patients did not show improvement in their Medical Research Council dyspnea scores nor functional status despite improvements in their pulmonary spirometry values. Two of these patients had a body mass index greater than 35 kg/m^2 and 3 had documented unilateral diaphragm paralysis for at least 4 years before plication.

Conclusions.—Plication of the hemidiaphragm produces improvement for the vast majority of patients in pulmonary spirometry, dyspnea, and functional status that endures over long-term follow-up. Patients who are morbidly obese or who have longstanding unilateral diaphragm paralysis may not realize the same benefits of plication.

▶ Adult patients with lifestyle-limiting dyspnea secondary to diaphragm paralysis have been shown to have an improvement in their dyspnea and functional status with diaphragm plication. It is unclear how long these improvements remain. Therefore, the authors examined the subjective and objective results of patients undergoing hemidiaphragm plication for symptomatic dyspnea. Between 2001 and 2007, 41 patients underwent hemidiaphragm plication for symptomatic paralysis. Most of them (24/41) underwent plication of their left diaphragm. The operative approach was a thoracotomy (N = 11) or video-assisted thoracoscopy (N = 30). The mean hospital stay was 3 days. The authors found that there was significant improvement at 6 months and 48 months following plication. The average improvement at 48 months was essentially equivalent to that which was seen at 6 months. There was roughly an improvement of 20% across all pulmonary spirometry values. Interestingly, of the 4 patients who did not report significant improvement in their dyspnea score, 2 suffered from morbid obesity with a body mass index greater than 35, and 3 of the 4 patients had a significant delay between the diagnosis of unilateral paralysis and diaphragm plication.

This study provides evidence of a prolonged beneficial effect to diaphragm plication in adult patients. The operation is simple and provides an improvement in dyspnea scores as well as objective pulmonary function studies over time. Referring physicians and pulmonologists need to be aware of the benefits of this operation.

D. R. Jones, MD

Surgical Management of Pulmonary and Mediastinal Sequelae of Histoplasmosis: A Challenging Spectrum

Hammoud ZT, Rose AS, Hage CA, et al (Henry Ford Hosp, Detroit, MI; Indiana Univ School of Medicine, Indianapolis)

Ann Thorac Surg 88:399-403, 2009

Background.—Histoplasmosis may result in a spectrum of complications that require thoracic surgical intervention. We reviewed our 17-year experience in the management of histoplasmosis to determine outcomes as well as gain insight into the distribution of complications requiring surgical intervention.

Methods.—The hospital records of patients who underwent surgical treatment for complications related to histoplasmosis from 1991 to 2008 were reviewed. Based on the predominant presentation, patients were categorized with complications secondary to broncholithiasis, granulomatous disease, or fibrosing mediastinitis. Patients who underwent diagnostic surgery and were found to have histoplasmosis were excluded.

Results.—Of the 49 patients who underwent surgery for histoplasmosis-related complications, 27 (55%) had granulomatous disease, 13 (27%) had broncholithiasis, and 9 (18%) had fibrosing mediastinitis. The most common clinical presentations were recurrent pneumonia (n = 16) and hemoptysis (n = 13); less common presentations included dysphagia (n = 3) and superior vena cava syndrome (n = 1). Two patients required cardiopulmonary bypass for resection; 1 of these died postoperatively (series mortality 2%). Seven patients (14%) had complications. Relief of symptoms was achieved in all surviving patients.

Conclusions.—Complications of histoplasmosis requiring thoracic surgical intervention are diverse with pulmonary complications predominating. Although surgically challenging, excellent short- and long-term outcomes may be expected (Fig 2).

► Histoplasmosis presents with a wide spectrum of complications, most of which do not require thoracic surgical intervention. When necessary, surgical intervention can be technically challenging and potentially hazardous, secondary to the normal tissue planes being obliterated. In this study from Indiana University the authors report on a 17-year experience in 49 patients who underwent surgery for histoplasmosis-related complications. The most common indication for surgery was for granulomas disease followed for broncholithiasis and fibrosing mediastinitis. All patients had significant symptoms before proceeding with surgery. As noted in the abstract above, all patients did well with the exception of 1 patient who required cardiopulmonary bypass. A relief of symptoms was achieved in all patients.

Despite the uncommon need to proceed with surgery for complications of histoplasmosis, it is important for surgeons to realize that these operations, although technically difficult, can be done with excellent results. It is appropriate to group the patients, as was done in this study, into 3 distinct categories: mediastinal granulomatous disease, fibrosing mediastinitis, and broncholithiasis

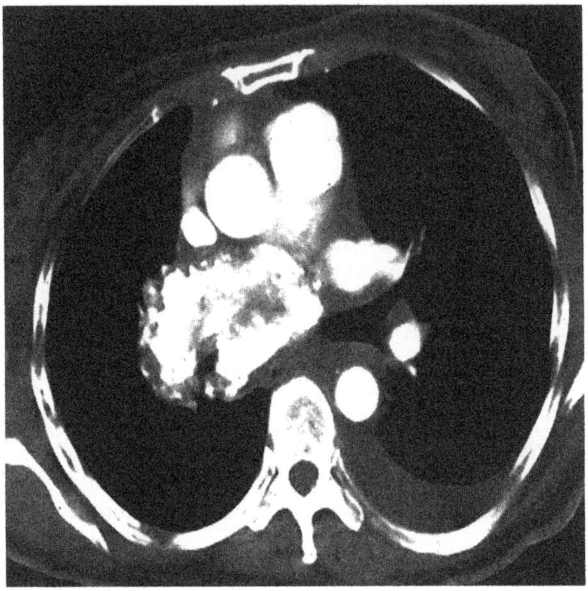

FIGURE 2.—Computed tomography showing extensive fibrosing mediastinitis. (Reprinted from Hammoud ZT, Rose AS, Hage CA, et al. Surgical management of pulmonary and mediastinal sequelae of histoplasmosis: a challenging spectrum. *Ann Thorac Surg.* 2009;88:399-403, with permission from The Society of Thoracic Surgeons.)

(see Fig 2). An important technical point related to the procedures is the need to obtain control of the proximal pulmonary artery. This clearly should be done in cases where fibrosis or granulomatous nodal disease involves the pulmonary artery or its segmental branches. Finally, although uncommon, the need for cardiopulmonary bypass is present in some cases, and therefore, the pump should be available on standby.

D. R. Jones, MD

The Influence of Surgeon Specialty on Outcomes in General Thoracic Surgery: A National Sample 1996 to 2005

Schipper PH, Diggs BS, Ungerleider RM, et al (Oregon Health and Science Univ, Portland, OR)

Ann Thorac Surg 88:1566-1573, 2009

Background.—While general thoracic surgical procedures are performed by several different surgical subspecialties, debate remains as to whether surgeon specialty impacts outcomes.

Methods.—The Nationwide Inpatient Sample (NIS) was queried for procedure codes for pneumonectomy, lobectomy, limited lung resection, and decortication. We constructed multivariate logistic regression models to calculate odds of hospital mortality or length-of-stay (LOS) greater than 14 days (a marker of morbidity), adjusted for age, sex, patient comorbidities, hospital setting, and surgeon specialty. A surgeon was considered general thoracic if they performed greater than 75% general thoracic operations and less than 10% cardiac operations, cardiac if greater than 10% cardiac operations, and general surgeon if less than 75% general thoracic and less than 10% cardiac operations. A second set of models additionally adjusted for procedure-specific hospital and surgeon volume.

Results.—From 1996 to 2005, the NIS estimates 41,808 pneumonectomies, 321,767 lobectomies, 75,200 limited lung resections, and 149,318 decortications were performed in the United States. For all procedures studied, general thoracic surgeons had significantly decreased odds-of-death and LOS greater than 14 days compared with general surgeons. Cardiac surgeons had significantly decreased LOS greater than 14 days for all operations and decreased odds-of-death for decortications, lobectomy, and limited lung resection compared with general surgeons. When further adjusted for surgeon volume, most differences in odds-of-death were no longer present; however, significantly decreased LOS greater than 14 days largely persisted for both general thoracic and cardiac surgeons.

Conclusions.—The majority of general thoracic surgical operations in the United States are performed by surgeons not specializing in thoracic surgery. Both general thoracic surgeons and cardiac surgeons achieve better outcomes than general surgeons. Differences in mortality may be more dependent on surgeon volume than subspecialty. Differences in morbidity are significantly impacted by surgeon specialty and volume.

▶ This study by the group from the Oregon Health Sciences Center examines the influence of surgeon speciality on outcome. Using the Nationwide Inpatient Sample survey the authors evaluated the results of 4 procedures (pneumonectomy, lobectomy, limited lung resection, and decortication) among general thoracic, cardiac, and general surgeons. Interestingly, the percent of patients operated on by the general thoracic surgeons for these 4 categories is never greater than 10% using the definition of a "general thoracic surgeon" proposed by the authors of the study. The conclusions are interesting in that even with multivariate analysis adjusting for surgeon volume and comorbid conditions, the differences in odds of death were significantly decreased for length of stay for both cardiac and general thoracic surgeons compared with general surgeons.

This study adds to an increasing number of articles suggesting that surgeon specialty does affect patient outcome. This is a complex, and frankly dynamic, issue in which confounders such as patient volume, years of experience, payor status, and other variables are also very important. Despite this complexity the authors have shown that at least for one important variable, length of stay, there is a significant difference among groups. There is no way to link survival using the Nationwide Inpatient Sample, so those results will need to come from other types of databases. The major limitation of this study is the use of this administrative data set, which is not designed to answer these types of questions but is more commonly used for claims, data collection, and billing and not health care research. In addition, the definitions proposed by the authors for what constitutes a general thoracic surgeon versus a general surgeon are arbitrary, and this too could impact the overall results of the article.

Despite these limitations this article adds to a growing body of literature suggesting that patient outcomes are linked to important factors such as experience, specialization, and hospital and surgeon volumes.

D. R. Jones, MD

Pre- and Postoperative Management

A Randomized Trial Evaluating Amiodarone for Prevention of Atrial Fibrillation After Pulmonary Resection

Tisdale JE, Wroblewski HA, Wall DS, et al (Purdue Univ, IN; Indiana Univ School of Medicine; Indiana Univ Hosp of Clarian Health Partners, Indianapolis)

Ann Thorac Surg 88:886-895, 2009

Background.—Atrial fibrillation (AF) occurs commonly after anatomic pulmonary resection. In this study, the efficacy of amiodarone for prevention of post–pulmonary resection AF was investigated.

Methods.—One hundred thirty patients undergoing lobectomy, bilobectomy, or pneumonectomy were randomly assigned prospectively to receive amiodarone (n = 65) or no prophylaxis (control group, n = 65). The amiodarone group received 1,050 mg by continuous intravenous infusion over 24 hours, initiated at the time of anesthesia induction, followed by 400 mg orally twice daily until hospital discharge or for a maximum of 6 days. The primary endpoint was AF requiring treatment during hospitalization. Secondary endpoints included postoperative length of hospital and intensive care unit stays.

Results.—There were no significant differences between the amiodarone and control groups in demographics, comorbid conditions, extent of pulmonary resection, or preoperative or postoperative use of beta-blockers or calcium-channel blockers. The incidence of AF was lower in the amiodarone group than in the control group (13.8% versus 32.3%, $p = 0.02$; relative risk reduction = 57%). There was no difference between the amiodarone and control groups in median length of hospital stay (7 versus 8 days, $p = 0.79$), but median length of intensive care unit stay was shorter in the amiodarone group (46 versus 84 hours, $p = 0.03$). There was no significant difference between the amiodarone and control groups in the incidence of pulmonary complications or other adverse effects.

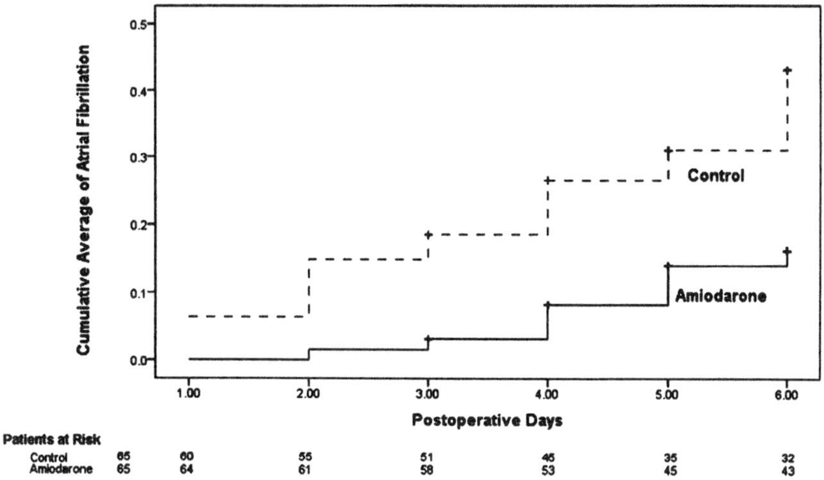

FIGURE 2.—Kaplan-Meier cumulative incidence of atrial fibrillation. Log rank p = 0.009. (Reprinted from Tisdale JE, Wroblewski HA, Wall DS, et al. A randomized trial evaluating amiodarone for prevention of atrial fibrillation after pulmonary resection. *Ann Thorac Surg*. 2009;88:886-895, with permission from The Society of Thoracic Surgeons.)

Conclusions.—Amiodarone prophylaxis significantly reduces the incidence of AF after anatomic pulmonary resection, and is associated with a significant reduction in length of intensive care unit stay (Fig 2).

▶ The incidence of atrial fibrillation following pulmonary resection has been reported to be 24% to 67% for pneumonectomy and 12% to 30% following lobectomy. Early results have suggested that patients undergoing video-assisted thoracoscopic (VATS) resections have a lower incidence of atrial fibrillation. Atrial fibrillation is a significant morbidity associated with these operations and has been shown to increase hospital length of stay and cost.

The group from the University of Indiana performed a prospective randomized trial of prophylactic amiodarone or no prophylaxis in 130 patients undergoing lobectomy, bilobectomy, and pneumonectomy. The authors found that the incidence of atrial fibrillation was lower in the amiodarone group than in the control group (14% vs 32%, $P = .02$). This is a relative risk reduction of 57% and is both statistically and clinically significant. Importantly, there was no significant difference in postoperative adverse events, morbidity, or mortality between the groups.

A potentially important clinical observation in this study was the incidence of bradycardia in those patients receiving amiodarone. This was 4-fold higher in the amiodarone group compared with the control group, but this did not result in any complication. This does mandate that all patients receiving amiodarone should be monitored electrocardiographically. Perhaps one of the most commonly held fears associated with amiodarone therapy has been pulmonary toxicity, specifically pulmonary fibrosis. The incidence of pulmonary fibrosis following oral amiodarone therapy has an incidence of less than 3%. In this study, as well as more contemporary studies with lower amiodarone dosing, the incidence of pulmonary toxicity has been decreased significantly. Importantly, patients in this study only took oral amiodarone for 6 days or until hospital discharge. Therefore, the likelihood that there would be pulmonary toxicity associated with such a short dosing of amiodarone is unlikely. In summary, this is a superb randomized clinical trial investigating a very common postoperative problem, atrial fibrillation following pulmonary resection. The results are intriguing, and the study was well done. Although the study was not double-blinded and placebo-controlled and a larger multicenter trial could be entertained, it is highly likely that this study is the definitive study in this patient population at present.

D. R. Jones, MD

Chest Tube–Delivered Bupivacaine Improves Pain and Decreases Opioid Use After Thoracoscopy

Demmy TL, Nwogu C, Solan P, et al (Roswell Park Cancer Inst and State Univ of New York, Buffalo)

Ann Thorac Surg 87:1040-1047, 2009

Background.—This study compared a simplified method of intrapleural bupivacaine administration with traditional analgesic therapy to decrease postoperative pain and opioid usage in patients after thoracoscopy.

Methods.—Thirty patients who had non-rib-spreading thoracoscopic operations under general anesthesia were prospectively randomized to no local anesthetic infusion (control), intermittent bolus (30 mL every 6 hours), or continuous infusion (5 mL/h). Bupivacaine (0.25%) was delivered through the pleural infusion channel of a specially designed single silicone 28F chest tube. Total intravenous fentanyl patient-controlled analgesia (boluses with basal rate) infused in the first 24 hours postoperatively was the designated primary study end point. Escalations of analgesic therapy, including ketorolac administration, were standardized across all groups. Nurses assessed pain control at onset and every 6 hours by visual analog pain scales (VAPS, 100 mm). VAPS were repeated 10 minutes later to assess any opioid or bupivacaine bolus effects.

Results.—No study-related adverse events occurred. Compared with controls, pooled VAPS scores and 24-hour fentanyl consumption were significantly lower for the intermittent and continuous administration groups (1753 vs 1180 vs 1177 μg/24 h, respective median; $p = 0.04$). Early (6-hour) VAPS analgesic responses were more certain for intermittent (10 of 10) and continuous (10 of 10) patients than controls (7 of 10, $p = .04$). Five continuous patients successfully maintained VAPS scores below 20 mm throughout the study vs 3 intermittent and 2 controls ($p = .045$).

Conclusions.—Intermittent or continuous intrapleural bupivacaine infused through the chest tube reliably reduces postoperative pain and 24-hour opioid usage in thoracoscopy patients.

▶ The number of thoracoscopic procedures being performed has increased dramatically. Despite no rib spreading, which is the hallmark of video-assisted thoracic surgery (VATS) and/or thoracoscopic procedures, patients still have a significant amount of pain, presumably from intracostal neuralgias. Local anesthetics, such as bupivacaine, administered intrapleurally have been used in a number of studies, although the results have been inconsistent or even conflicting. This prospective randomized controlled trial attempted to address the use of intrapleural bupivacaine administered through an intrapleural catheter and its ability to affect postoperative pain. Thirty patients were randomized to intravenous fentanyl only intermittent to bupivacaine only or continuous bupivacaine only. The study shows that a simple chest tube device to administer local anesthetic can reduce narcotic consumption and decrease pain after thoracoscopic operations. No isolated method of pain control was completely effective, but clearly both intermittent and continuous bupivacaine administered through the intrapleural catheter resulted in decreased narcotic use.

The strength of this study is that it was randomized and prospective. Although the study numbers were small and clearly not adequately powered to address the question completely, the results are intriguing and suggest that surgeons need to consider incorporating the use of intrapleural bupivacaine administered by chest tubes in their clinical practice. Given that pain is now considered to be the "fifth vital sign," surgeons need to take the opportunity to conduct clinical trials such as the one reported by these authors. Studies such as these will impact the overall quality and experience that our patients have even when undergoing the most minimally invasive approaches to their disease.

D. R. Jones, MD

Impact of Smoking Cessation Before Resection of Lung Cancer: A Society of Thoracic Surgeons General Thoracic Surgery Database Study

Mason DP, Subramanian S, Nowicki ER, et al (Heart and Vascular Inst; Res Inst, Cleveland, OH; Duke Univ, Durham, NC)

Ann Thorac Surg 88:362-371, 2009

Background.—Smoking cessation is presumed to be beneficial before resection of lung cancer. The effect of smoking cessation on outcome was investigated.

Methods.—From January 1999 to July 2007, in-hospital outcomes for 7990 primary resections for lung cancer in adults were reported to the Society of Thoracic Surgeons General Thoracic Surgery Database. Risk of hospital death and respiratory complications was assessed according to timing of smoking cessation, adjusted for clinical confounders.

TABLE 2.—Outcome After Resection for Lung Cancer According to Smoking Status

Category	Overall No. (% of 7990)	Hospital Mortality No. (%)	Overall No. (% of 7965)[a]	Pulmonary Complications No. (%)
Current smoker	1595 (20)	24 (1.5)	1590 (20)	110 (6.9)
Pre-op smoking cessation interval				
>14 d–1 mo	404 (5.1)	7 (1.7)	402 (5.0)	25 (6.2)
1–12 mo	940 (12)	12 (1.3)	938 (12)	60 (6.4)
>12 mo	4026 (50)	62 (1.5)	4011 (50)	234 (5.8)
Never smoked[b]	1025 (13)	4 (0.39)	1024 (13)	27 (2.6)
Total	7990 (100)	109 (1.4)	7965 (100)	456 (5.7)

[a]Excludes 25 patients who died on the day of operation.
[b]Includes patients who smoked fewer than 100 cigarettes in their lifetime.

Results.—Hospital mortality was 1.4% (n = 109), but 1.5% in patients who had smoked (105 of 6965) vs 0.39% in those who had not (4 of 1025). Compared with the latter, risk-adjusted odds ratios were 3.5 ($p = 0.03$), 4.6 ($p = 0.03$), 2.6 ($p = 0.7$), and 2.5 ($p = 0.11$) for those whose timing of smoking cessation was categorized as current smoker, quit from 14 days to 1 month, 1 to 12 months, or more than 12 months preoperatively, respectively. Prevalence of major pulmonary complications was 5.7% (456 of 7965) overall, but 6.2% in patients who had smoked (429 of 6941) vs 2.5%% in those who had not (27 of 1024). Compared with the latter, risk-adjusted odds ratios were 1.80 ($p = 0.03$), 1.62 ($p = 0.14$), 1.51 ($p = 0.20$), and 1.29 ($p = 0.3$) for those whose timing of smoking cessation was categorized as above.

Conclusions.—Risks of hospital death and pulmonary complications after lung cancer resection were increased by smoking and mitigated slowly by preoperative cessation. No optimal interval of smoking cessation was identifiable. Patients should be counseled to stop smoking irrespective of surgical timing (Table 2).

▶ Although smoking cessation is intuitively obvious before a planned surgical resection for lung cancer, this issue has not been adequately addressed in the medical literature. In this study from the Cleveland Clinic, the authors used the Society of Thoracic Surgeons General Thoracic Surgical Database to examine whether smoking cessation had an effect on postoperative morbidity and hospital mortality. The authors found that hospital mortality was 1.5% in those patients who had smoked compared with 0.4% in patients who had no smoking history. As expected, patients who had smoked had a higher incidence of pulmonary complications relative to those patients who had not (see Table 2). Unfortunately in this study, the authors were unable to identify an optimal interval of smoking cessation. Of patients undergoing a resection for lung cancer, 87% had a smoking history and 13% had never smoked. Of the nearly

7000 patients with a history of smoking, 58% had quit more than 12 months preoperatively.

The results of this study are important for several reasons. First, the findings of this study provide the best evidence we have to date that surgeons need to strongly counsel their patients to stop smoking before surgery. Second, patients who have any history of smoking have a higher instance of pulmonary complications and in-hospital death. This is important information to convey to our patients. It also may be important in designing care-specific pathways for those patients who have a smoking history. One could envision enhanced pulmonary physiotherapy, early mobilization, and enhanced deep breathing techniques. Other important information from this study is that although hospital mortality is higher for smokers after pulmonary resection, the risk appears to be modified by cessation and improved with a longer interval of cessation. This again highlights the importance of surgeons counseling the patients to stop smoking as soon as possible.

D. R. Jones, MD

Predictors of Prolonged Postoperative Endotracheal Intubation in Patients Undergoing Thoracotomy for Lung Resection

Cywinski JB, Xu M, Sessler DI, et al (Cleveland Clinic, OH)

J Cardiothorac Vasc Anesth 23:766-769, 2009

Objective.—The aim of this study was to identify predictors of delayed endotracheal extubation defined as the need for postoperative ventilatory support after open thoracotomy for lung resection.

Design.—An observational cohort investigation.

Setting.—A tertiary referral center.

Participants.—The study population consisted of 2,068 patients who had open thoracotomy for pneumonectomy, lobectomy, or segmental lung resection between January 1996 and December 2005.

Interventions.—Not applicable.

Measurements and Main Results.—Preoperative and intraoperative variables were collected concurrently with the patient's care. Risk factors were identified using logistic regression with stepwise variable selection procedure on 1,000 bootstrap resamples, and a bagging algorithm was used to summarize the results. Intraoperative red blood cell transfusion, higher preoperative serum creatinine level, absence of a thoracic epidural catheter, more extensive surgical resection, and lower preoperative FEV_1 were associated with an increased risk of delayed extubation after lung resection.

Conclusion.—Most predictors of delayed postoperative extubation (ie, red blood cell transfusion, higher preoperative serum creatinine, lower preoperative FEV_1, and more extensive lung resection) are difficult to modify in the perioperative period and probably represent greater severity of underlying lung disease and more advanced comorbid conditions. However, thoracic epidural anesthesia and analgesia is a modifiable factor

TABLE 3.—Risk Factors for Delayed Extubation From the Multivariable Regression Model

Factor	Odds Ratio (CI)	*p* Value
Intraoperative RBC transfusion (yes/no)	2.68 (1.92, 3.74)	<.001
Preoperative serum creatinine	1.42 (1.20, 1.69)	<0.001
Presence of thoracic epidural	0.44 (0.33, 0.58)	<0.001
Lower preoperative measured FEV1	1.47 (1.23, 1.72)	<0.001
Type of procedure		<0.001
	SLR v CP: 0.33 (0.20, 0.56)	<0.001
	LOL v CP: 0.70 (0.52, 0.95)	0.022
	SLR v LOL: 0.47 (0.30, 0.75)	0.001

Abbreviations: LOL, lobectomy of lung; SLR, segmental lung resection; CP, complete pneumonectomy; RBC, red blood cell; CI, confidence interval.

that was associated with reduced odds for postoperative ventilatory support. Thus, the use of epidural analgesia may reduce the need for post-thoracotomy mechanical ventilation (Table 3).

▶ Most of the patients undergoing a thoracotomy for lung resection are able to be extubated in the operating room (OR). Furthermore, they rarely require reintubation. Delayed postoperative extubation has been shown to prolong the duration of recovery, increase cost, and is associated with increased postoperative morbidity. There have been limited studies addressing which patients may be at risk for delayed extubation. This study examined over 2000 patients who had undergone anatomic lung resection from 1996 to 2005. Most of the patients were able to be extubated, but there were several predictors of delayed postoperative extubation. These include red blood cell transfusion, elevated creatine, a low preoperative forced expiratory volume in 1 second (FEV_1), and more extensive lung resections (see Table 3). A functional thoracic epidural catheter was found to be predictive of successful extubation.

An ability to identify modifiable preoperative predictors could certainly help clinicians design interventions to reduce this phenomenon. Unfortunately, several of the factors cannot be modified. One could envision a short course of pulmonary rehabilitation improving FEV_1, but it is unlikely that the need for red blood cell transfusions intraoperatively, creatine level, or the type of resection can be modified. Perhaps what is most important about this study is that identification of these variables preoperatively may help with resource allocation with respect to intensive care unit (ICU) bed utilization. The other important aspect is that intraoperative activation of an epidural catheter spares opioid use, which should improve postoperative respiratory function. Consistent with this, authors found that use of a thoracic epidural catheter improved the odds of OR extubation significantly.

D. R. Jones, MD

The analysis of a prospective surgical database improves postoperative fast-tracking algorithms after pulmonary resection

Bryant AS, Cerfolio RJ (Univ of Alabama at Birmingham)

J Thorac Cardiovasc Surg 137:1173-1179, 2009

Objective.—We evaluated our results from our prospective database to identify possible modifications that may improve our fast-tracking protocols in selected high-risk patients.

Methods.—We conducted a retrospective study of a prospective database. Using multivariable regression, we identified several patient characteristics that predicted failure to fast-track owing to increased morbidity. We modified our fast-tracking algorithm by substituting pain pumps for epidurals in elderly patients (>70 years). In addition, patients with a body mass index greater than 35 had increased aspiration precautions. Patients with poor pulmonary function (ratio of forced expiratory volume in 1 second to forced vital capacity and/or diffusing capacity/alveolar volume < 45%) underwent increased respiratory treatments and more aggressive ambulation. Differences in outcomes between groups were compared after adjusting for differing baseline patient characteristics, including use of a propensity score.

Results.—A total of 2895 patients underwent elective pulmonary resection before the algorithm modifications (January 1997–December 2001) and 3252 patients afterward (January 2002–July 2007) by one surgeon. The length of stay was reduced by the protocol changes from 6.7 to 4.9 days ($P = .024$) in elderly patients, from 5.7 to 4.8 days in obese patients, and from 6.2 to 4.3 days ($P = .008$) in those with poor pulmonary function. Morbidity was reduced from 26% to 17% in elderly patients ($P = .046$), from 29% to 20% ($P = .027$) in obese patients, and from 45% to 23%in those with poor pulmonary function. Overall mortality was also reduced 4.0% to 2.1% ($P = .014$).

Conclusion.—A prospective database provides important information that can lead to improvement in patient care by identifying specific complications. High-risk patients such as the elderly, the obese, and those with poor pulmonary function can safely undergo pulmonary resection and have a shorter hospital stay.

▶ The postoperative care of patients undergoing general thoracic surgical procedures is increasingly complicated by the multiple comorbidities of these patients and increasing pressures on the patient care team to discharge these patients in a timely manner without sacrificing safety or quality. This study from the University of Alabama at Birmingham uses the findings identified retrospectively in their prospectively maintained database to improve postoperative algorithms following pulmonary resection.

The authors note that several groups did not respond well to fast-tracking algorithms. Specifically, patients with poor pulmonary function studies, obese patients, and the elderly all have higher incidences of failing to stay on the post-operative clinical care pathways. Simple changes in care plans, such as altering pain management strategies, being more attentive to risk of aspiration, and increasing patient mobilization, resulted in significant decreases in morbidity and mortality. It is unclear whether these changes were solely responsible for the improved results. Furthermore, the enhanced experience of a dedicated team and that of the surgeon who may have improved patient selection are all possible reasons for the improvement.

In my opinion, the most important point of this article is that the authors made important clinical decisions about patient care pathways based on prior experiences. The authors are to be highly commended for maintaining and tracking their data in order to make adjustments to the clinical care pathway. This is perhaps the best example of how surgeons can most directly affect the quality of their results at a local level. The observations and the specific changes made to their postoperative care plans need to be considered by general thoracic surgeons as well as nursing and ancillary care teams in order to maximize the number of patients who can safely undergo pulmonary resection, despite being at relatively high risk.

D. R. Jones, MD

Staging of Non-small Cell Lung Cancer

A thoracic surgery clinic dedicated to indeterminate pulmonary nodules: Too many scans and too little pathology?

Veeramachaneni NK, Crabtree TD, Kreisel D, et al (Washington Univ School of Medicine, St Louis, MO)

J Thorac Cardiovasc Surg 137:30-35, 2009

Objective.—Widespread application of computed tomographic scans has increased detection of asymptomatic pulmonary nodules. A dedicated clinic was established to encourage referral and manage large numbers of patients with such nodules.

Methods.—Patients were evaluated periodically by a nurse practitioner with surgeon oversight, and follow-up imaging was centralized. Patients were rescanned at intervals on the basis of radiologist recommendation.

Results.—A total of 414 patients, 189 male and 225 female with a median age of 60.2 years (20.7–84.1 years), were evaluated since April 2000. Median follow-up was 1.51 years (0–6.65 years). Thirty-seven percent (153/414) were older than 60 years with at least 10 pack-years of tobacco use, whereas 30% (123/414) had never smoked. A total of 286 patients completed at least 2 years of follow-up computed tomographic evaluation. After 2 years, 24.2% (69/286) were deemed in stable condition and were discharged from further follow-up, whereas 22.4% (64/286) of patients were followed up longer than 2 years owing to the development of new nodules. Forty-five percent (127/286) of patients did not complete their recommended follow-up at our clinic. Overall, 3% (13/414) of our patients have been shown to have a malignant tumor. Only 5 patients underwent curative resection of a primary lung cancer.

Conclusion.—In a population of patients with indeterminate nodules in routine clinical practice, few patients required intervention and few cancers were detected. Although the benefits of a "nodule" clinic may include patient reassurance and convenience to referring physicians, a significant number of patients did not complete their follow-up in our clinic.

▶ The widespread application of computed tomography (CT) technology has certainly increased the detection of otherwise asymptomatic lung nodules. Many of these nodules are subcentimeter in size and there is no documentation of how long they have been present. The group from Washington University implemented a clinic dedicated to following these patients. The authors report their experience on 414 patients with asymptomatic pulmonary nodules. Interestingly, only 37% of the patients were older than 60 years and had at least a 10-pack-year history of tobacco use. This group of patients would be expected to have the highest incidence of an occult malignancy. Overall, 3% (13/414) of the patients in this study were found to have a malignant tumor. Only 5 of these patients underwent curative resection.

Both the Fleischner Society and the American College of Chest Physicians use the 2-year stability of a solitary pulmonary nodule as a suggestion for a benign etiology. In this study, 70% of patients completed at least 2 years of follow-up CT evaluation for their nodule(s). The median nodule size was 6 mm. Seven patients presented with masses greater than 3 cm in size. Ten percent of patients underwent fluorodeoxyglucose positron emission tomography (FDG-PET) imaging, which suggested malignances in 8 of 42 (19%) patients.

This study suggests that indeed there are too many scans and too little pathology in follow-up of small indeterminate pulmonary nodules. Going forward, an alternative strategy may be to only follow patients who fall into high-risk categories (older age, significant smoking history, history of a previous malignancy, etc) in such a clinic. Interestingly, the authors only made a pathological diagnosis of the pulmonary nodule in 20 patients (5%). This suggests that in the absence of a larger lesion with a suspicious clinical history these nodules can be followed with serial imaging studies and patients do not need to undergo attempts to obtain a tissue diagnosis.

D. R. Jones, MD

Safety and efficacy of video-assisted versus conventional lung resection for lung cancer

Farjah F, Wood DE, Mulligan MS, et al (Univ of Washington, Seattle)
J Thorac Cardiovasc Surg 137:1415-1421, 2009

Objective.—We sought to evaluate the use of video-assisted thoracoscopy among patients with lung cancer and its safety and effectiveness relative to conventional resection.

Methods.—A cohort study (1994–2002) was conducted by using the Surveillance, Epidemiology, and End-Results Medicare database. Video-assisted thoracoscopy and conventional resection were hypothesized to be equivalent in terms of risks of death. Equivalency was defined by a confidence interval of 0.72 to 1.28 for the odds of 30-day death and 0.89 to 1.11 for the hazard of death, corresponding to a difference of no more than 1%for 30-day mortality and 5% for 5-year survival, respectively.

Results.—Among 12,958 patients who underwent segmentectomy or lobectomy (mean age, 74 ± 5 years), 6% underwent video-assisted thoracoscopy. The use of video-assisted thoracoscopy increased from 1% to 9% between 1994 and 2002. Compared with those who underwent conventional resection, patients who underwent video-assisted thoracoscopy more frequently had smaller tumors ($P < .001$) and stage I disease ($P = .03$), underwent lymphadenectomy ($P < 001$), and were cared for by higher-volume surgeons ($P < 001$) and at higher-volume hospitals ($P < 001$). After adjusting for differences in patient, cancer, management, and provider characteristics, the odds of early death were not significantly different between patients undergoing video-assisted thoracoscopy and those undergoing conventional resection, although equivalency was not demonstrated (adjusted odds ratio, 0.93; 95% confidence interval, 0.57–1.50). The hazard of death was equivalent for video-assisted thoracoscopy and conventional resection (adjusted hazard ratio, 0.99; 95% confidence interval, 0.90–1.08).

Conclusions.—Video-assisted thoracoscopy was uncommonly used to manage lung cancer, although its use has increased over time. Video-assisted thoracoscopy and conventional resection were equivalent in terms of long-term survival.

▶ The purpose of this study was to assess, using a noninferiority-based analysis of observational data, whether the use of video-assisted thoracoscopic surgery (VATS) for lung cancer was equivalent to conventional open thoracotomy resection. The authors used the Surveillance, Epidemiology, and End-Results (SEER) database to examine nearly 13 000 patients with lung cancer over an 8-year period. Only 6% of the patients underwent VATS by 7% of the surgeons and at 13% of the hospitals. While the frequency of VATS increased over the time of the study, its overall use was still significantly less than that of an open thoracotomy. Despite this, the unadjusted analysis demonstrated that VATS was associated with a significantly higher 5-year overall survival rate compared with open thoracotomy. In the fully adjusted model evaluating survival, the hazard of death for VATS and open resection was equivalent, suggesting that VATS may not be superior, but it was certainly not less of a cancer operation.

As with any new technology, VATS is slowly increasing in use by general thoracic surgeons. The adoption of VATS into a clinical practice has been slow likely for several reasons. Surgeons may be uncomfortable performing VATS because of insufficient training or experience. Alternatively, some surgeons may believe that there are insufficient levels of evidence to confirm the safety and the oncologic efficacy of VATS compared with standard resections. This study does much to allay the latter concerns of safety and oncologic efficacy. Several other smaller single-institution trails have shown that VATS is at least equivalent to an open pulmonary resection and almost informally results in decreased morbidity and decreased length of stay. An interesting, although not quite statistically significant, observation is that the stratified analysis suggested that the risk of death associated with VATS procedures was more commonly associated with low-volume VATS surgeons. The likely explanation for this observation is that it is a surrogate for appropriately performed VATS and not overall volume in isolation.

In summary, the study supports the use of VATS for lung cancer provided that it is done by well-trained and reasonably high-volume VATS surgeons.

D. R. Jones, MD

Tumor Biology and Prognostic Variables

Differentiation of Lung Adenocarcinoma, Pleural Mesothelioma, and Nonmalignant Pulmonary Tissues Using DNA Methylation Profiles

Christensen BC, Marsit CJ, Houseman EA, et al (Brown Univ, Providence, RI; et al)

Cancer Res 69:6315-6321, 2009

Pathologic differentiation of tissue of origin in tumors found in the lung can be challenging, with differentiation of mesothelioma and lung adenocarcinoma emblematic of this problem. Indeed, proper classification is essential for determination of treatment regimen for these diseases, making accurate and early diagnosis critical. Here, we investigate the potential of epigenetic profiles of lung adenocarcinoma, mesothelioma, and nonmalignant pulmonary tissues ($n = 285$) as differentiation markers in an analysis of DNA methylation at 1413 autosomal CpG loci associated with 773 cancer-related genes. Using an unsupervised recursively partitioned mixture modeling technique for all samples, the derived methylation profile classes were significantly associated with sample type ($P < 0.0001$). In a similar analysis restricted to tumors, methylation profile classes significantly predicted tumor type ($P < 0.0001$). Random forests classification of CpG methylation of tumors—which splits the data into training and test sets—accurately differentiated mesothelioma from lung adenocarcinoma over 99% of the time ($P < 0.0001$). In a locus-by-locus comparison of CpG methylation between tumor types, 1266 CpG loci had significantly different methylation between tumors following correction for multiple comparisons ($Q < 0.05$); 61% had higher methylation in adenocarcinoma. Using the CpG loci with significant differential methylation in a pathway analysis revealed significant enrichment of methylated gene-loci in Cell Cycle Regulation, DNA Damage Response, PTEN Signaling, and Apoptosis Signaling pathways in lung adenocarcinoma when compared with mesothelioma. Methylation profile–based differentiation of lung adenocarcinoma and mesothelioma is highly accurate, informs on the distinct etiologies of these diseases, and holds promise for clinical application.

▶ It is well recognized that histopathologic differentiation between adenocarcinoma and malignant mesothelioma can be difficult despite cytologic advances and use of immunohistochemical panels containing both epithelial and mesothelial markers. In this study, the authors explore the ability to examine promoter DNA methylation as a mechanism to differentiate between lung adenocarcinoma and malignant mesothelioma. Using tissue from malignant mesotheliomas, nontumorigenic partial pleural, as well as non-small cell lung cancer/adenocarcinoma, the authors provide an analysis of methylation of specific promoters of approximately 773 genes. Interestingly, subsequent analysis of the most methylation-variable autosomal CpG loci reveals readily apparent differences in the epigenetic profiles among lung adenocarcinoma, mesothelioma, and nonmalignant tissues.

This study highlights advances in molecular profiling of tumors such that the diagnosis of specific tumors can be facilitated. While thoracic surgeons are not typically involved in these analyses, it is important to understand that new proteomic, genomic, and epigenetic analyses of tumors are available and will be part of our everyday practice in the future. The fact that several surgeons were part of this important study highlights the need for appropriate interaction between researchers and clinicians. It is also possible that beyond the classification of lung adenocarcinoma and malignant mesothelioma, the methods described in this article are likely to be used for a range of other clinical scenarios.

D. R. Jones, MD

Fluorodeoxyglucose positron emission tomography and tumor marker expression in non–small cell lung cancer

Taylor MD, Smith PW, Brix WK, et al (Univ of Virginia, Charlottesville)

J Thorac Cardiovasc Surg 137:43-48, 2009

Objective.—The best current noninvasive surrogate for tumor biology is fluorodeoxyglucose positron emission tomography (FDG–PET). Both FDG–PET maximal standardized uptake values and selected tumor markers have been shown to correlate with stage, nodal disease, and survival in non–small cell lung cancer (NSCLC). However, there are limited data correlating FDG–PET with tumor markers. The purpose of this study was to determine the correlation of tumor marker expression with FDG–PET maximal standardized uptake values in NSCLC.

Methods.—FDG–PET maximal standardized uptake values were calculated in patients with NSCLC (n = 149). No patient had induction chemoradiotherapy. Intraoperative NSCLC tissue was obtained and tissue microarrays were created. Immunohistochemical analysis was performed for 5 known NSCLC tumor markers (glucose transporter 1, p53, cyclin

TABLE 3.—FDG–PET SUV_{max} and Tumor Marker Expression

SUV_{max}	No.	Node Positive (%)	Immunohistochemistry Percent Scores (mean ± SEM) GLUT-1 (%)	EGFR (%)
0–2.5	25	1/25 (4%)	28 ± 6 reference	10 ± 4 reference
2.5–5.0	37	10/37 (27%)	39 ± 6 $P = .25$	27 ± 6 $P = .02$*
5–10	53	20/53 (38%)	44 ± 5 $P = .06$	34 ± 5 $P = .0003$*
10 or greater	34	14/34 (41%)	65 ± 6 $P = .0001$*	37 ± 7 $P = .002$*

SUV_{max}, Maximal standardized uptake values; *SEM*, standard error of the mean; *GLUT-1*, Glucose transporter 1; *EGFR*, epidermal growth factor receptor.
*Two-tailed Student t test, $P < .05$.

D1, epidermal growth factor receptor, and vascular endothelial growth factor). Each tumor marker was assessed independently by two pathologists using common grading criteria. Subgroup analysis based on histologic characteristics and regional nodal status was performed.

Results.—FDG–PET correlated with T classification ($P < .0001$), N stage ($P = .002$), and greatest tumor dimension ($P < .0001$). In addition, increasing maximal standardized uptake values correlated with increased expression of glucose transporter 1 ($P < .0001$) and p53 ($P = .04$) in adenocarcinoma. Epidermal growth factor receptor expression correlated with maximal standardized uptake values without predilection for histologic subtype ($P = .004$).

Conclusion.—FDG–PET maximal standardized uptake values correlate with an increased expression of glucose transporter 1 and p53 in lung adenocarcinoma, but not squamous cell cancer. Future studies attempting to correlate FDG–PET with tumor biology will need to consider the effect of different tumor histologic types (Table 3).

► Fluorodeoxyglucose positron emission tomography (FDG-PET) is an important diagnostic and staging imaging modality for patients suspected of having non-small cell lung cancer. In addition, the maximal standardized uptake values (SUV-max) of FDG-PET have been shown to predict survival in patients with non-small cell lung cancer. In this study the authors examined the correlation of selective tumor marker expression to FDG-PET, which currently is the best noninvasive surrogate marker of tumor biology. Tissue microarrays were created from approximately 150 patients with non-small cell lung cancer. Immunohistochemical analyses of p53, vascular endothelial growth factor (VEGF), epidermal growth factor receptor (EGFR), cyclin-D1, and glucose transporter 1 (GLUT-1) were performed. The results show that tumor marker expression varies between tumor histology with adenocarcinoma having an increased expression of GLUT-1 and p53. In addition, tumor marker expression correlated with SUV-max by nodal status with node-positive patients having significantly more cyclin-D1, p53, and GLUT-1 expressions.

These studies support the clinical use of FDG-PET as a means of assessing response to EGFR inhibitor therapy. This has also been suggested by other groups. Interestingly, there was no significant difference in EGFR expression based on tumor nodal status. The lack of correlation between FDG-PET activity and VEGF expression in the tumor suggests a limited use of this imaging modality to assess clinical response of adenocarcinomas to anti-VEGF therapies. Studies such as these will be important as thoracic, surgical, and medical oncologists continue to examine the role of noninvasive imaging modalities to assess the response to molecularly targeted therapies.

D. R. Jones, MD

Article Index

Chapter 1: General Considerations

Chapter 2: Trauma

Chapter 3: Burns

Chapter 4: Critical Care

Chapter 5: Transplantation

Chapter 6: Surgical Infection

Chapter 7: Endocrine

Chapter 8: Nutrition

Chapter 9: Wound Healing

Chapter 10: Gastrointestinal

Chapter 11: Oncology

Chapter 12: Vascular Surgery

Chapter 13: General Thoracic Surgery

Author Index

S

T

U

V

W

X

Y

Z